普通高等教育"十一五"国家级规划教材

全国高等医药院校药学类专业第二轮实验双语教材

药理学实验与指导

（第 4 版）

U0286257

主　　编　龚国清
副 主 编　陈　真　钱之玉
编　　委　何　玲　皋　聪　胡　梅
　　　　　孙继红　戴　丽　孙　逸
　　　　　王文辉

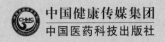

中国健康传媒集团
中国医药科技出版社

内 容 提 要

　　《药理学实验与指导》第4版是在上版的基础上全面修订完成的，内容覆盖了药理学科的经典实验。实验部分包括实验目的、实验原理、实验材料、实验方法和实验结果等内容；实验指导部分主要由注意事项、方法评价及思考题等组成。教材体例设计合理，特别强调了技能训练、关键性操作和对学生举一反三能力的培养，有助于学生实验能力的提高。

　　本次修订增加了近年来药理学新发展的一些前沿实验，目的是由经典药理学实验即整体、器官、组织水平向细胞、分子药理水平深入，以拓展学生思路。本书为书网融合教材，即纸质教材有机融合电子教材、教学配套资源（PPT、微课、视频、图片等）、题库系统、数字化教学服务（在线教学、在线作业、在线考试），使教学资源更加多样化、立体化。本书适合高等医药院校药学类专业师生使用。

图书在版编目（CIP）数据

药理学实验与指导／龚国清主编 . —4 版 . —北京：中国医药科技出版社，2019. 12

全国高等医药院校药学类专业第二轮实验双语教材

ISBN 978 – 7 – 5214 – 1369 – 4

Ⅰ. ①药…　Ⅱ. ①龚…　　Ⅲ. ①药理学—实验—医学院校—教学参考资料　　Ⅳ. ①R965. 2

中国版本图书馆 CIP 数据核字（2019）第 298350 号

美术编辑　陈君杞
版式设计　南博文化

出版　**中国健康传媒集团** | 中国医药科技出版社
地址　北京市海淀区文慧园北路甲 22 号
邮编　100082
电话　发行：010 – 62227427　邮购：010 – 62236938
网址　www. cmstp. com
规格　889 × 1194mm $\frac{1}{16}$
印张　22 ½
字数　550 千字
初版　2003 年 8 月第 1 版
版次　2019 年 12 月第 4 版
印次　2020 年 12 月第 2 次印刷
印刷　三河市万龙印装有限公司
经销　全国各地新华书店
书号　ISBN 978 – 7 – 5214 – 1369 – 4
定价　**58. 00 元**

获取新书信息、投稿、为图书纠错，请扫码联系我们。

教学是学校人才培养的中心环节，实验教学是这一环节的重要组成部分。"全国高等医药院校药学类专业实验双语教材"是中国药科大学坚持药学实践教学改革，突出提高学生动手能力、创新思维，通过承担教育部"世行贷款21世纪初高等教育教学改革项目"等多项教改课题，逐步建设完善的一套与药学各专业学科理论课程紧密结合的高水平双语实验教材。

本轮修订，适逢"全国高等医药院校药学类专业第五轮规划教材"及《中国药典》（2020年版）、新版《国家执业药师资格考试大纲》出版，整套教材的修订强调了与新版理论教材知识的结合，与《中国药典》（2020年版）等新颁布的法典法规结合。为更好地服务于新时期高等院校药学教育与人才培养的需要，在上一版的基础上，进一步体现了各门实验课程自身独立性、系统性和科学性，又充分考虑到各门实验课程之间的联系与衔接，主要突出了以下特点。

1. 适应医药行业对人才的要求，体现行业特色，契合新时期药学人才需求的变化，使修订后的教材符合《中国药典》（2020年版）等国家标准及新版《国家执业药师资格考试大纲》等行业最新要求。

2. 更新完善内容，打造教材精品。在上版教材基础上进一步优化、精炼和充实内容。紧密结合"全国高等医药院校药学类专业第五轮规划教材"，强调与实际需求相结合，进一步提高教材质量。

3. 为适应信息化教学的需要，本轮教材全部打造成为书网融合教材，即纸质教材与数字教材、配套教学资源、题库系统、数字化教学服务有机融合，为读者提供全免费增值服务。

4. 坚持双语体系，强调素质培养教材以实践教学为突破口，采用双语体系编写有利于加快药学教育国际接轨，提高学生的科技英语水平，进一步提升学生整体素质。

"全国高等医药院校药学类专业第二轮实验双语教材"历经15年4次建设，在各个时期广大编者的努力下，在广大使用教材师生的支持下日臻完善。本轮教材的出版，必将对推动新时期我国高等药学教育的发展产生积极而深远的影响。希望广大师生在教学实践中对本套教材提出宝贵意见，以便今后进一步修订完善，共同打造精品教材。

吴晓明

全国高等医药院校药学类专业第五轮规划教材常务编委会主任委员

2019年10月

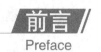

　　《药理学实验与指导》自 2003 年 3 月出版以来，受到了高等医药院校药学类及相关专业师生的广泛欢迎。它不仅可以帮助学生掌握药理学实验基本操作技术，提高实验动手能力，树立实践第一的观点，养成严谨、求实的科学作风，而且在提高学生的科技英语水平，训练"听、读、写"的能力方面，起到了"授人以渔，一生足食"的教学效果。

　　随着药理学的发展，实验内容不断更新，实验教学条件大幅度改善，实验教学也应与时俱进；在教学过程中，我们也发现了原版中存在的一些问题和不足，尤其是在英文准确表达方面存在的不足。因此，在前几版教材的基础上，进行《药理学实验与指导》第 4 版修订，并经过一年的努力终于编写完成。

　　本书与全国高等医药院校药学类专业第五轮规划教材《药理学》（第 5 版）和《药理学学习指导》构成完整的药理学教学体系。这是药理学教材建设系列化，努力提高立体化的教学效果的一种尝试。通过努力培养学生的合理知识结构和能力结构，满足社会对高素质复合型药学人才的需要。

　　本书为书网融合教材，即纸质教材有机融合电子教材、教学配套资源（PPT、微课、视频、图片等）、题库系统、数字化教学服务（在线教学、在线作业、在线考试），使教学资源更加多样化、立体化。

　　本书适用于高等医药院校药学类各专业的本科、研究生教学，也可作为医药行业科研人员的参考书。由于水平有限，书中难免有疏漏和不足之处，敬请读者批评指正。

编　者

2019 年 11 月

中 文 部 分

英 文 部 分

中 文 部 分

第一章 药理学实验的基本知识和技术

一、药理学实验课的目的和要求

药理学实验是药理学的基本实践，对药理学的发展起着推动作用，对寻找新药及临床医学的发展也有着直接的影响。药理学实验课是药理学教学的一个重要组成部分。它的目的如下。

（1）验证药理学中的某些重要的基本理论，巩固和加强对理论知识的理解，更牢固地掌握药理学的基本概念。

（2）训练基本技术操作，掌握进行药理学实验的基本方法，培养严肃认真的科学态度和实事求是的科学作风。

（3）培养学生对事物进行观察、比较、分析、综合和解决实际问题的能力。

（4）学习新药临床前药理学研究方法，为从事新药的药理学、毒理学研究打下基础。

为了使实验结果正确可靠，必须在实验过程中认真操作，仔细观察，详细记录，最后进行科学的分析。

实验前，应作好预习，明确实验目的、方法、步骤和原理，做到心中有数，避免实验中出现忙乱和差错。

实验过程中，要在教师指导下，培养独立操作能力，克服对教师的依赖性。实验器材妥善安排，正确装置，按照实验步骤进行操作，准确给药，细致地观察实验现象，随时记录，认真思考。

实验后，整理实验器材，并洗净、擦干；无论死活，动物都应按老师要求送往指定处，做好清洁卫生工作；整理实验结果，经过分析思考，写出实验报告，交指导教师评阅。

写实验报告是培养文字表达能力和综合分析问题能力的重要训练。实验结束后要求用统一实验报告本写好报告。实验报告要求列出实验题目、实验方法、实验结果，并对实验结果加以讨论，进行综合分析和理论说明。

二、实验动物的捉持和给药方法

实验1.1 小鼠的捉持和给药方法

【目的】

学习小鼠的捉持和给药方法。

【材料】

小鼠3～4只，体重18～22g，雌雄不限。

鼠笼、天平、注射器、针头、小鼠尾静脉注射用固定箱、生理盐水。

【方法】

1. **捉持法** 以右手捉小鼠尾，将小鼠放于粗糙面上，向后轻拉小鼠尾部，使小鼠固定于粗糙面上。用左手的拇指、示指和中指捏住小鼠两耳及头部皮肤，无名指、小指和掌心夹住其背部皮肤和尾部，使头部朝上，颈部拉直但不宜过紧，以免窒息（图1-1）。

另一种捉持法是只用左手，先用示指和拇指抓住小鼠尾巴，后用手掌及小指和无名指夹住其尾部，再以拇指及示指抓住两耳和头部皮肤（图1-2）。前者易学，后者便于快速捉拿给药。

2. **灌胃** 以左手捉持小鼠，头部朝上，使其头颈部充分拉直。右手拿起装有灌胃针头的注射器，自口角插入口腔，再从舌面紧沿上腭进入食管（图1-3）。如插入正确，灌胃针头容易进入；如遇阻力，可能插入气管，则应退出再插。灌胃液最多不超过1.0ml。

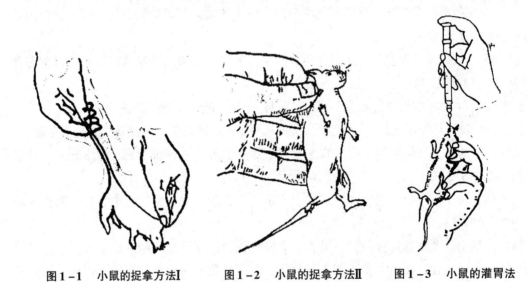

图1-1 小鼠的捉拿方法Ⅰ　　图1-2 小鼠的捉拿方法Ⅱ　　图1-3 小鼠的灌胃法

3. **皮下注射** 将小鼠置于铁丝网上，左手抓住小鼠，以拇指扣示指捏起背部皮肤，右手持注射器刺入背部皮下注射药液（图1-4）。另一种方法可由两人合作，一人左手抓住小鼠头部皮肤，右手拉住尾巴；另一人左手捏起背部皮肤，右手持注射器（针头不宜过粗，选用5号或6号针头）将针头刺入背部皮下。旋转注射器出针，否则药液将会从针眼处漏出。

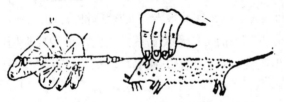

图1-4 小鼠的皮下注射法

4. **肌内注射** 左手拇指和示指抓住小鼠头部皮肤，小指、无名指和手掌夹住鼠尾及一侧后肢，将针头刺入后肢外侧部肌肉。如两人合作，一人左手抓住小鼠头部皮肤，右手拉住鼠尾，另一人持注射器（选用4号或5号针头）。注射量每腿不宜超过0.2ml。

5. **腹腔注射** 左手持小鼠（方法同灌胃），腹部朝上，头部下斜，右手持注射器（选用5号或6号针头），以10°角从下腹左或右侧（避开膀胱）朝头部方向首先刺入皮下，然后再以 45°角刺入腹腔，注射药液（图 1-5）。分两次进针，防止漏液；针头与腹腔的角度不宜太小，否则易进入皮下；正下腹部进针，易刺破膀胱；穿刺部位不宜太深或太近于上腹部，避免刺破内脏。常用注射量为 0.5ml，不宜超过 1.0ml。

　　6. **尾静脉注射**　将小鼠置于小鼠专用固定器内，露出尾巴，涂擦 75% 乙醇，使血管扩张。将鼠尾拉直，选择一条扩张最明显的血管，用拇指及中指拉住尾尖，示指压迫尾根保持血管充血扩张，用 4 号注射针头以 3°～5°（几乎平行）刺入尾静脉内，缓缓将药液注入（图 1-6）。如针头没有插入静脉内，推注药液遇阻力，而且局部变白，此为注入皮下的表现，应重新穿刺。因此，尾静脉注射时，必须从近尾端静脉开始，这样可以重复注射数次，以便失败后可在前一次穿刺点的上方重新进行，小鼠尾静脉注射的药液量一般为 0.2～1.0ml。

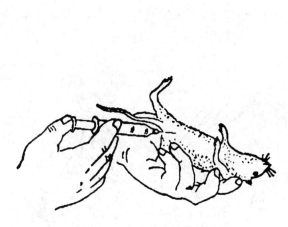 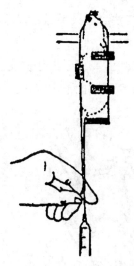

图 1-5　小鼠的腹腔注射法　　　　　　图 1-6　小鼠的尾静脉注射法

实验 1.2　大鼠的捉持和给药方法

【目的】

学习大鼠的捉持和各种给药方法。

【材料】

大鼠 2 只，体重 180～250g，雌雄不限。

鼠笼、天平、注射器、针头、灌胃针头、大鼠尾静脉注射用固定箱、加厚帆布手套一副、生理盐水。

【方法】

　　1. **捉持法**　左手戴防护手套，一般可按与小鼠相同方式捉持，对较大者可用左手的拇指和中指分别放在大鼠的左右腋下，示指放于颈部，使大鼠伸开前肢，握住大鼠。

　　2. **灌胃**　与小鼠相似。一次给药量不超过 2ml。

　　3. **腹腔注射**　同小鼠。

　　4. **静脉注射**　麻醉后大鼠可从舌下静脉或尾静脉注射给药。要充分加温或用二甲苯涂擦使尾静脉扩张，尾静脉注射才易成功。

实验1.3　家兔的捉持和给药方法

【目的】

学习家兔的捉持和各种给药方法。

【材料】

家兔1~2只，体重2~3kg，雌雄不限。

兔箱、兔开口器、磅秤、导尿管、注射器、生理盐水。

【方法】

1. **捉持法**　一只手抓颈背部皮肤，轻轻将兔提起，另一只手托住臀部，使兔呈坐位姿势（图1-7）。

将兔仰卧，一只手抓住颈皮，另一只手顺其腹部摸至膝关节。另外一人用绳带捆绑兔的四肢，使兔腹部向上固定在兔手术台上。头部则用兔头固定夹固定。

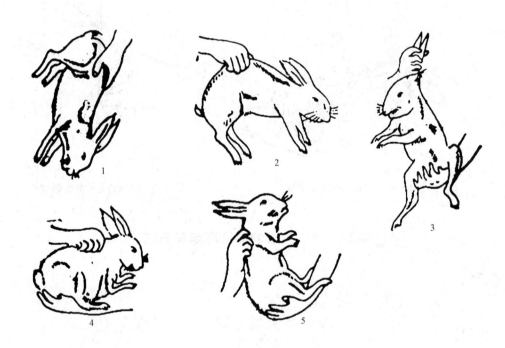

图1-7　兔的捉持方法

注：1，2，3均为不正确的捉持方法：其中1可损伤两肾脏；2可造成皮下内出血；3可损伤两耳；4，5为正确的捉持方法：颈后部的皮厚可以抓，并用手托住兔体

2. **灌胃**　将兔固定于兔箱内，用木制开口器由齿列间横插入口内，并向内上方转动直至兔舌被掩压出为止，然后将导尿管从开口器中的小孔插入，沿上腭后壁轻轻地送入食管15~20cm，以达胃部（图1-8）。注意不能插入气管，可将导尿管的外端浸入水内，观察有无气泡放出。无气泡方能注入药液，药液推完后再注入4~5ml水或少许空气，以便将导尿管中的药液全部推至胃中。而后紧捏导尿管迅速拔出，否则水可由导尿管滴至气管内。最后移去开口器。

3. **静脉注射**　将兔固定于兔箱内，先拔去耳背面外侧静脉处的毛（便于辨认静脉），然后用左手拇指和中指捏住耳尖部，示指垫在兔耳注射处的下面。右手持注射器（选用6号针头），先从耳尖端开始注射，约以5°角刺入，刺入后用左手拇指、示指及中指捏住针头接头处及兔耳加以固定，以防兔突然挣扎时针尖脱出血管（图1-9）。注射时，注意不能有气泡注入，否则有可能造成兔子死亡。常用注射量为10ml以下（等渗溶液可达10ml以上），应缓缓注射药液；如插入血管，药液推进容易；如插在血管外，则有丘状突起，应拔出针头，在近心端重新注射。针头拔出时，须用棉球压住注射部位，以防出血。

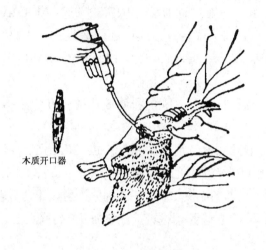

图1-8 家兔的灌胃法

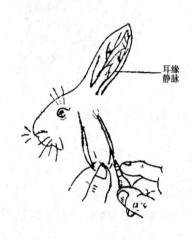

图1-9 家兔的耳静脉注射法

4. **皮下、肌内、腹腔注射** 方法与小鼠同。唯针头选用粗的，给药量增加（灌胃：5~10ml；皮下注射：2ml；肌内注射：2ml；腹腔注射：5ml）。

【附】豚鼠的捉持和给药方法

1. **捉持法** 以右手抓住豚鼠，将前肢夹在右手拇指和示指之间，抓住整个颈胸部（不要抓得太紧以免窒息），左手抓住两后肢，使腹部向上进行操作。

2. **灌胃、腹腔注射、皮下注射和肌内注射** 方法基本上同小鼠，给药量需稍多。

3. **静脉注射** 可选用后脚掌外侧的静脉或外颈静脉进行注射。进行后脚掌外侧静脉注射时，由一人捉豚鼠并固定一条后腿，另一人剪去注射部位的毛，用酒精棉球涂擦后脚掌外侧，使皮肤血管显露，将连在注射器上的小儿头皮静脉输液针头刺入血管。外颈静脉注射时需先剪去一点皮肤，使血管暴露，然后将连在注射器上的小儿头皮静脉输液针头刺入。豚鼠的静脉血管壁比较脆弱，操作时需特别小心。

实验1.4 犬的捉持和给药方法

【目的】
学习犬的捉持和各种给药方法。

【材料】
犬一条，体重5~10kg，雌雄不限。

特制铁钳、犬开口器、磅秤、导尿管、注射器、针头、绳索、生理盐水。

【方法】

对于未经驯服的犬，需先以特制铁钳夹住头颈，将其按倒，以绳索捆扎犬嘴。用粗绳带从下颌绕到上颌打一结，然后绕向下颌再打一结，最后将绳带索引到头后，在颈项上打第三结，在这一结上再打一活结（图1-10）。捆绑过程中要求动作轻巧、迅速。捆绑犬嘴的目的只是避免其咬人。已驯服（一般经一周左右训练）做实验的犬，不必施以暴力，只需将犬嘴绑好，即可进行给药或其他操作，不宜用铁钳夹头，否则，犬的性情将由此变坏而不易驯服。

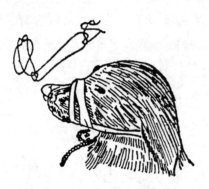

图1-10 犬嘴的捆绑方法

1. **灌胃、皮下、肌内和腹腔注射** 方法基本上同家兔。用具和给药量相应增大。

2. **静脉注射** 常用的注射部位是后肢小隐静脉（图1-11），该血管由外踝前侧走向外上侧。也可选用前肢的皮下静脉（图1-12），该血管在脚爪上方背侧的正前位。注射时先局部剪毛，以酒精涂擦皮肤，一人捏紧注射肢体的上端，阻断血液回流，使静脉充盈，以便看清走向；另一人持注射器进行静脉穿刺，将药液注入。

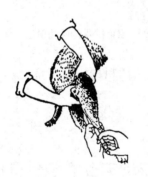

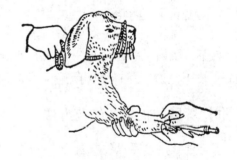

图1-11 犬后肢外侧小隐静脉注射法　　　图1-12 犬前肢背侧皮下静脉注射法

三、常用实验动物的麻醉

动物麻醉，在急性实验和慢性实验中经常采用。麻醉药除了有抑制中枢神经系统的作用外，还会引起其他生理功能变化。因此麻醉药的选择，对于保证实验的顺利进行和获得良好的实验结果是十分重要的。由于实验目的和动物种类不同，可采用不同的麻醉药和麻醉方法。

（一）乙醚

乙醚（ether）是吸入法中最常用的麻醉药，各种动物皆可应用。其麻醉量和致死量相差大，所以安全度大。但乙醚局部刺激作用大，可刺激上呼吸道使黏液分泌增加，易引起手术后肺炎；通过神经反射可以对呼吸、血压和心脏活动产生扰乱，并且容易引起窒息，在麻醉过程中应注意。总的说来，乙醚麻醉的优点多，麻醉深度易于掌握，麻醉后恢复比较快，适用于时间不太长的手术。在麻醉前给予一定量的吗啡和阿托品，通常在麻醉前20~30min，皮下注射盐酸吗啡或硫酸吗啡（5~10mg/kg）及阿托品（0.1mg/kg），前者可降低中枢神经系统兴奋性，提高痛阈，降低乙醚用量及避免乙醚麻醉过程中的兴奋期；后者可对抗乙醚刺激呼吸道引起的黏液分泌作用，可防止麻醉过程中发生呼吸道堵塞或手术后发生吸入性肺炎。

使用乙醚麻醉大鼠、小鼠、蛙类时，可将动物放在玻璃钟罩或烧杯中，把沾有乙醚的棉球或纱布投入容器内，动物吸入容器内的乙醚蒸气后，很快进入麻醉状态，即可进行操作。

使用乙醚麻醉鸽和鸡时，可取 25ml 烧杯一个，内装沾乙醚棉球，将动物用小手术巾包裹固定，把头部放入烧杯内吸取乙醚蒸气，动物很快进入麻醉状态，即可进行操作。

使用乙醚麻醉猫和兔时，可将动物放入玻璃麻醉箱内，不断打气，使乙醚蒸气由乙醚瓶输入麻醉箱，当动物倒下后，可把盛乙醚的插管从麻醉箱中取出。如动物四肢紧张度明显减低，角膜反射迟钝，皮肤痛觉消失，则动物已进入麻醉，可进行手术和操作。

使用乙醚麻醉犬时，应先将犬嘴绑好，以免麻醉初期动物兴奋时咬人。按照犬的大小，选好合适的麻醉口罩，并在口罩内放入纱布，加上乙醚。一人用手固定犬的前后肢，另一人用右膝压犬的胸颈部，一手捏住头颈，但不能引起窒息，一手将口罩套在犬嘴上，使其吸入乙醚。开始麻醉时乙醚量可稍多，后逐渐减少。吸入乙醚后，可出现兴奋、挣扎、呼吸不规则，有时甚至发生窒息，一旦发生窒息应暂停吸入乙醚，待动物呼吸恢复后再继续吸入，加深麻醉。每呼吸数次乙醚后，取去口罩呼吸一次空气，此后呼吸则渐趋稳定，肌肉紧张度渐渐消失，角膜反射迟钝，呈深睡状态，则表示动物已进入麻醉状态，应即解去犬嘴绑绳，开始手术。

（二）巴比妥类

巴比妥类是巴比妥酸的衍生物，呈弱酸性，白色结晶，难溶于水但其钠盐易溶于水，可作静脉注射用。因其钠盐溶液不稳定，久置易分解沉淀，故一般多于临用时溶解配制。

巴比妥类对动物有良好的麻醉作用，手术时间较长者可用苯巴比妥钠或异戊巴比妥钠。若要动物手术后恢复者宜用作用较短的戊巴比妥钠、硫喷妥钠。

用法用量见表 1 - 1 至表 1 - 6。

表 1 - 1　巴比妥钠

动物	给药途径	浓度和剂量	作用
犬	静脉	10%，1.8~2.2ml/kg	麻醉
猫	灌胃	10%，2.5~4ml/kg	麻醉
猫	腹腔	10%，5ml/kg	麻醉
兔	静脉	10%，1.2~1.5ml/kg	麻醉
兔	灌胃	0.1~0.12g/kg	最小麻醉量
大鼠	皮下	0.2g/kg	麻醉
鸽	腹腔	0.182g/kg	麻醉
蛙	淋巴囊	0.18~0.2g/kg	最小麻醉量

表 1 - 2　苯巴比妥

动物	给药途径	浓度和剂量	作用
犬、猫	静脉	10%，0.8~1.0ml/kg	麻醉
猫	腹腔	10%，1.5ml/kg	麻醉
兔	腹腔	10%，1.5~2.0ml/kg	麻醉
鸽	肌内	10%，3.0ml/kg	麻醉
蛙	皮下	13mg/kg	麻醉

表 1 - 3　戊巴比妥钠

动物	给药途径	剂量	作用
犬、猫、兔	静脉、腹腔	25 ~ 40mg/kg	麻醉
兔	静脉	10mg/kg	睡眠
大鼠	灌胃	60mg/kg	麻醉
豚鼠	腹腔	40 ~ 50mg/kg	麻醉

表 1 - 4　异戊巴比妥

动物	给药途径	剂量	作用
犬	腹腔	60mg/kg	睡眠
犬	静脉	30mg/kg	最小麻醉量
猫	皮下	100mg/kg	麻醉
兔	静脉	40 ~ 50mg/kg	麻醉
大鼠	灌胃	70mg/kg	最小麻醉量
大鼠	腹腔	100mg/kg	麻醉
大鼠	静脉	20mg/kg	最小麻醉量

表 1 - 5　硫喷妥钠

动物	给药途径	浓度和剂量	作用
犬、猫	静脉	20 ~ 30mg/kg	麻醉
犬、猫	腹腔	30 ~ 50mg/kg	麻醉
兔	静脉	1%，1 ~ 1.8ml/kg	麻醉

表 1 - 6　环己巴比妥钠

动物	给药途径	剂量	作用
犬	静脉	30mg/kg	麻醉
犬	静脉	25mg/kg	睡眠
犬	皮下	120mg/kg	麻醉
猫	静脉	25mg/kg	麻醉
兔	静脉	15mg/kg	睡眠
兔	静脉	25mg/kg	麻醉
兔	腹腔	70mg/kg	麻醉

（三）氨甲酸乙酯

氨甲酸乙酯（Urethane）亦称乌拉坦，是脲的衍生物，无色结晶，易溶于水，是一种温和的催眠药，对动物的作用强而迅速，可用于动物麻醉。该药可引起大鼠和猫血压下降，呼吸中枢 CO_2 阈稍提高，需氧量减少，大量给药可致各种损害。

（四）氯醛糖

氯醛糖（Chloralose）是氯醛与糖的化合物，用于动物麻醉。对某些实验颇适用，例如心肺装置，一定剂量的氯醛糖，可麻醉运动感觉脊髓中枢而不影响反射作用，增强肾上腺素兴奋子宫作用，而降低副交感神经的作用。血压变化不一致。

猫、兔，可采用1%氯醛糖和3%乌拉坦混合麻醉，7ml/kg，静脉或腹腔注射。

四、实验动物的取血方法

（一）大鼠、小鼠取血方法

1. **尾静脉取血**　将鼠装入固定盒内，盖上盒盖，露出尾巴，用手揉擦或用温水（45～50℃）加温，亦可用二甲苯等擦鼠尾，使鼠尾静脉充分充血，揩干后剪去尾尖（大鼠5～10mm，小鼠1～2mm），尾静脉血即可流出，用手轻轻从尾根部向尾尖部挤压，可以取到数滴血。取血后，先用棉球压迫止血，并立即用6%火棉胶涂于伤口处，使伤口外结一层火棉胶薄膜，保护伤口。

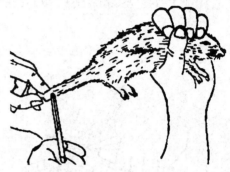

另外可采用交替切割尾静脉方法取血。用一锋利的刀片在尾巴上切破一段尾静脉，静脉血即由伤口流出，每次可取0.3～0.5ml，可供一般血常规等实验（图1-13）。三根尾静脉可以交替切割，由尾尖部向尾根部方向切割，切割后棉球压迫止血，约3天伤口结痂痊愈。这种方法对大鼠较适用。

清醒时取血常未能达到所需血量就停止出血，过多剪去尾尖也无效。可用硫喷妥钠（50mg/kg）麻醉后，按上述方法尾尖取血。由于鼠血易凝，需

图1-13　鼠尾静脉取血方法

要全血时，应事先将抗凝剂置于采血管中，如用血细胞混悬液应立即与生理盐水混合。

2. **眼眶动脉和静脉取血**　用左手抓住大鼠，拇指和示指尽量将鼠头部皮肤捏紧，使鼠眼突出，右手取一无钩弯头小镊子在右侧眼球部将眼球摘出。将鼠倒置，头部向下，此时眼眶很快流血，将血滴入预先加有抗凝剂的玻璃器皿内，直至流血停止。此法由于取血过程中动物末死，心脏不断跳动，一般可取鼠体重4%～5%的血液量，是一种较好的取血方法，但只适用于一次性取血。

3. **后眼眶静脉丛连续穿刺取血**　这种方法适用于小动物采血。采用后眼眶静脉丛穿刺，穿刺的部位是位于眼球和眼眶后界之间的后眼眶静脉丛。穿刺采用一根特制的硬玻璃吸管，管长7～10cm，前端拉成毛细管，内径0.1～1.5mm，长为1cm，后端的管径为0.6cm。取血时用左手从背部抓住动物，用示指和拇指握住两耳之间的头部皮肤使头固定，并轻轻向下压迫颈部两侧，引起头部静脉血液回流困难，使眼球充分突出。右手持预先浸入1%的肝素溶液并干燥的毛细玻璃管，将其尖端从内侧插入眼睑和眼球之间后，轻轻向眼底部方向移动，深4～5mm，就达到眼眶静脉丛，略加捻转，血自然进入毛细玻璃管内，得到所需的血量后，除去加于颈部的压力，将毛细玻璃管拔出，即停止出血（图1-14、图1-15）。根据实验需要，可在数分钟后在同一穿刺孔重复取血。

4. **断头取血**　实验者带上棉纱手套，用左手小指、无名指和掌部握住鼠背部，用拇指和示指固定头部，右手持剪刀在鼠颈部将鼠头剪掉，立即将鼠颈向下，对准已准备好的盛血容器（内放抗凝剂），鼠血即可从颈部很快滴入容器内（图1-16）。

5. **心脏内取血**　动物仰卧，固定鼠于固定板上，用剪刀将心前区的毛剪去，用碘酒、酒精消毒此处皮肤，在左侧第3～4肋间，用左手示指摸到心搏，右手持连有4～5号针头

的注射器，选择心搏最强处穿刺。当针头正确刺到心脏时，鼠血液由于心脏跳动的力量，自然进入注射器，即可进行取血（图1-17）。

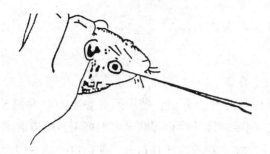

图1-14　小鼠眼底静脉丛取血方法

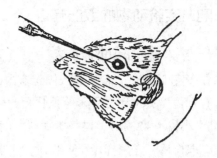

图1-15　大鼠眼底静脉丛取血方法

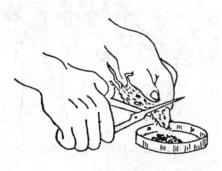

图1-16　小鼠断头取血方法

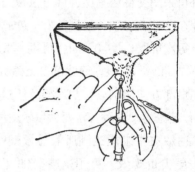

图1-17　小鼠心内取血方法

6. 颈动脉和静脉取血　将动物仰卧固定于鼠固定板上，将一侧颈外侧的毛剪去，作一般颈静脉或颈动脉分离手术。颈静脉或颈动脉暴露清楚后，即可用注射针沿颈静脉或颈动脉平行方向刺入抽取血量。采用此种取血方法，体重20g小鼠可取血0.6ml左右。体重300g大鼠可取血8ml左右。也可将颈静脉和颈动脉挑起来，用剪刀剪断，以注射器（不带针头）吸取流出来的血液或用试管接血。

（二）兔、豚鼠取血方法

1. 兔心脏内取血　兔心脏穿刺是一项容易掌握的操作方法。将动物仰卧固定在手术台上，把心前区的毛剪去，用碘酒、酒精消毒皮肤，用左手触摸左侧第3~4肋间，选择心跳最明显处。一般由胸骨左缘外3mm处，将注射针头插入第三肋间腔，当注射针头接近心脏时，就会感觉到心脏的跳动，将针头再向里穿刺即可进入心室。穿刺时最好用左手触诊心跳，在触诊的配合下进行穿刺。当针头正确地刺入心脏内时，兔血由于心跳的力量就自然地进入注射器，可行取血。经6~7天后可重复行心脏穿刺术。家兔一次可取全血量1/6~1/5。

2. 兔耳中央动脉取血　将家兔置于兔箱内，用手揉擦兔耳或用灯泡烘烤，片刻后可见到兔耳充血，在兔耳中央有一条较粗、颜色较鲜红的中央动脉。用左手固定住兔耳，右手持注射器，在中央动脉的末端，沿着动脉向心方向穿刺入动脉，动脉血立即进入针筒，取完血后注意止血。中央动脉抽血容易发生痉挛性收缩，故必须让兔耳充分充血。在动脉扩张，未发生痉挛性收缩前立即抽血。取血的针头一般用6号针头；针刺的部位从中央动脉的末端开始。

另一种方法，待兔耳中央动脉充血后，在靠耳尖中央动脉分支处，用一把锋利的小刀，轻切一个小口，兔血即由血管破口处流出，立即取装有抗凝剂、有刻度的试管，在血管破口处接血。取血后注意压迫伤口止血。

3. 兔耳缘静脉取血 以小血管夹夹紧耳根部，并以二甲苯涂局部使血管扩张，涂后酒精拭净。然后以粗大针头插入耳缘静脉取血（图1-18）。

另外，做一般常规检查时，只需取少量血液。可在耳缘静脉充血后，用5½号针头刺破靠近耳尖部血管，即收集从刺破口流出的血液。

4. 兔后肢胫部皮下静脉取血 将兔仰卧固定于固定板上，拔去胫部被毛，在胫部上端股部扎橡皮管，在胫部外侧浅表皮下即可清楚看到皮下静脉。用左手两指固定好静脉，右手取带有5½号针头注射器，由皮下静脉平行方向刺入血管。抽一下针栓，如血进入注射器，表示针头已进入血管，即可取血，一次可取2～5ml。取完血必须用棉球压住取血

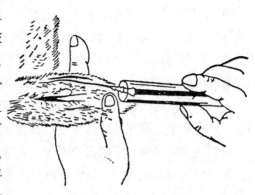

图1-18 兔耳缘静脉取血方法

部位止血，时间要略长一些。如止血不好，可造成皮下血肿，影响连续多次抽血。

5. 兔股静脉、颈静脉取血 首先做股静脉和颈静脉暴露分离手术，取股静脉血时，用连有5½号或6号针头的注射器，平行于血管，从股静脉下端向心方向刺入，徐徐抽动针筒即可取血。抽完血后注意止血，一般用干纱布轻压取血部位即可止血。如要连续多次取血，尽量选择离心端部位取血。

外颈静脉取血时，用连有6号针头的注射器，由近心端（距颈静脉分支2～3cm处）向头侧端沿血管平行方向刺入，使注射针头一直引深至颈静脉分枝分叉处，即可取血。该处血管较粗，容易取血，取血量较多，一次可取10ml以上。取血完毕，拔出针头，用干纱布轻轻压住取血部位也易止血。

6. 兔股动脉、颈总动脉取血 先做股动脉、颈总动脉暴露分离手术。血管分离后，在主动脉下穿一根线备提起用。取血时提起血管，用左手示指垫于血管下面，取连有6号针头的注射器，与血管平行向心方向将注射针刺入血管，稍向前引深一段，即可见动脉血进入针筒，用左手拇指和示指将注射针头和血管一起固定好，便可进行取血。如要从颈动脉抽取多量血液时，可在颈总动脉上剪一小口，插入软塑料管，用细胶皮管连接在大注射器上（胶皮管和注射器内要加抗凝剂），先将注射器针筒向外抽，使注射器内呈半真空状态，然后打开塑料管，动脉血即很快进入注射器。

7. 兔眼底取血 将注射针头或毛细管沿眼球眼眶间的眼内角刺入眼底静脉，可见血自动进入毛细滴管。或用注射器抽吸，一般一次可取血1～2ml以上。

豚鼠的各部位取血方法，基本和上述兔取血方法相同。

（三）犬、猫取血方法

1. 犬心脏内取血 这种取血方法最好在麻醉情况下进行。将犬仰卧固定于固定台上，前肢向背侧方向固定好，暴露胸部，将左侧第3～5肋间的被毛剪去，用碘酒、酒精消毒，用左手触摸左侧3～5肋间处，选择心跳最明显处穿刺。一般选择胸骨左外缘1cm第4肋间处，取连有8号针头的注射器，由上述位置进针，向背侧方向垂直刺入心脏，穿刺者可根

据针头接触心脏跳动时的感觉，调整刺入方向和深度。当针头正确刺入心脏时，血液即可进入注射器，可抽取多量血液。但应注意不能让针头在胸腔内乱搅，摆动的角度尽量小，避免刺破心脏造成胸腔大出血。一般犬的血量为80ml/kg。

2. 犬后肢外侧小隐静脉和前肢内侧皮下的头静脉取血 对未经驯服的犬，需先用特制铁钳夹住头颈，再以绳索捆扎犬嘴；但对已驯服的犬，不宜用铁钳夹头，仅以绳索捆扎犬嘴即可。

常用的取血部位是前肢内侧皮下的头静脉，也可选用后肢外侧小隐静脉。取血时，先局部剪毛，然后用碘酒、酒精消毒，一人捏紧取血肢体的上方，阻断血液回流，使静脉充盈，以便看清静脉走向；另一人持注射器进行静脉穿刺，由皮下静脉平行方向刺入血管，抽一下针栓，如血进入注射器，表示针头已进入血管，并用左手两指固定好静脉，右手持注射器，进行取血。取完血后，用棉球压迫止血。如需取较多血量时，则可用注射器直接抽取，抽取速度要稍慢，否则血液不能进入注射器。抽血时应解除静脉上端加压的手或橡皮管，取完血后注意止血。如只需采取少量血液，则不必用注射器抽取，用5½号针头直接刺入静脉，接住滴下的血液，即可作血常规检查。一般取血量为10～20ml，并不困难（图1－19～图1－21）。

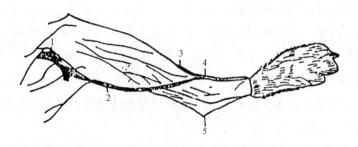

图1－19 犬后肢外侧小隐静脉行走方向
注：1. 膝动脉；2. 小隐静脉；3. 大隐静脉；4. 小隐及大隐静脉之间的侧枝；5. 跗关节

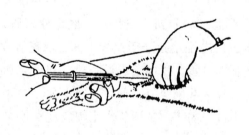

图1－20 犬后肢外侧小隐静脉取血方法

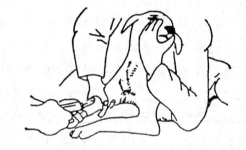

图1－21 犬前肢内侧皮下的头静脉取血方法

3. 犬颈静脉取血 取侧卧位，剪去颈部被毛约10cm×3cm范围，用碘酒、酒精消毒。将动物颈部拉直，头尽量后仰，用左手拇指压住颈静脉入胸部位的皮肤使颈静脉怒张，右手取连有6½号针头的注射器，针头沿血管平行方向向心端刺入血管。由于此静脉在皮下容易滑动，针刺时除用左手固定好血管外，刺入要准确，取血后压迫止血，此法可取较多血量（图1－22）。

4. 犬股动脉取血 动物可不用麻醉。仰卧后固定好动物，伸展后肢向外拉直，暴露腹股沟三角区动脉搏动的部位，剪去被毛，用碘酒、酒精消毒。左手中指、示指探摸股动脉

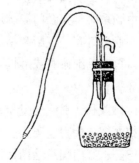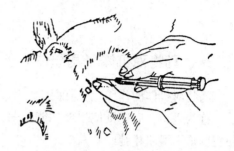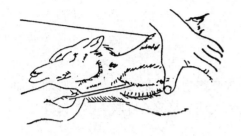

跳动部位并固定好血管，右手取连有5½号针头的注射器，针头由动脉跳动处直接刺入血管，当血液进入注射器内时，可根据需要量抽取血液（图1-23）。取完血后用纱布压迫止血2~3min。

图1-22 犬颈静脉取血方法

图1-23 犬股动脉取血方法

5. 犬耳缘静脉取血 此种方法适用取少量血作常规检查。经过训练的犬可不必绑嘴，让犬跳上手术台，剪去耳尖部短毛，可见到耳缘静脉。揉擦耳朵，使静脉充盈，皮肤涂少许凡士林，用5½号针头刺破静脉，用右手顺静脉走向由头端向耳尖部轻轻挤压，血液即由破口流出。取完血后用干棉球压迫止血。

6. 犬颈动脉取血方法 取血方法基本同兔颈动脉取血方法。

猫的各种取血方法和操作基本上同犬。

（四）羊的取血方法

羊常采用颈静脉取血。颈静脉粗大，容易抽取，取血量较多，一般一次可抽取50~100ml血，也可在前后肢皮下静脉取血。

将羊蹄捆缚压倒在地，由助手双手握住羊下颌，向上固定住头部。在颈部一侧外缘剪去羊毛约5cm²范围，碘酒、酒精消毒。用左手拇指固定颈静脉，使之怒张，右手持连有粗针头的注射器，沿静脉一侧以30°倾斜，由头端向心方向刺入血管，然后缓缓抽至所需量。取血完毕，拔去针头，采血部位以酒精棉球压迫片刻，同时迅速将血液注入盛有玻璃珠的灭菌烧瓶内，振荡数分钟，脱去纤维蛋白，防止凝血。或将血液直接装入有抗凝剂的烧瓶内。

如一次需要的血量较多，可在避免污染的情况下，采用密闭采血法。

储血瓶：可用500ml或200ml三角烧瓶，内装玻璃珠，瓶口橡皮塞中央钻孔，孔的大小以正好能插入采血玻管为宜，瓶口严密包扎，高压消毒后备用。此种储血瓶为去纤维蛋白用，也可采用普通血库用的储血瓶加入抗凝剂（10%枸橼酸钠生理盐水4ml可抗凝100ml羊血），此血可保存一周。

采血器：可用普通血库采血用的玻管，橡皮管和玻璃连通管，按上采羊血的针头，高压灭菌后备用。羊采血瓶见图1-24。

采血方法：①用羊固定架将羊固定好（固定方法类似犬的固定方法）。②颈部剪毛，以碘酒及酒精消毒。③于颈部近心端处缚以橡皮带，使颈静脉怒张。④装好储血瓶。⑤刺入羊颈静脉，采血瓶放置较羊身稍低处，血即可自动流入采血瓶，随时摇动，直至达到所需量后拔出针头，取下采血管封闭瓶口，如用抗凝剂则稍加摇匀即可。如用作脱纤维蛋白血液，必须持续振摇5min。

图1-24 羊采血瓶

13

第二章　药理学总论实验

一、药物对机体（病原体）的作用

药物对机体的作用主要有两类，即兴奋和抑制。有些药物可使机体原有的生理功能加强，称为兴奋；有些则使生理功能减弱，称为抑制。如戊四氮可兴奋呼吸中枢，阿托品可使胃肠道平滑肌松弛。

同时，一种药物对于机体各器官组织的作用并不是一样的，对某一个或几个器官组织的某些功能影响特别明显，对其他器官组织则影响较小，这就是药物的选择作用。如洋地黄对心脏、苯巴比妥对中枢神经系统具有高选择作用。选择性高的药物往往疗效好，不良反应少。

药物作用于机体时，根据其作用部位的不同，可分为局部作用和全身作用。前者系指药物在用药部位所呈现的作用，如普鲁卡因的局部麻醉作用；后者则指被机体吸收以后所呈现的作用，如服普萘洛尔后出现心率减缓。

药物之所以能够发挥作用，是由于它与机体效应器的某一部位相结合，这一部位称为受体（receptor）。除肾上腺素受体和胆碱受体外，目前还发现了许多受体种类，一般认为大多数药物是通过与受体结合而产生作用的。但也有一些药物的作用是通过其他机制实现的，如乙醚和三氯甲烷产生麻醉作用，可能是由于其易溶于类脂质，浓集于富含脂质的神经组织，使神经细胞膜的通透性发生改变，引起神经冲动传导障碍。

实验2.1　药物的局部作用和全身作用

【目的】

通过本实验，了解药物的局部作用和全身作用。

【原理】

药物在吸收入血液之前，在用药部位发挥的直接作用称为局部作用，如口服硫酸镁在肠道内不易吸收，有导泻作用；局麻药注射于神经末梢或神经干可阻断神经冲动的传导等。药物进入血液循环后，分布到机体各部位发挥的作用称为全身作用，如药物从胃肠道吸收后由肠系血管膜经门静脉进入肝脏，再进入血液循环；少数药物可用舌下给药或直肠给药，分别通过口腔、直肠和结肠黏膜直接吸收入血液；皮下或肌内注射，药物先沿结缔组织扩散，再经毛细血管或淋巴内皮细胞进入血液；静脉注射，药物不经吸收，直接进入血液循环。

口服和注射给药分别属于消化道和注射部位的吸收。局部用药主要是引起局部作用，例如涂擦、撒粉、喷雾、含漱、湿敷、洗涤、滴入等，灌肠、吸入、植入、离子透入、舌下给药、肛门阴道给药等方法，虽用于局部，目的多在于引起吸收作用。

【材料】

小鼠2只，体重18～22g，雌雄不限。

鼠笼，烧杯，玻璃平皿，止血钳等。

氯乙烷喷射剂（或瓶装氯乙烷试剂）。

【方法与步骤】

取小鼠 2 只，标记编号，观察两鼠的活动情况和尾部皮肤色泽。分别以止血钳夹小鼠的尾部和后肢，观察其痛反应，然后再作下列处置。

鼠甲，以氯乙烷喷其尾部或尾部滴加氯乙烷约 1ml，观察尾部皮肤的色泽变化，立即用止血钳夹该鼠的尾部和后肢，观察其痛反应，活动能力有无改变，并与用药前的情况作比较。

鼠乙，将该鼠放入烧杯内，放入吸有氯乙烷（约 1ml）的棉球，用玻璃皿盖上，如见小鼠麻醉翻倒，即将它从烧杯中取出，检查其尾部是否有与鼠甲相似的色泽变化，并以止血钳夹该鼠的尾部和后肢，观察其痛反应。

【结果处理】

将观察到的现象填入表 2 - 1。

表 2 - 1 氯乙烷局部作用和全身作用的实验结果

小鼠编号	用氯乙烷的方式	用药后的反应				是局部作用还是全身作用
		尾部皮肤色泽变化	夹尾部的痛反应	夹后肢时的痛反应	全身活动能力	

【注意事项】

1. 以止血钳夹小鼠尾部或后肢测试痛反应，必须轻重适度，前后一致，不要用力过大以致夹伤组织。

2. 密切观察小鼠的反应，氯乙烷的局部作用和全身作用在停止给药后都易消失，因此应迅速检查小鼠用药后的反应。

【方法评价】

本实验目的在于初步了解药物的局部作用和全身作用，观察的指标为阳性或阴性反应，实验简单，结果可靠。为进一步说明其作用类别，在给药后测定血药浓度则更为准确。

【思考题】

1. 何谓药物的局部作用和全身作用？它们各有何特点，进一步举例说明。

2. 试从氯乙烷在甲、乙两鼠身上所产生的作用中，分析哪些属于局部作用，哪些属于全身作用，并推测氯乙烷的药理作用。

实验 2.2 药物的间接作用

【目的】

了解药物的间接作用。

【原理】

药物对所接触的组织器官直接产生的作用称为直接作用，由直接作用所引起的其他器官的效应称为间接作用。例如，抗酸药→胃酸减少（直接作用）→胃痛减轻（间接作用）；强心苷→心力加强（直接作用）→循环改善（间接作用）→利尿（间接作用）等。

【材料】

家兔1只，体重1.8~2.2kg，雌雄不限。

生理信号采集记录系统，兔手术台，滑轮，肌力换能器，铁架台，蛙心夹，棉线。

10%浓氨溶液，2%盐酸丁卡因溶液。

【方法与步骤】

取家兔1只，仰缚于手术台上，用兔头夹固定兔头，用蛙心夹夹住腹壁呼吸运动最明显处的皮肤；以棉线通过滑轮连接肌力换能器，并与生理信号采集记录系统相连，记录家兔的呼吸。

记录一段时间的正常呼吸，然后将蘸有氨水的棉球置于家兔鼻孔附近，令其吸入氨气，观察对呼吸频率和幅度的影响。

撤去氨水棉球，待家兔呼吸恢复正常后，用棉球蘸2%盐酸丁卡因溶液，涂抹其两个鼻孔的黏膜，5min后用同样方法给家兔嗅氨水，观察对呼吸的影响。比较用盐酸丁卡因前后家兔吸入氨气时不同的反应。

【结果处理】

记录下呼吸曲线，并加文字说明。

【注意事项】

1. 要固定住家兔，使其不能挣扎，否则会影响呼吸曲线的描记。

2. 前后两次嗅氨水的条件尽可能相同，如蘸氨水的量和嗅的时间以及棉球与鼻子的距离。

3. 盐酸丁卡因需均匀地涂抹在家兔两个鼻孔的黏膜上，深度约1cm。

【方法评价】

本实验方法简单，但易于说明药物的间接作用及其影响环节。

二、机体对药物的作用

机体对药物的作用即我们常说的药代动力学，它研究药物在体内吸收、分布、代谢和排泄过程，对临床设计用药有重要的参考价值。药代动力学以动物为实验对象的研究方法大致可分两类，一是离体实验（*in vitro*），如肝药酶与药物代谢、血浆蛋白结合率研究；二是在体实验（*in vivo*），如血药浓度测定，根据各时间点的浓度值，拟合出药浓时程曲线，求得一系列药动学参数。

实验2.3　磺溴酞钠的药代动力学参数估算

【目的】

以磺溴酞钠（BSP）为例，学习估算药代动力学参数的基本方法。

【原理】

某些药物，在动物体内按一房室模型处置，静脉注射后，血药浓度－时间方程为一级动力学方程，即：

$$C = C_0 e^{-kt}$$

式中 k 为药物消除速率常数，C_0 为 $t = 0$ 时的血药浓度。

上式经对数变换得：

$$\lg C = \lg C_0 - \frac{k}{2.303} \times t，即血药浓度对时间 t 在半对数坐标纸上呈直线。$$

有关药代动力学参数的求算：

消除速率常数 $k = -2.303 \times b$（时间$^{-1}$）

半衰期 $t_{1/2} = 0.693/k$（时间）

表观分有容积 $V = X_0/C_0$（体积/体重）

消除率 $Cl = kV = 0.693 \times V/t_{1/2}$（体积/时间/体重）

【材料】

家兔 1 只。

离心管，试管，吸管，注射器，静脉插管，兔手术台，722 分光光度计。

2% 磺溴酞钠溶液，肝素化生理盐水（10U/ml），草酸钾，2.5mol/L NaOH 溶液，0.01mol/L HCl 溶液，1% 盐酸普鲁卡因。

【方法与步骤】

取家兔 1 只，称重，背位固定于手术台上，在一侧腹股沟部搏动处剪毛，用 1ml 1% 盐酸普鲁卡因作皮下局麻。纵切皮肤 3~4cm，分离股静脉，在静脉下穿双线，结扎远心端，作静脉切口，插入与注射器相连的静脉插管（内充满肝素化盐水），结扎固定，检查取血是否顺利。静脉注射 BSP（20mg/kg），分别于注射后第 2，4，6，10，15，20 分钟由股静脉取血 1.5~2ml 置于盛有草酸钾试管中，轻轻摇动试管，使草酸钾均匀地溶解于血液中。每次取血样时，先舍去 0.2ml 左右血液，取后，补充等量生理盐水。将各试管离心（3000r/min，5min），分别取血浆 0.5ml，转移入另一试管中，加入 0.01mol/L HCl 溶液 5.5ml，混匀后在 722 分光光度计于波长 540nm 处测吸光度。测定后，加 2.5mol/L NaOH 溶液 1 滴，混匀后再进行吸光度测定，计算吸光度差值，利用差值从标准曲线上求出相应的血药浓度，利用 $\ln c \sim t$ 作直线回归，求得斜率和截距，利用前面公式求出相应的药代动力学参数。

标准曲线绘制：以蒸馏水配制浓度为 200μg/ml 的 BSP 标准溶液，取 7 支试管，以 1，2，3……7 编号，按表 2-2 进行操作。

利用吸光度差及对相应的 BSP 浓度作图即得标准曲线。

表 2-2 BSP 标准曲线绘制

试管编号	1	2	3	4	5	6	7
加 200μg/ml 的 BSP（ml）	0.025	0.05	0.075	0.10	0.15	0.20	0.30
加 0.01mol/L HCl（ml）	5.975	5.95	5.925	5.90	5.85	5.80	5.70
测吸收度 A_{H^+}							
加 2.5mol/L NaOH 的 A_{OH^-}							
计算 $\Delta A = A_{OH^-} - A_{H^+}$							
相当于血浆浓度（μg/ml）	5	10	15	20	30	40	60

【注意事项】

1. 实验过程中，动作要轻，注意采血器用生理盐水吸洗，应尽量避免样品溶血，影响测定。

2. 每次取血样时，应先取 0.2ml 血弃去，采血过程尽可能轻快，确保血样时间准确。

3. 样品离心前必须平衡，转速适中。

【方法评价】

股静脉取血较其他途径如耳缘静脉取血有迅速、方便且不易溶血等优点。此法仅是一种粗略估算药代动力学参数的方法。

实验 2.4　药物血浆蛋白结合率测定

【目的】

了解血浆蛋白结合率的测定方法。

【原理】

蛋白结合率是重要的药代动力学参数，药物与蛋白高度结合时（一般指 80% 以上），具有很重要的临床意义。研究药物与蛋白结合的实验方法很多，目前以平衡透析、超过滤和凝胶过滤等法最为常用，这里对平衡透析作较详细介绍。将蛋白溶液装入半透膜内，然后置于含有药物的缓冲液中，让药物分子通过半透膜自由扩散，待扩散达到平衡后，测定袋内外的药物浓度。将袋内浓度减去袋外浓度，再除以袋内浓度即得蛋白结合率。

【材料】

管状半透膜（周长 5cm，长 10cm 左右），pH 7.4 的 0.2mol/L 磷酸缓冲液（内含 0.15mol/L NaCl），3% 磺基水杨酸溶液。

【方法与步骤】

1. 将管状半透膜一端折叠，用线扎紧，用吸管加入血浆样本 2.5ml，折叠并结扎袋口，袋内保留少量空气。

2. 将半透膜袋置于盛有 10ml 磷酸缓冲液的 30ml 广口瓶中，用袋两端线段调节袋内外液面，使其保持同一水平。

3. 置广口瓶于冰箱中（4℃），平衡 60h 以上，达到平衡时间后，吸出袋外磷酸缓冲液少许，加等量 3% 磺基水杨酸溶液，检查有无血浆蛋白漏出。

测定袋外和袋内溶液中的药物浓度。

【结果处理】

计算 β_p 及 K_{dp} 值的算式如下：

$$[D] = \beta_p \times \frac{P[D]}{[D] + [PD] - [D]W} - K_{dp}$$

式中：$[D]$ 和 $P[D]$ 为游离和已结合的药物摩尔浓度，P 为蛋白浓度，以 g/L 表示，W 为血浆含水率，β_p 为蛋白结合药物的表观最大能力，以 μmol/g 表示，K_{dp} 是药物 – 蛋白复合物的解离常数，以 μmol/L 表示。令 $[D]$ 为纵坐标，$\dfrac{P[D]}{[D] + [PD] - [D]W}$ 为横坐标，利用直线回归求得斜率 β_p 及纵截距 K_{dp}。再利用下列方程可求出任一浓度时的蛋白结合率

$$蛋白结合率 = 1 - \left(W + \frac{P\beta_p}{[D] + K_{dp}} \right)$$

【方法评价】

本法简便，适于多个样品同时测定，缺点是达到平衡的时间较长。

三、影响药物作用的因素

影响药物作用的因素，包括药物和机体两个方面。

（一）药物方面

（1）药物的化学结构和理化性质不仅直接决定药物的作用性质和强度，而且也决定药物在体内的吸收、分布、代谢和排泄。化学结构相似的药物往往有相似的药理活性。

（2）药物的剂量不仅可以产生强度的变化，也能产生质的变化，因此对一些治疗窗窄的药物应严格控制剂量，必要时个体化用药，以确保用药安全。

（3）给药途径不同可以直接影响药物吸收的量和速度，也会影响到药物分布和排泄，从而影响药物的作用。

（二）机体方面

不同年龄、性别、体重、种族间对药物反应存在差异，尤其是婴幼儿和老年人，他们对同剂量药物的反应与正常人相比，有显著不同。此外，如遗传因素、病理因素以及对一些药物的认识程度都有可能影响到药效的发挥。

实验 2.5 影响药物作用的因素

（一）剂型对药物作用的影响

【目的】

比较两种剂型的二甲弗林（回苏灵）对蟾蜍作用的差异。

【原理】

二甲弗林为中枢兴奋药。随给药剂量的增加，动物会产生惊厥，甚至死亡。药理作用强度与药物吸收的快慢有关。

【材料】

蟾蜍 2 只，同一性别。

0.2% 二甲弗林水溶液，0.2% 二甲弗林胶浆液（含羧甲基纤维素 2.5%）。

【方法与步骤】

1. 取蟾蜍 2 只，称重，以棉线系足做记号。

2. 胸淋巴囊内注射给药，1 只为 0.2% 二甲弗林水溶液，剂量 10mg/kg；另 1 只为 0.2% 二甲弗林胶浆液，剂量亦为 10mg/kg。

3. 注射后把蟾蜍置于手术灯下，经常加以触动，直至出现强直性惊厥。

4. 记录 2 只蟾蜍二甲弗林作用的潜伏期以及惊厥的严重程度。

【结果处理】

将上述观察到的结果填入表 2 - 3 和表 2 - 4，并对全班各组的潜伏期数据进行统计分析。

表 2 - 3　两种剂型对蟾蜍惊厥的影响

剂型	性别	体重（g）	潜伏期（min）	惊厥程度
水溶液				
胶浆液				

表 2 - 4　不同剂型对蟾蜍惊厥潜伏期的影响

剂型	组号								$\bar{x} \pm SD$
	1	2	3	4	5	6	7	8	
水溶液									
胶浆液									

（二）给药途径对药物作用的影响

【目的】

观察不同给药途径对药物作用的影响。

【原理】

二甲弗林（回苏灵）为中枢兴奋药，可引起动物兴奋、惊厥或死亡。

【材料】

小鼠 3 只，体重 18 ~ 22g，同一性别。

0.04% 二甲弗林水溶液。

【方法与步骤】

动物称重，标记。各鼠给药剂量均为 8mg/kg。甲鼠灌胃给药，乙鼠皮下注射，丙鼠则为腹腔注射。仔细观察动物反应，记录下各鼠二甲弗林作用的潜伏期和最终结果。

【结果处理】

将上述观察到的结果填入表 2 - 5、表 2 - 6，并结合全班的实验结果，比较三种给药途径与药物反应的出现时间和作用程度，最好能进行统计分析。

表 2 - 5　不同给药途径对药物作用的影响

鼠号	剂量（mg/kg）	给药途径	潜伏期（min）	惊厥程度
甲				
乙				
丙				

表 2 - 6　不同给药途径对小鼠惊厥潜伏期的影响

给药途径	组号								$\bar{x} \pm SD$
	1	2	3	4	5	6	7	8	
灌胃									
皮下注射									
腹腔注射									

（三）肝脏功能状态对药物作用的影响

【目的】

观察肝脏病理功能状态对药物作用的影响。

【原理】

四氯化碳是一种肝脏毒物，其中毒动物常被作为中毒性肝炎的动物模型，用于筛选保肝药物。

【材料】

小鼠2只，体重18～22g，同一性别。

四氯化碳原液，0.3%戊巴比妥钠，生理盐水。

【方法与步骤】

1. 取性别相同、体重相近的2只小鼠，在实验前24h，分别皮下注射四氯化碳原液0.1ml和生理盐水0.1ml。

2. 2只小鼠分别腹腔注射戊巴比妥钠（30mg/kg）。

3. 观察动物的翻正反射消失情况，记录药物作用的潜伏期和持续时间。

4. 实验结束后，解剖小鼠，比较2只小鼠的肝脏外观有何不同。

【结果处理】

将上述观察到的结果填入表2－7、表2－8，并结合全班的实验结果，比较不同肝功能状态对药物作用影响，最好能进行统计分析。

表2－7　不同肝功能状态对药物作用的影响

鼠号	剂量（mg/kg）	肝脏状态	潜伏期（min）	睡眠时间（min）	肝脏解剖情况
甲					
乙					

表2－8　不同肝功能状态对动物产生睡眠的潜伏期的影响

肝脏状态	组号								$\bar{x} \pm SD$
	1	2	3	4	5	6	7	8	
生理盐水									
四氯化碳									

第三章　中枢神经系统药物实验

中枢神经系统药物包括全身麻醉药、镇静催眠药、镇痛药、抗癫痫药和抗惊厥药、抗精神失常药、中枢兴奋药等。

全身麻醉药传统上分为吸入麻醉药（乙醚、氟烷类、氧化亚氮等）、静脉麻醉药（硫喷妥钠、氯胺酮、γ-羟基丁酸等）等。吸入麻醉药和静脉麻醉药能广泛抑制中枢神经系统的脑电活动，麻醉可达第三期，从而意识、痛觉反射消失，肌肉松弛，故称为抑制性麻醉药。个别麻醉药，如氯胺酮，能选择性地阻断痛觉，而对网状结构和边缘系统呈现兴奋作用，因而也称之为兴奋性麻醉药，麻醉时，患者意识不完全丧失而痛觉却完全消失，意识和感觉分离，称此为"分离麻醉"。

镇静催眠药为能抑制中枢神经系统的药物，根据对中枢抑制程度的不同分为镇静作用和催眠作用。其中包括巴比妥类（苯巴比妥等）、苯二氮䓬类（氯氮䓬、地西泮等）以及其他镇静催眠药。这些药物小剂量时产生镇静作用，中等剂量产生催眠作用，故称为镇静催眠药。此外，抗组胺药（如苯海拉明、异丙嗪等）、抗精神病药（如氯丙嗪等）、镇痛药和一些中草药亦有镇静、催眠作用。

镇痛药能选择性地缓解疼痛，可分为强镇痛药和弱镇痛药。强镇痛药是指抑制中枢痛觉区的镇痛药，包括成瘾性镇痛药或称麻醉性镇痛药（如阿片类镇痛药：哌替啶、芬太尼、美沙酮等），弱镇痛药是指作用于外周痛觉感受器的镇痛药，常称为解热镇痛抗炎药（如阿司匹林等）。

癫痫是由于脑部神经兴奋性过高，产生异常放电而出现大脑功能失调的综合征，可分为大发作、小发作、精神运动性发作和局限性发作等类型。临床上常选用对大脑皮质异常放电具有抑制作用或阻止其扩散的药物进行控制性治疗。惊厥是各种原因引起的中枢神经过度兴奋的一种症状，表现为全身骨骼肌不自主、不协调、强直性和阵挛性抽搐。常见于小儿高热、子痫、破伤风和急性中毒等情况，可用中枢性运动抑制药，或某些外周性肌松药加以控制。

精神失常是由各种原因引起的思维、情感、行为等精神活动异常的疾病，包括精神分裂症、躁狂症、抑郁症、焦虑症等。抗精神失常药物是对精神分裂症、躁狂症、抑郁症及焦虑症等有治疗作用的药物。这类药物可分为以下几类：①抗精神分裂症（或抗精神病）药；②抗躁狂抑郁药；③抗焦虑药等。

凡能提高中枢神经系统机能活动的药物称为中枢兴奋药。按作用部位的不同，分为大脑兴奋药（如咖啡因、尼可刹米、洛贝林，二甲弗林、贝美格、戊四氮等）及脊髓兴奋药（士的宁）等类。此类药物在治疗量时，主要作用于延髓呼吸中枢，故又称延髓兴奋药；亦兴奋延髓血管运动中枢引起血压升高，能改善呼吸及循环功能。临床主要用于各种原因引起的呼吸衰竭。但剂量过大或应用过频时，由于大脑和延髓的过度兴奋，可产生惊厥；过度兴奋后，由于大脑能量耗竭，又容易转化为超限抑制，甚至危及生命。

一、全身麻醉药实验

实验 3.1　挥发性液体麻醉药活性测定

【目的】

观察乙醚麻醉的特点，了解全身性麻醉药活性测定的方法。

【原理】

一般采用小动物翻正反射消失和大动物的垂头（头正位反射消失）作为麻醉药活性测定的指标。

当在一已知容量的容器内，加入已知分子量和相对密度的挥发性液体麻醉药时，则可按下式算出容器内的麻醉药蒸气浓度：

$$蒸气百分浓度 = \frac{液体体积（ml）×相对密度×22.4（L）×100}{药物分子量×容器容积（L）}$$

按上式算出的浓度系在标准状态时的体积。上式中的体积 22.4L 为理想气体在标准状态即 1 个标准大气压、0°C 时的体积。实际体积尚需按试验时情况用下式校正：

$$PV/T = P'V'/T'$$

注：P、V、T 为气体在标准状态时的压强、体积和温度。P'、V'、T' 为试验时气体的压强、体积和温度。

【材料】

小鼠，体重 18~22g，雌雄不限。

动物麻醉箱，乙醚。

【方法与步骤】

1. 动物麻醉箱为一玻璃制成的密闭小箱，小箱容量为 4~10L（图 3-1）。小箱中置有盛钠石灰的小盘，以吸收箱中的二氧化碳和水分。箱的上方为可开启的顶盖。箱内亦可装一小电扇，以加快药物的蒸发。

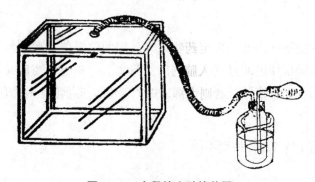

图 3-1　小鼠的麻醉箱装置

2. 按小箱中所需药物蒸气浓度，算出应注入箱中的药量，振摇麻醉箱使药液挥发，然后投入小鼠。如欲求出半数有效麻醉浓度（AD_{50}），可将药液蒸气百分浓度按等比级数递增 4~6 个剂量，动物每组 5~10 只，即可求出量效反应曲线，并算出 AD_{50} 值。

3. 麻醉诱导期应为 0.5~5min，如不在此范围内，应调整麻醉药蒸气浓度。

4. 采用翻正反射消失和痛觉消失作为麻醉指标。若动物群集和互相倾倚，难以判定结果时，应将可疑小鼠置于仰卧位观察。测痛觉时可用大头针刺后足或用小鳄鱼夹夹小鼠尾根部近肛门处。

5. 麻醉后继续观察 10～30min，观察麻醉过程是否平稳。

【结果处理】

计算 AD_{50} 值。

【注意事项】

1. 乙醚易燃易爆，且比重较空气重，试验时严禁明火。

2. 试验前应检查麻醉箱有无漏气。

3. 严格掌握麻醉指标——翻正反射消失与否。

【方法评价】

全身麻醉药实验主要有两种方法，即小动物法和大动物法。前者方法简单、经济，适用于初筛实验，后者多用来进行复试观察。常用小鼠进行的小动物法，可以从麻醉浓度与致死浓度或麻醉剂量与致死剂量之间的差距，初步估计药物的安全性，并可用于同类麻醉药效价的比较。但是大动物法观察所得的结果较接近于临床患者的反应情况，参考价值较大，同时便于准确测定麻醉药的诱导期、麻醉过程、恢复期以及对呼吸、血压和心电图、各种反射、肌松程度等的影响。故大、小动物法宜结合进行。

【思考题】

乙醚麻醉有何优缺点？现在在临床上地位如何？

二、镇静催眠药实验

实验 3.2　巴比妥类药物作用的比较

【目的】

比较几种巴比妥类药物的作用强度、潜伏期和药效维持时间。

【原理】

巴比妥类药物的脂溶性高低是决定药物进入脑组织快慢的主要因素，脂溶性越高越易穿透血脑屏障，不但潜伏期短而且进入脑内的药量也大。脂溶性高的药物主要由肝药酶代谢，作用维持时间短，而脂溶性低者则大部分以原形由肾脏排泄，故作用维持时间较长。

【材料】

小鼠 3 只，体重 18～22g，性别不限。

天平、注射器。

0.6% 苯巴比妥钠、0.2% 戊巴比妥钠、0.2% 硫喷妥钠、苦味酸。

【方法与步骤】

取小鼠 3 只，称重标号，分别腹腔注射下列药物：

鼠甲：0.6% 苯巴比妥钠 150mg/kg（即 0.25ml/10g）。

鼠乙：0.2% 戊巴比妥钠 50mg/kg（即 0.25ml/10g）。

鼠丙：0.2%硫喷妥钠 50mg/kg（即 0.25ml/10g）。

观察各鼠用药后的行为活动有何改变，翻正反射是否消失，记录翻正反射的消失时间和恢复时间。

【结果处理】

按表 3 – 1 记录实验结果。

表 3 – 1　巴比妥类药物作用的比较

鼠号	体重（g）	药物与剂量（mg/kg）	行为活动变化	翻正反射		作用特点
				消失时间（min）	恢复时间（min）	

【注意事项】

1. 进行本实验时必须保持环境安静。

2. 翻正反射消失是指：将小鼠轻轻置于仰卧位，如松手后仍能保持仰卧状态，即为翻正反射消失。

3. 小鼠翻正反射消失后应保持环境温度。

【方法评价】

镇静药、催眠药和安定药均可不同程度地改变动物的行为，如使小鼠产生安静、群聚、闭眼、嗜睡及翻正反射消失等现象。根据这类药物的作用特点、强度、潜伏期和维持作用时间的长短可比较药物作用的强弱。虽然该方法简单，但中枢抑制药物均有上述作用，因此，该法特异性较差，只能作初步的定性观察。如要进一步探讨药物作用的性质，应选用特异性较高的方法，如驯服实验、对抗中枢兴奋药的作用及条件反射实验等。

【思考题】

根据实验结果讨论上述各种巴比妥类药物作用强度、起效快慢及作用时间的差异及其原因。

实验 3.3　镇静催眠药的协同作用和对抗中枢兴奋药的作用

【目的】

通过认识药物相互作用的协同作用和拮抗作用，学习镇静催眠药的筛选方法。

【原理】

镇静催眠药随剂量的递增依次表现为镇静和催眠作用，巴比妥类药物还会出现麻醉作用。镇静催眠药合用作用加强，且可对抗中枢兴奋药引起的惊厥行为。

【材料】

小鼠 5 只，体重 18～22g，性别不限。

注射器、天平、钟罩。

0.04% 地西泮、0.2% 戊巴比妥钠、0.04% 二甲弗林。

【方法与步骤】

取性别相同、体重相近的小鼠 5 只，编号、称重，然后作下述处置：

鼠甲腹腔注射 0.04% 地西泮 8mg/kg（即 0.2ml/10g）。

鼠乙皮下注射 0.2% 戊巴比妥钠 40mg/kg（即 0.2ml/10g）。

鼠丙先腹腔注射 0.04% 地西泮 8mg/kg（即 0.2m1/10g），10min 后再皮下注射 0.2% 戊巴比妥钠 40mg/kg（即 0.2ml/10g）。

鼠丁皮下注射 0.04% 二甲弗林 8mg/kg（即 0.2ml/10g）。

鼠戊先腹腔注射 0.04% 地西泮 8mg/kg（即 0.2ml/10g）。10min 后再皮下注射 0.04% 二甲弗林 8mg/kg（即 0.2ml/10g）。

将 5 鼠分别置于钟罩内，比较所出现的药物反应及最终结果。观察小鼠预先注射地西泮对于戊巴比妥钠和二甲弗林的药理作用各有何影响。

【结果处理】

按表 3 - 2 记录实验结果。

表 3 - 2　药物协同作用和拮抗作用实验结果

鼠号	性别	体重（g）	第一次给药		第二次给药		两药相互作用类型
			药物与剂量（mg/kg）	给药后反应	药物与剂量（mg/kg）	给药后反应	

【注意事项】

1. 注射药物比较多，每次注射之前应充分洗净注射器，以免药物相互作用影响实验结果。

2. 镇静催眠药均属于中枢抑制药，故动物实验时其作用往往不能区分。镇静作用的指标主要是自发活动减少；催眠作用的指标是动物的共济失调，当环境安静时，可以逐渐入睡。翻正反射的消失既可代表催眠作用，又可反映巴比妥类催眠药的麻醉作用。

3. 实验环境需安静，室温以 15～20℃ 为宜。

【方法评价】

镇静催眠药的初筛方法常用行为学实验，如与阈下剂量的戊巴比妥合用，可以促使小鼠入睡。常以翻正反射消失的小鼠数作为指标来衡量药效。另外，也可以用减少中枢兴奋药所致的过度活动来筛试，或以对抗中枢兴奋药的毒性、提高半数致死量的幅度来衡量药效。但这些方法特异性均不高，难以区分药物的作用性质，常用来初筛定性分析。

【思考题】

在合并用药过程中各药可以通过哪几种方式发生相互作用，引起哪几种后果？

实验 3.4　药物对动物自发活动的影响

【目的】

观察地西泮对小鼠自发活动的影响，学习镇静催眠药的筛选方法。

【原理】

自发活动是动物的生理特征，自发活动的多少往往表现其中枢兴奋或抑制状态。镇静催眠药等中枢抑制药均可明显减少小鼠的自发活动。自发活动减少的程度与中枢抑制药的作用强弱成正比。

【材料】

小鼠 3 ~ 4 只，体重 18 ~ 22g，同一性别。

小鼠自发活动记录仪、注射器、鼠笼、天平。

0.05% 地西泮溶液、生理盐水、苦味酸溶液。

【方法与步骤】

将自发活动记录仪通电，设定记录时间为 5min。取活动度相近的小鼠 2 只，称重，编号。

取鼠甲置于自发活动记录仪的盒内，使其适应环境约 5min。然后开始计算时间，观察并记录 5min 的活动数，作为给药前的对照值。将小鼠取出，然后腹腔注射 0.05% 地西泮 10mg/kg（即 0.2ml/10g）。给药后将小鼠放回盒内，给药后 15min、30min、60min、90min 和 120min 按上述方法测定 5min 的自发活动数。

鼠乙先按上述方法测试 5min 内的自发活动数，然后腹腔注射生理盐水 20ml/kg（0.2ml/10g），同样观察、记录 120min 内的活动情况，与甲鼠作比较。

【结果处理】

收集全实验室的数据，填入表 3 - 3。

表 3 - 3　地西泮对小鼠自发活动的影响

组别	药物及剂量（mg/kg）	5min 内自发活动数					
		给药前	给药后				
			15min	30min	60min	90min	120min
生理盐水							
地西泮							

【注意事项】

1. 实验环境要求安静，有条件可在隔音室内进行。

2. 动物活动与饮食条件、昼夜及生活环境等有密切关系，观察自发活动最好多方面条件相近。

3. 动物宜事先禁食 12h，以增加觅食活动。

【方法评价】

镇静催眠药和神经安定药的作用，常以动物自发活动减少程度来衡量。常用的方法是将小鼠置于特制笼内，以抖动、遮断光径等方法记录其自发活动数，比较给药前后的变化。但动物自发活动易受环境因素影响，变化较大，因而须有严格的对照观察。

【思考题】

用本方法测定小鼠自发活动应注意哪些问题？适用于哪几类药物？

三、抗癫痫药和抗惊厥药实验

实验 3.5　药物抗电惊厥作用

【目的】

观察苯妥英钠和苯巴比妥对电惊厥的保护作用。

【原理】

以一强电流刺激小鼠头颅可引起全身强直性惊厥，若药物预防强直性惊厥发生，可初步推测该药有抗癫痫大发作的作用。

【材料】

小鼠 3~4 只，体重 18~22g，雌雄不限。

钟罩、天平、注射器，药理生理多用仪。

0.5% 苯妥英钠溶液、0.5% 苯巴比妥溶液，生理盐水。

【方法与步骤】

1. 调机：将药理生理多用仪的刺激方式旋钮置于"单次"位置，"A"频率置于"8Hz"，后面板上的开关拨向"电惊厥"一边，电压调至最大。

2. 将输出线前端的两鳄鱼夹用生理盐水浸湿，分别夹在小鼠的两耳上。接通电源，按下"启动"按钮，即可使小鼠产生前肢屈曲，后肢伸直的强直惊厥（如未产生强直惊厥，可将"频率"旋钮拨到"4Hz"试之，否则另换小鼠）。

3. 选择 3 只典型强直惊厥小鼠，称重标记。分别腹腔注射 0.5% 苯妥英钠 75mg/kg（即 0.15ml/10g）、0.5% 苯巴比妥 75mg/kg（即 0.15ml/10g）及生理盐水 0.15ml/10g。

4. 给药后 40min，再以各鼠的原惊厥阈值给予刺激，观察并记录各鼠是否出现挣扎反应或强直惊厥。

【结果处理】

收集全实验室的数据，填入表 3-4。

表 3-4　药物对小鼠电惊厥的拮抗作用

药物		各组的反应强度							
		1	2	3	4	5	6	7	8
生理盐水	给药前 给药后								
苯妥英钠	给药前 给药后								
苯巴比妥	给药前 给药后								

【注意事项】

1. 引起惊厥的刺激电流参数因动物的个体差异，须通过试验而测得，不宜过大，以免引起死亡。

2. 夹住两鼠耳的鳄鱼夹严防短路，以免引起刺激器的损坏。

3. 动物惊厥可分为五个时期：潜伏期、僵直屈曲期、后肢伸直期、阵挛期（有的动物无）以及恢复期。

【方法评价】

惊厥是由中枢神经系统过度兴奋而引起的骨骼肌不自主和不协调的抽搐。用电刺激或声刺激等引起的实验性惊厥来筛选抗癫痫药。目前广泛应用的电惊厥法有最大电休克发作和精神运动性发作两种方法。前者被认为是很好的癫痫大发作实验模型，后者相当于精神运动性发作。因此本法主要是用来筛选抗大发作药物。

【思考题】

试从用药后动物活动改变情况及电刺激后的反应，比较苯巴比妥与苯妥英钠作用的异同。

实验 3.6 药物对抗中枢兴奋药惊厥的作用

【目的】

观察丙戊酸钠对二甲弗林惊厥的保护作用。

【原理】

二甲弗林是直接兴奋呼吸中枢的中枢兴奋药，剂量过大时可引起惊厥反应。药物对二甲弗林所致惊厥反应的保护作用可用来初筛抗惊厥药和抗癫痫药。

【材料】

小鼠 2 只，体重 18～22g，雌雄不限。

钟罩、天平、注射器。

0.04% 二甲弗林溶液、2% 丙戊酸钠溶液、生理盐水。

【方法与步骤】

1. 取小鼠 2 只，编号，称重。

2. 分别腹腔注射 2% 丙戊酸钠 600mg/kg（即 0.3ml/10g）和生理盐水 0.3ml/10g。

3. 30min 后，再皮下注射 0.04% 二甲弗林溶液 8mg/kg（即 0.2ml/10g）。观察各鼠反应的快慢和强度（痉挛、跌倒、强直或死亡）。

【结果处理】

记录小鼠注射二甲弗林后各种症状出现的时间和强弱，判断丙戊酸钠的作用。

【注意事项】

条件许可的情况下，最好以戊四氮代替二甲弗林。戊四氮的惊厥反应较典型，所用剂量为 120mg/kg，皮下注射。

【方法评价】

化学物质引起惊厥法操作简单，不需要特殊仪器设备，这种方法可以在一定程度上进行作用原理分析。目前将戊四氮惊厥发作试验作为筛选癫痫小发作有效药物的常用方法。

【思考题】

试从以上结果讨论各药的作用及临床应用。

四、抗精神失常药实验

实验 3.7　氯丙嗪的安定作用

【目的】

观察氯丙嗪对小鼠激怒反应的影响。

【原理】

小鼠足部持续受到一定强度电刺激后可出现激怒反应，即逃避、吱吱叫、格斗、对峙、互咬。抗精神病药可抑制此种激怒反应。

【材料】

小鼠 4 只，体重 20～24g，雄性，异笼喂养。

药理生理多用仪附激怒刺激盒、注射器、针头、天平。

0.04% 盐酸氯丙嗪溶液，生理盐水。

【方法与步骤】

1. 调节刺激器，刺激参数为：工作状态——激怒；输出电压——最小；刺激方式——连续 B；时间——1s；频率——8Hz。把交流电压输出线插入后面板的"交流电压输出"插座中，另一端的两个鳄鱼夹分别夹在附件盒的红、黑接线柱上。

2. 选择激怒的小鼠：放 2 只雄性异笼小鼠于附件盒内。接通电源，调节交流电压输出强度，逐渐由小增大，直至小鼠出现激怒反应为止（激怒反应指标：两鼠竖立，对峙，互相撕咬）。如小鼠不互相撕咬，则弃去。选两对有明显激怒反应的小鼠，记录阈电压(图 3-2)。

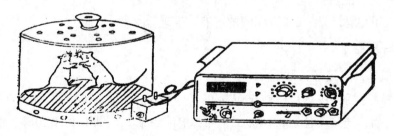

图 3-2　小鼠激怒试验装置

3. 一对腹腔注射 0.04% 盐酸氯丙嗪 4mg/kg（即 0.1ml/10g），另一对腹腔注射生理盐水 0.1ml/10g。

4. 给药后 20min，分别再以给药前的阈值电压进行刺激，观察两对小鼠给药前后的反应差异。

【结果处理】

按表 3-5 记录实验结果。

表 3-5　氯丙嗪对小鼠激怒反应的影响

组别		激怒阈值电压（V）	潜伏期（S）
生理盐水组	给药前		
	给药后		
氯丙嗪组	给药前		
	给药后		

【注意事项】

1. 在 3min 内每对鼠典型格斗不少于 3 次者选做实验。给药后以原刺激参数刺激，典型格斗少于 3 次者称抑制。

2. 刺激盒应保持干燥，随时擦净小鼠尿液和粪便，以免引起短路，影响正常电压输出。

3. 出现典型格斗反应后应立即关闭电源，取出刺激盒中小鼠时应仔细检查有无电压输出，以免发生意外。

【方法评价】

由于抗精神病药作用于脑内多巴胺能系统，因此出现许多与多巴胺能系统有关的行为反应，如僵直症、抗呕吐反应、抗阿扑吗啡等作用。这些反应虽然是抗精神病药的副作用或次要作用，但是许多实验证明它们与治疗作用有一定的平行关系。抗精神病药对实验性诱发激怒反应的作用具有重要的临床意义。该法简单，适用于大量初筛。如有条件者可进行放射配基受体结合分析与行为试验相结合的方法来筛选抗精神病药。预测抗精神病药的作用强度主要依赖于以上两项实验结果。

【思考题】

试从上述结果讨论氯丙嗪的安定作用特点与用途。

实验 3.8　氯丙嗪对小鼠基础代谢的影响

【目的】

以耗氧量为指标，观察氯丙嗪对小鼠基础代谢的影响。

【原理】

小鼠在密闭容器中的存活时间可以反映动物消耗氧的能力。降低机体代谢（如中枢抑制药）可延长小鼠在密闭容器中的存活时间。

【材料】

小鼠 20 只，体重 18~22g，雌性。

广口瓶、凡士林、钠石灰。

0.1% 盐酸氯丙嗪溶液，生理盐水。

【方法与步骤】

1. 取 20 只体重相近的雌性小鼠分为 2 组，每组 10 只。

2. 腹腔注射给药。甲组：0.1% 盐酸氯丙嗪 15mg/kg（即 0.15ml/10g）。乙组：生理盐水 15ml/kg。

3. 给药后 20min，分别将各小鼠置于含 25g 钠石灰的磨口广口瓶（125ml）中。

4. 瓶口用涂以凡士林的瓶盖密封。

5. 观察和记录小鼠的死亡时间，并收集全实验室的结果进行统计，用 t 检验法检验是否有显著性差异。

【结果处理】

按表 3-6 记录实验结果。

表 3 - 6　氯丙嗪对小鼠耐缺氧的影响

组别	存活时间（min）										$\bar{x} \pm SD$
	1	2	3	4	5	6	7	8	9	10	
对照组											
氯丙嗪组											

【注意事项】

1. 钠石灰需新鲜，装置应密封，等容量。

2. 各小鼠体重应尽量接近，因为能量代谢率正比于体表面积。

3. 观察瓶内小鼠死亡时间应观察到呼吸停止后 5min，以确证小鼠已经死亡。

4. 注意实验环境温度的恒定与一致。

【方法评价】

密闭容器小动物存活时间的测定是观察中枢抑制药增加脑血流量、提高中枢神经元摄氧能力等作用的常用初筛方法。该法简单，但特异性较差。

【思考题】

从氯丙嗪对基础代谢的影响，联系其降温作用，讨论该药在这方面的临床应用。

实验 3.9　药物的镇痛作用（热板法）

【目的】

了解用热板法筛选镇痛药并比较药物镇痛效价的方法。

【原理】

各种伤害如热刺激引起的疼痛性刺激通过感觉纤维传入脊髓，最后到达大脑皮质感觉区而引起疼痛。中枢性镇痛药（如吗啡等）和外周性镇痛药（如水杨酸等），通过痛感觉中枢整合作用以及抑制或减少痛觉的传入而达到镇痛作用。中枢性镇痛药的镇痛作用较易在动物实验中加以证实，但某些外周性镇痛药如水杨酸类的镇痛作用不易测定。

【材料】

小鼠 3 ~ 4 只，体重 18 ~ 22g，雌性。

电热板、鼠笼、天平、注射器、针头、烧杯。

0.1% 盐酸吗啡溶液、2% 水杨酸钠溶液，生理盐水。

【方法与步骤】

1. 将热板温度调节至 55℃ ± 0.5℃，置小鼠于热板上，测定各小鼠的正常痛反应（舔后足或抬后足并回头）时间，共测 2 次，每次间隔 5min，以平均值不超过 30s 为合格，共选出 3 只小鼠，编号。

2. 甲鼠腹腔注射 0.1% 盐酸吗啡 15mg/kg（即 15ml/kg）；乙鼠腹腔注射 2% 水杨酸钠 300mg/kg（即 15ml/kg）；丙鼠腹腔注射生理盐水 15ml/kg。

3. 给药后 15、30、45、60min 同前分别测定痛反应时间 1 次。如小鼠在热板上 60s 无痛反应，按 60s 计算。

4. 按下列公式计算痛阈提高百分率。

$$痛阈提高百分率 = \frac{用药后痛反应时间 - 用药前痛反应时间}{用药前痛反应时间} \times 100\%$$

（如用药后痛反应时间减去用药前痛反应时间为负数，则以零计算）

【结果处理】

按表 3 – 7、图 3 – 3 记录处理实验结果。

表 3 – 7　吗啡和水杨酸钠的镇痛作用

鼠号	体重（g）	药物与剂量（mg/kg）	痛反应潜伏期（s）						
			给药前			给药后			
			第1次	第2次	半均	15min	30min	45min	60min
甲									
乙									
丙									

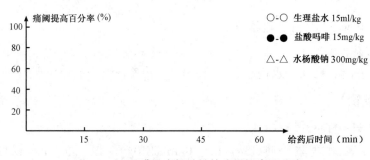

图 3 – 3　吗啡和水杨酸钠的痛阈提高百分率

【注意事项】

1. 测定痛反应时一旦小鼠表现出典型痛反应即应移离热板，60s 无痛反应也立即移离热板，以免造成烫伤。

2. 本实验不能使用雄性小鼠，因雄性小鼠受热后阴囊下坠，阴囊皮肤对痛敏感。

3. 室温对此实验有一定影响，以 15～20℃为宜。过低时小鼠反应迟钝，过高则过于敏感，易引起跳跃，均会影响结果的准确性。

4. 正常小鼠一般在放到受热平板上 10～15s 内出现不安、举前肢、舔前足、踢后肢、跳跃等现象，但这些动作均不作为痛指标，只有舔后足才作为疼痛的指标。

【方法评价】

筛选镇痛药的常用致痛方法包括物理性（热、电、机械）和化学性刺激法。这些方法各有其优缺点，其中以热、电刺激及钾离子皮下透入致痛法使用居多。常用的动物有小鼠、大鼠、豚鼠、家兔、犬等。动物实验中常用的痛反应指标为嘶叫、舔足、甩尾、挣扎及皮肤、肌肉抽搐等。

热板法装置简便，指标明确，对组织损伤小，动物可反复利用，并且痛反应潜伏期较长，便于观察及测出药物之间的较小差异，以利于比较药物镇痛作用的强弱、快慢及持续时间，故为目前比较常用的方法之一。缺点是具有镇静、肌松或拟精神病表现的药物常出现假阳性。

由于致痛原因各异，其适用场合也有所不同。机械刺激法与电刺激法适用于筛选麻醉性镇痛药，而不适于筛选解热镇痛药。热刺激法主要也用于筛选麻醉性镇痛药。化学刺激法比较适用于筛选解热镇痛药的镇痛作用。

【思考题】

联系吗啡和水杨酸钠的镇痛实验结果讨论两类镇痛药的作用和应用。

实验 3.10　药物的镇痛作用 （化学刺激法）

【目的】

了解用腹腔注射刺激性物质，引起扭体反应来筛选镇痛药的方法。

【原理】

腹腔注射一些化学物质如醋酸等刺激腹膜引起深部的、大面积而较持久的疼痛刺激，致使小鼠产生扭体反应，表现为腹部内凹，躯干与后肢伸展，臀部高起。

【材料】

小鼠 3 只，体重 20～25g，雌雄兼用。

天平、注射器、小鼠笼。

0.1% 盐酸吗啡溶液、4% 水杨酸钠溶液、0.8% 醋酸溶液、生理盐水。

【方法与步骤】

1. 取小鼠 3 只，称重并编号。

2. 鼠甲皮下注射盐酸吗啡 15mg/kg（0.15ml/10g），鼠乙灌胃水杨酸钠 400mg/kg（0.15ml/10g），鼠丙皮下注射生理盐水 15ml/kg。

3. 30min 后，各鼠分别腹腔注射 0.8% 醋酸 0.2ml，观察 15min 内发生扭体反应的小鼠数或各小鼠发生的扭体次数。

4. 汇集全实验室的结果，评价两药的镇痛作用。

【结果处理】

按表 3 – 8 记录、处理实验结果。

表 3 – 8　盐酸吗啡和水杨酸钠对小鼠腹腔注射醋酸引起疼痛的作用

组别	剂量 （mg/kg）	实验鼠数 （只）	扭体反应鼠数 （只）	扭体反应百分率 （%）	扭体反应数 （$\bar{x} \pm SD$）	扭体抑制率 （%）
生理盐水						
盐酸吗啡						
水杨酸钠						

【注意事项】

1. 可用酒石酸锑钾溶液代替醋酸溶液，但必须新鲜配制，放置过久易致作用减弱。醋酸亦需临时配制，以免挥发后浓度不准。

2. 室温最好恒定于 20℃，温度过低时小鼠扭体次数减少。小鼠体重过轻，扭体反应出现率亦低。

3. 结果可采用扭体或不扭体小鼠数统计，也可用小鼠扭体次数统计。

【方法评价】

本法适用于中枢和外周镇痛药的筛试，尤其适合解热镇痛药的筛选，具有敏感、简便和重复性好的特点。缺点是缺乏特异性，不仅镇痛药有效，许多非镇痛药也可以出现阳性结果。如 H_1 受体阻断剂、拟胆碱药、抗胆碱药、可乐定和氟哌啶醇等，必须结合其他实验结果，才能确定其镇痛作用。有报道认为扭体抑制率低于 70% 的药物无镇痛作用。

$$扭体抑制率 = \frac{对照组平均扭体次数 - 给药组平均扭体次数}{对照组平均扭体次数} \times 100\%$$

【思考题】

试从本实验及实验 3.9 的结果，讨论热板法和化学刺激法的区别。

五、中枢兴奋药实验

实验 3.11 士的宁和印防己毒素惊厥类型及作用部位的比较

【目的】

观察士的宁和印防己毒素所致的不同惊厥类型，学习从惊厥类型及分段破坏中枢神经系统来分析药物作用部位的方法。

【原理】

士的宁和印防己毒素均作用于中枢神经系统。前者主要作用于脊髓，惊厥类型是对称性的，是不协调性强直型惊厥，表现为双侧肢体同时产生持续性的强直性痉挛，脊髓以上部位对惊厥无影响；后者主要作用于中脑，惊厥类型呈不对称性，协调性阵挛型惊厥，表现为两侧肢体交互伸张、屈曲的阵发性痉挛，当中脑破坏时惊厥消失（图 3-4）。

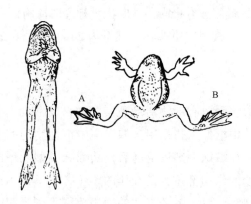

图 3-4 士的宁、印防己毒素所致惊厥类型的比较

注：A. 士的宁所致之惊厥；B. 印防己毒素所致之惊厥

【材料】

蟾蜍 2 只，体重 70g 以上，雌雄不限。

玻璃分针、注射器、烧杯、小镊子、探针、剪刀、天平、棉线。

0.03% 硝酸士的宁溶液、0.3% 印防己毒素溶液。

【方法与步骤】

1. 取蟾蜍 2 只,分别背位固定于蛙板上,剪开右侧大腿皮肤,由半膜肌与股二头肌之间分离坐骨神经,并在其下穿过一粗线,除该神经外将该腿的肌肉血管全部扎紧,以阻断血流。

2. 将蟾蜍自蛙板上取下,甲蟾蜍自胸淋巴囊注射 0.03% 硝酸士的宁 3mg/kg(即 0.1ml/10g),乙蟾蜍注射 0.3% 印防己毒素 30mg/kg(即 0.1ml/10g)。15min 后给予下列各种刺激,观察并比较两只蟾蜍产生惊厥和惊厥类型的差异:①突然触其皮肤;②以口吹风于其皮肤;③击掌发声;④拉动后肢。

3. 作用部位分析的步骤如下。

(1) 剪断一腿的坐骨神经,惊厥发生时该腿表现与正常腿有何区别?

(2) 从眼后缘剪去大脑,惊厥是否停止?

(3) 从鼓膜后缘剪去延脑,惊厥是否停止?

(4) 刺毁脊髓,惊厥是否停止?

【结果处理】

按表 3-9 仔细记录实验结果。

表 3-9   士的宁和印防己毒素所致惊厥类型的比较

蟾蜍号	体重 (g)	药物与剂量 (mg/kg)	对各种刺激的反应和类型				剪断一侧坐骨神经		去大脑后变化	去延脑后变化	毁脊髓后变化	主要作用部位
			轻触	吹风	击掌	拉后肢	断神经腿	保留神经腿				
甲												
乙												

【注意事项】

1. 分离坐骨神经应尽量靠近脊椎端,剪断坐骨神经时应将侧支一并剪断。

2. 如无印防己毒素,可改用二甲弗林,剂量为 24mg/kg(0.2% 溶液 0.12ml/10g),可得类似结果。

【方法评价】

中枢兴奋药的筛选方法主要有动物活动观察,如自发活动、条件反射活动、呼吸描记及反射时间测定等;拮抗中枢抑制药作用,如提高中枢抑制药的 LD_{50} 值或对抗呼吸抑制药中毒等;作用部位分析,如蟾蜍大剂量给药后,从惊厥类型及逐段破坏中枢神经系统对药物作用的影响来判断药物的作用部位,是经典的定位方法。作用部位分析法适用于中枢兴奋药的原理和致惊剂的研究。以上各种方法的适用范围不同,应根据具体的实验要求和实验的进行阶段来进行选择。

【思考题】

试从实验结果分析士的宁和印防己毒素的中枢作用部位。

实验 3.12   尼可刹米对抗吗啡的呼吸抑制作用

【目的】

学习常用的呼吸活动记录法,观察尼可刹米对抗吗啡的呼吸抑制作用。

【原理】

大剂量吗啡可抑制延髓呼吸中枢，呼吸中枢兴奋药则可对抗吗啡引起的呼吸抑制。

【材料】

家兔 1 只，体重 1.8~2.2kg，雌雄不限。

手术台、手术缝针、丝线、张力换能器、生理信号采集记录系统、注射器、针头。

1.5% 盐酸吗啡溶液、2% 尼可刹米溶液。

【方法与步骤】

1. 家兔称重后背位固定于兔手术台上，用手术缝针在剑突处穿线结扎，连接张力换能器，并与生理信号采集记录系统连接，进行呼吸曲线描记。

2. 待呼吸平稳，通过记录仪记录一段正常呼吸曲线。

3. 静脉快速注射 1.5% 盐酸吗啡 45mg/kg（即 3ml/kg），记录呼吸变化，注意呼吸频率。当出现明显呼吸抑制时，立即缓慢静脉注射 2% 尼可刹米 50mg/kg（即 2.5ml/kg），观察动物反应并记录呼吸变化。

【结果处理】

按表 3-10 记录结果。

表 3-10 尼可刹米对吗啡呼吸抑制的拮抗作用

观察项目	给药前	注射盐酸吗啡后	注射尼可刹米后
呼吸幅度（mm）			
呼吸频率（次/分）			

【注意事项】

1. 快速注射盐酸吗啡，以便血浆药物浓度迅速达到引起呼吸抑制的浓度。

2. 注射尼可刹米的速度宜稍慢，否则可致惊厥。

【方法评价】

呼吸兴奋作用观察法和对中枢抑制药的拮抗作用主要用于解除抑制状态、选择性兴奋呼吸功能的苏醒剂的筛选和研究。中枢兴奋药有不同类型，具体实验时可根据研究的目的选用一定的方法。

【思考题】

为什么尼可刹米较适用于吗啡急性中毒的解救？使用时应注意什么？

实验 3.13 尼莫地平对小鼠获得记忆的促进作用

【目的】

观察 Y 型迷宫训练小鼠产生获得记忆的过程，了解影响学习记忆药物的常用实验方法。

【原理】

Y 型迷宫装置内设起步区、电击区和安全区。给动物电击刺激，由于非条件反射的存在，使它逃避并获得找到安全区的记忆力，由此来观察药物对这种记忆力的影响。

【材料】

小鼠 8 只，体重 18~22g。

鼠笼、注射器、小鼠 Y 型电迷宫实验装置。

0.1% 尼莫地平溶液、生理盐水。

【方法与步骤】

1. 连接好仪器，固定起步点后对每只实验小鼠分别进行训练。训练时将小鼠放入规定的起步区，使之适应环境 1min，打开闸门并按下电击按钮给小鼠以电刺激。根据小鼠反应调节电压，以能引起小鼠奔跑、逃避为度（如鼠吱吱嘶叫表示电压过高，如鼠无运动反应，说明电压太低）。如小鼠在奔跑中最后窜到安全区（无电击），让其在此停留 10s 以巩固记忆。

2. 将小鼠从安全区取出放回起步点，休息 1min 后再给予第二次电击刺激，鼠又逃到安全区，如此反复训练。以小鼠在电击后能从起步点直接进入安全区的反应为"正确"，通过其他区域或乱窜后再进入安全区为"错误"，直至小鼠在连续 10 次电击中有 9 次"正确"为训练成功（或称获得记忆）。记录小鼠达 9/10 次正确反应时所需电击总次数。

3. 将已训练成功的小鼠 4 只给予尼莫地平（10mg/kg，腹腔注射），另 4 只给予等体积生理盐水后再连续给予电击，直至小鼠出现 9/10 次正确反应。记录此时电击刺激的总次数，计算记忆保存率，并比较 2 个实验组的结果，从而对药物的作用作出评价。

$$记忆保存率 = \frac{A - B}{A} \times 100\%$$

A 为给药前连续 10 次电击中有 9 次"正确"时所需电击总次数；

B 为给药后连续 10 次电击中有 9 次"正确"时所需电击总次数。

【结果处理】

按表 3-11 统计实验结果。

表 3-11　尼莫地平对小鼠学习记忆能力的影响

组别	编号	剂量（mg/kg）	动物数（只）	电击总数（次）给药前	电击总数（次）给药后	记忆保存率（%）
生理盐水组	1					
	2					
	3					
	4					
尼莫地平组	1					
	2					
	3					
	4					

【注意事项】

1. 一般用成年鼠进行实验，并测量两前肢皮肤电阻，电阻在 150~300kΩ 之间比较合适。

2. 电刺激以快速断续为宜，不能持续通电。

3. 每次电击后，不要将小鼠从安全区经迷路赶回起步点，而须从安全区取出，直接放回起步点。

4. 实验室要安静，光线不宜太强，室温最好为 18～30℃。

5. 亦可以吡拉西坦代替尼莫地平进行实验，其剂量为 20～40mg/kg，灌胃给药。

【方法评价】

学习和记忆是脑的重要功能之一。但人和动物的内部心理过程无法直接观察到，只能通过可观察到的刺激反应来推测脑内发生的过程。对脑内记忆过程的研究只能从人类或动物学习或执行某项任务后间隔一定时间，测量他们的操作成绩或反应时间来衡量。学习记忆的主要实验方法有跳台法、避暗法、穿梭箱法和迷宫法等。啮齿类动物是空间辨识学习中的高手，它们通常只需几次训练即可掌握，而迷宫法中的 Y 型迷宫法属最简单的、一次性训练的空间辨别反应试验，常作为促智药的初步筛选方法。但动物的行为反应易受体内各种生理因素的影响而发生改变，因此这种实验仅是以一种非特异指标来评价药物对动物全身生理功能的综合作用。同时，实验结果又易受多种外界因素的干扰，所以实验时一定要严格控制实验条件以减少实验误差。需与其他学习记忆实验结果一起综合评价一种药物的促智作用。

【思考题】

小鼠 Y 型迷宫训练时的正确方法是什么？

第四章　传出神经系统药物实验

传出神经系统包括自主神经和运动神经。自主神经主要支配心脏、平滑肌和腺体等效应器，根据产生效应的不同，自主神经又可分为交感神经和副交感神经。副交感神经兴奋时，心脏受到抑制，血管扩张，血压下降，胃肠道和支气管平滑肌兴奋，腺体分泌增加，瞳孔缩小。交感神经兴奋时，产生的效应与上述相反。一般地说，交感神经对心肌和小血管影响占优势，而副交感神经对平滑肌、腺体影响较明显。运动神经自中枢发出后，不更换神经元，直接到达所支配的骨骼肌。

由于传出神经系统涉及的面较广，使得其药理实验方法繁多，在方法和原理上，主要是围绕神经递质、受体及由此产生的效应而进行。交感神经节后纤维末梢释放去甲肾上腺素作为其递质，通过靶细胞或突触后膜上的 α、β 受体起作用。副交感神经末梢释放乙酰胆碱作用于后膜的 M 受体。

药物对受体方面作用的研究，常用的方法有药物效应方法和放射配基结合分析法。前者往往采用整体或离体动物实验模型，观察药物对之产生的效应，如对肾上腺素受体，兴奋 α 受体，血压上升；兴奋 β 受体，血压下降，心率加快；若要确切区分药物对 α、β 受体的作用，还可采用 α 受体阻断药酚妥拉明，β 受体阻断药普萘洛尔等为工具药，所用的实验方法如猫瞬膜、猫（犬）在体血压和肠管活动等实验。体外实验可分析药物的拟交感作用，如大鼠胃底条、离体兔耳、豚鼠气管链、回肠实验等。与乙酰胆碱有关的 M、N 受体，M 受体兴奋，心率减慢，心肌收缩力减弱，血压下降，胃肠道平滑肌收缩，瞳孔缩小等。N 受体又分 N_1 和 N_2 受体，N_1 受体兴奋，自主神经节兴奋及肾上腺髓质分泌，在阿托品化的猫身上，凡不具有血管收缩作用而能使血压上升的药物即为 N_1 受体激动药。

放射配基结合分析法，是通过药物放射性标记配基与受体结合的相互作用，分析药物与何种受体结合，结合强弱，为动物器官实验提供进一步依据。

药物对神经递质的研究。药物影响传出神经递质的主要环节有递质的合成、释放、摄取和转化，这类的实验方法亦很多，原理不外是利用工具药（递质或拟递质物质）观察药物是否阻断了神经兴奋引起的反应，但并不影响工具药的作用，并由此分析药物对递质的作用环节。

总之，传出神经系统的药理实验方法很多，在这里主要要求学生掌握和了解一些常用的实验。

实验 4.1　传出神经系统药物对麻醉犬血压、肠蠕动和腺体分泌的影响

【目的】

学习急性麻醉犬血压、肠蠕动和腺体分泌实验装置和方法，观察传出神经系统药物对上述生理现象的影响，加深对这类药物相互作用关系的理解。

【原理】

传出神经系统中的自主神经系统有以乙酰胆碱为递质的副交感神经系统和以去甲肾上

腺素为递质的交感神经系统，它们互相协调，互相对抗，维持机体的正常生理功能。药物影响副交感和交感神经系统的作用环节主要是递质和受体，通过对动物血压、平滑肌舒缩和腺体分泌的影响，间接地定性分析药物的作用机理。

【材料】

犬，1只，体重6~10kg，雌雄不限。

手术台、手术器械、生理压力监测仪、生理信号采集记录系统、压力换能器、滴定管、注射器。

肝素生理盐水、生理盐水、3%戊巴比妥钠溶液，试验用药物。

【方法与步骤】

1. **麻醉**　犬称重后，前肢皮下头静脉注射3%戊巴比妥钠30mg/kg，使之麻醉，背位固定于手术台上。

2. **手术**　分三部分进行。

（1）颈部　剪去颈部的毛，正中切开颈部皮肤，分离气管，在气管上作一"⊥"形切口，插入气管插管，结扎固定。分离一侧颈总动脉，插入与压力换能器相连的动脉插管（内充满肝素化生理盐水），待生理压力监测仪之零点和量程调试好后，打开动脉夹，记录正常血压。

（2）腹部　剪去腹部的毛，于剑突下正中切开上腹部皮肤5~8cm，沿腹白线切开腹肌，暴露腹腔，找到十二指肠与空肠，在空肠处作一荷包缝合，在待缝处作一小切口，向十二指肠方向插入水囊（预先抽去空气），收紧荷包，于水囊中充满水，将水囊出口连接于与生理信号采集记录系统相连的另一生理压力监测仪及滴定管，记录正常肠蠕动情况。

（3）腹股沟　在任意侧的腹股沟部位，用手触得股动脉搏动处，剪去毛，纵切皮肤3~4cm，分离出股静脉，结扎远心端，向近心端插入与输液装置相连的静脉插管，检查静脉插管是否畅通。

3. **给药**　上述手术完成后，先描记一段正常血压和肠蠕动曲线，观察腺体分泌情况，然后依次注射下列药物，每次给药后立即由输液管中注入生理盐水2ml，将药液全部进入血液循环，观察血压、肠蠕动和腺体分泌情况，待上述情况恢复正常或平稳后，再给下一药物。

A. 观察拟肾上腺素药对血压、肠蠕动及腺体分泌的影响

（1）盐酸肾上腺素10μg/kg或0.1ml/kg（10^{-4}，W/V）。

（2）重酒石酸去甲肾上腺素10μg/kg或0.1ml/kg（10^{-4}，W/V）。

（3）盐酸异丙肾上腺素25μg/kg或0.05ml/kg（$5×10^{-4}$，W/V）。

B. 观察α受体阻断药对拟肾上腺素药作用的影响

（4）酚妥拉明5mg/kg或0.2ml/kg（$2.5×10^{-2}$，W/V）。

（5）重复（1）。

（6）重复（2）。

（7）重复（3）。

C. 观察β受体阻断药对拟肾上腺素药作用的影响

（8）盐酸普萘洛尔0.1mg/kg或0.1ml/kg（10^{-3}，W/V）。

（9）重复（1）。

（10）重复（2）。

（11）重复（3）。

D. 观察拟胆碱药对血压、肠蠕动及腺体分泌的影响及 M 受体阻断药对拟胆碱药作用的影响

（12）毛果芸香碱 0.1mg/kg 或 0.1ml/kg（10^{-3}，W/V）。

（13）乙酰胆碱 1μg/kg 或 0.1ml/kg（10^{-5}，W/V）。

（14）阿托品 0.5mg/kg 或 0.1ml/kg（5×10^{-3}，W/V）。

（15）重复（13）。

（16）乙酰胆碱 10μg/kg 或 0.1ml/kg（10^{-4}，W/V）。

【结果处理】

复制血压、肠蠕动曲线，标明血压值，所给药物的名称和剂量，分析各药的相互作用，解释给药前后出现的各种生理现象的变化。

实验结果填入表 4 – 1。

表 4 – 1 传出神经药物对麻醉犬血压、肠蠕动和腺体分泌的影响

动物		体重		性别		麻醉	

药 品	剂 量	血压		肠蠕动		腺体分泌	
		用药前	用药后	用药前	用药后	用药前	用药后
肾上腺素 去甲肾上腺素 异丙肾上腺素	10μg/kg 10μg/kg 50μg/kg						
酚妥拉明 肾上腺素 去甲肾上腺素 异丙肾上腺素	5mg/kg 10μg/kg 10μg/kg 50μg/kg						
普萘洛尔 肾上腺素 去甲肾上腺素 异丙肾上腺素	0.1mg/kg 10μg/kg 10μg/kg 50μg/kg						
毛果芸香碱 乙酰胆碱 阿托品 乙酰胆碱 乙酰胆碱	0.05mg/kg 1μg/kg 0.5mg/kg 1μg/kg 10μg/kg						

【注意事项】

1. 颈部手术部位不宜靠近甲状腺部位，否则易出血，切勿损伤颈部迷走神经和交感神经。

2. 当血压较低时，应夹闭动脉插管，从防过多抗凝剂倒流入动物体内。

3. 本实验中药物的剂量按盐类计算，可根据实际情况做适当调整。

【方法评价】

血压、腺体分泌实验是检验传出神经药物作用极其敏感的方法，一般采用犬、猫、兔和大鼠的急性试验。用犬做实验优点较多，如血压恒定，较大鼠、家兔等小动物更接近人体，对药物反应灵敏，并与人基本一致，血管和神经较粗，管壁弹性强，便于手术操作，

心搏动力量强，能描绘出较好的血压曲线，适用于分析药物对循环系统的作用机制，用作药物筛选试验可反复应用；缺点是成本较高，不适用于需要动物数量较多的实验。

实验 4.2　药物对离体兔主动脉条的作用

【目的】

观察拟肾上腺素药和抗肾上腺素药对离体兔主动脉条的作用。

【原理】

兔主动脉条上含有 α 受体，对儿茶酚胺类药物非常敏感，它是筛选作用于 α 受体药物的良好标本。

【材料】

家兔 1 只，体重 1.8~2.2kg，雌雄不限。

麦氏浴槽、超级恒温水浴、生理信号采集记录系统、温度计、铁支架、双凹夹、剪刀、眼科镊、烧杯、培养皿、缝针、棉线、克氏液。

0.01% 去甲肾上腺素、0.01% 肾上腺素、1% 酚妥拉明。

【方法与步骤】

用木棒猛击家兔头部处死，迅速暴露心脏，分离主动脉，尽量靠近心脏处剪取胸主动脉，置于饱和氧的克氏液中。去除血管周围的结缔组织，将血管套在细玻棒上（直径 3~4mm），用眼科剪剪成宽 4mm，长 3~4cm 的螺旋形条片。将两端分别穿线结扎，一端固定在通气钩上，另一端连接于换能器并与生理信号采集记录系统相连，前负荷 1g，浴槽体积 20ml，温度 37℃ ±0.5℃，通氧，放置稳定 2h 后观察下列药物的作用，每次加药后，均用克氏液冲洗 2~3 次。

（1）0.01% 去甲肾上腺素 10μg（0.1ml）。

（2）0.01% 肾上腺素 10μg（0.1ml）。

（3）1% 酚妥拉明 1mg（0.1ml）加入 15min 后，重复上述（1），（2）。

【结果处理】

复制描记曲线，标明药物和剂量。

【注意事项】

（1）标本勿用手拿，应用镊子取，亦不能在空气中暴露过久，以免失去敏感性。

（2）克氏液须新鲜配制。余下的主动脉条放入 4℃ 冰箱中保存，1~2 天内仍可用作实验。

（3）本标本对拟交感药的收缩反应发生较缓慢（1~15min），松弛亦慢。

（4）本实验也可采用大鼠主动脉条。

【方法评价】

该法是筛选 α 受体激动药和拮抗药经典方法之一，因为兔主动脉条上主要存在 α 受体，标本可做成环、片及条状，其中螺旋条最合适，而且一个主动脉可制作 3~4 个标本，供配对实验。标本对低浓度的激动药和拮抗药都很敏感，重现性好，且能维持较长时间。若研究激动药和拮抗药的竞争关系时，可以通过不同的剂量效应曲线分析，呈平行右移且最大效应保持不变，视为竞争性拮抗，其作用强度可以用 pA_2 表示。

实验 4.3　药物对离体肠管的作用

【目的】

学习离体动物平滑肌器官的学习方法，观察拟胆碱药和抗胆碱药对离体豚鼠回肠的作用。

【原理】

胃肠道平滑肌的收缩反应主要由副交感神经控制，肠道平滑肌上富含 M 受体，M 受体激动药和拮抗药均可明显影响肠道平滑肌的收缩反应。因豚鼠回肠标本加负荷后已完全松弛，所以，本法可用来观察乙酰胆碱和拟胆碱药的作用。

【材料】

豚鼠 1 只，体重 200~300g，雌雄不限，最好空腹 6h 以上。

麦氏浴槽、恒温水浴、温度计、肌力换能器、生理信号采集记录系统、铁支架、双凹夹、剪刀、眼科镊、10ml 量筒、注射器、烧杯、培养皿、缝针、棉线、台氏液、氧气瓶。

10^{-4}、10^{-5} 的氯化乙酰胆碱溶液（W/V），0.1% 硫酸阿托品，1% 氯化钡溶液。

【方法与步骤】

猛击头部将豚鼠处死，打开腹腔，取出回肠，放入盛有台氏液的培养皿内。取豚鼠回肠 1.5~2cm，在肠段两端从里向外各穿 1 线，将肠段固定在浴槽中，负荷约 0.5g。在浴槽中加入 10ml 台氏液，标记液面高度，浴槽恒温在 38℃±0.5℃。插入通气管，供气以 2 个小气泡/秒为宜。连接肌力换能器，经生理信号采集记录系统记录肠肌蠕动情况，一般经平衡 15min 以上，待基线平稳后，即可进行下列实验。

1. 在浴槽中加入 10^{-5} 的氯化乙酰胆碱溶液 0.1ml。

2. 当肠段收缩明显时，加入 0.1% 硫酸阿托品 0.05ml。

3. 当出现预期作用时，加入 10^{-5} 的氯化乙酰胆碱溶液 0.1ml，观察 3min，如肠管无明显变化，再加入 10^{-4} 的氯化乙酰胆碱溶液 0.1ml。

4. 更换浴槽中的台氏液 3 次，待基线稳定后，加入 1% 氯化钡溶液 0.5ml，观察其作用。

5. 再次更换浴槽中的台氏液 3 次，待基线稳定后，加入 0.1% 硫酸阿托品 0.05ml，接着加入 1% 氯化钡溶液 0.5ml，观察其作用。

【结果处理】

复制描记曲线，注明药物和剂量。

【注意事项】

1. 回肠位于小肠的末端，平滑肌层较薄，自律性较低，越靠近回盲部自律性越低，基线越平稳。

2. 注意控制浴槽的水温和前负荷的大小，否则会影响到标本的收缩功能和对药物的反应。

3. 结扎肠两端时切勿扎闭肠腔，否则会影响到药物的作用强度。

【方法评价】

多种动物的离体肠肌可用来试验传出神经系统药物，一般采用豚鼠或兔的肠道。豚鼠回肠由于其自发活动较少，描记基线稳定和对乙酰胆碱和拟胆碱药敏感，反应明显，因此是筛选、检定拟胆碱药的常用实验方法。兔空肠因具有规则的摆动运动，适用于观察药物对此运动的影响。作为离体实验，它具有简明快速可大量筛选药物等优点，但要考虑体内的吸收和代谢等因素的影响，正确分析药物的作用情况。

实验4.4　药物对在体豚鼠下腹神经输精管的作用

【目的】

学习用在体豚鼠下腹神经输精管制备进行实验的方法，观察几种 α 受体激动药、阻断药、肾上腺素能神经阻断药在该模型上的作用。

【原理】

下腹神经是支配输精管等脏器的一个交感神经分支，输精管平滑肌上有 α 受体，刺激下腹神经或给予 α 受体激动药，均能引起输精管平滑肌收缩，而 α 受体阻断药、肾上腺素能神经阻断药则通过影响受体或神经传导对此产生作用。

【材料】

豚鼠1只，体重 $400 \sim 450g$，雄性。

生理药理多用仪、保护电极、肌力换能器、生理记录系统、保温手术台、铁支架、头皮静脉注射针头、滑轮、手术剪刀、止血钳、气管插管、棉线、纱布、注射器。

10^{-3}、10^{-5}重酒石酸去甲肾上腺素溶液（W/V），3×10^{-3}硫酸胍乙啶溶液（W/V），10^{-3}甲磺酸酚妥拉明溶液（W/V），乌拉坦，生理盐水。

【方法与步骤】

豚鼠称重后腹腔注射乌拉坦 $1.2g/kg$ 麻醉，背部固定于保温手术台上，切开颈部皮肤，在气管上剪口，气管插管，暴露颈外静脉，插入连接于注射器的小儿头皮静脉注射针头，结扎固定，以备注射药物。

在下腹正中切开皮肤，将肠管推向右上方，在肠系膜中央部靠后腹壁处寻找到两条与输尿管大致平行、白色、纤细状的下腹神经。任选一侧下腹神经，用线结扎其中枢端，在结扎处之下安置保护电极，以备刺激。分离同侧输精管，在接近睾丸处将输精管剪断，用线结扎其残端，将输精管提起，系于肌力换能器，记录其舒缩活动（图 4-1）。

用生理药理多用仪对下腹神经进行刺激时采用下列参数：波宽 $1ms$，频率 $50 \sim 80Hz$，电压从 $3V$ 试起，以能引起输精管明显收缩为度，每次刺激持续 $5s$。

装置安妥后按照下述次序进行实验：

（1）重酒石酸去甲肾上腺素 $10\mu g/kg$（10^{-5}

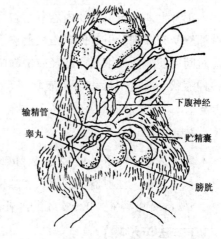

图 4-1　豚鼠下腹神经和输精管的位置

输精管

睾丸

下腹神经

贮精囊

膀胱

溶液 1ml/kg）静脉注射。

（2）刺激下腹神经 5s，观察输精管的反应，直至作用消失。

（3）硫酸胍乙啶 6mg/kg（3×10^{-3} 溶液 2ml/kg）静脉注射，给药后等待 45min。

（4）刺激下腹神经 5s，观察此时输精管的反应如何。

（5）重酒石酸去甲肾上腺素 10μg/kg（10^{-5} 溶液 1ml/kg）静脉注射。

（6）甲磺酸酚妥拉明溶液 2mg/kg（10^{-3} 溶液 2ml/kg）静脉注射。

（7）重酒石酸去甲肾上腺素 2mg/kg（10^{-3} 溶液 2ml/kg）静脉注射。

【结果处理】

复制输精管收缩曲线，标明前后处置，并解释实验结果。

【注意事项】

1. 本实验最好用刚到性成熟期的豚鼠，小于 2 个月的动物输精管太细，不便于记录，大于 5 个月的动物对药物不敏感。

2. 下腹神经较细，较难寻找，一般先找到双侧输尿管，把输尿管向外侧推开，便可见发丝粗的白色纤维，即下腹神经。

3. 在整个实验过程中应注意防止输精管的受冷与干燥。

4. 由于所给药物均可引起血压剧烈波动，注射速度必须缓慢。

【方法评价】

下腹神经是交感神经节后纤维，支配输精管，输精管平滑肌上有 α 受体，刺激下腹神经能引起输精管平滑肌收缩。该法对于追踪肾上腺素能神经阻断药的作用点较为方便，而且输精管收缩迅速，是分析 α 受体激动药、阻断药、肾上腺素能神经阻断药的常用方法之一。

实验 4.5　有机磷药物中毒及解救

【目的】

观察有机磷药物中毒的症状及血液胆碱酯酶的抑制情况。根据阿托品和碘解磷定对有机磷中毒的解救效果，初步分析两药的解毒机制。

【原理】

正常生理情况下，体内乙酰胆碱含量的维持依赖于神经突触部位的乙酰胆碱酯酶。胆碱酯酶受到抑制会引起体内乙酰胆碱含量明显积聚，产生中毒症状。胆碱酯酶复活药能在短时间内使酶活性恢复，减轻或消除中毒表现。M 受体阻断药可直接对抗由 M 受体介导的各种症状。通过中毒表现及症状缓解情况分析两类药物对治疗有机磷中毒的协同作用和差异。

【材料】

家兔 2 只，体重 2.0~2.5kg，雌雄不限。

兔固定箱、注射器、测瞳尺、酒精棉球、干棉球、血清乙酰胆碱酯酶活性测定盒。

5% 敌百虫溶液、0.1% 硫酸阿托品、2.5% 碘解磷定。

【方法与步骤】

1. 取家兔 2 只，称其体重，固定于兔箱中，观察并记录下列指标：呼吸频率与幅度、瞳孔大小、唾液分泌、尿粪排泄及肌震颤情况，并于耳缘静脉采集血样 1ml，离心取血清，进行乙酰胆碱酯酶活性测定。

2. 用酒精棉球涂擦兔耳，使耳缘静脉扩张，耳缘静脉注射 5% 敌百虫 120mg/kg（2.4ml/kg）。观察上述各项指标变化情况，待中毒症状明显时，记录各症状，如给敌百虫 20~25min 后无中毒症状出现或症状不明显，再追加初始剂量的 1/3，并于耳缘静脉采集血样 1ml，离心取血清，进行乙酰胆碱酯酶活性测定。

3. 立即给其中一只家兔耳缘静脉注射 0.1% 硫酸阿托品 4.0mg/kg（4ml/kg），另一只静脉注射 2.5% 碘解磷定 50mg/kg（2.0ml/kg），观察两兔中毒症状是否减轻，待中毒症状明显减轻，记录以上各指标。若给药后中毒症状未见明显减轻，可再按初剂量的 1/3 追加，并于耳缘静脉采集血样 1ml，离心取血清，进行乙酰胆碱酯酶活性测定。

【结果处理】

将各种结果按表 4-2 格式记录，并进行分析对比。

表 4-2 有机磷药物中毒及解救情况

	呼吸	瞳孔	唾液分泌	尿粪排泄	肌震颤	胆碱酯酶活性
给药前						
给敌百虫后						
给阿托品后						
给药前						
给敌百虫后						
给碘解磷定后						

【注意事项】

1. 敌百虫为剧毒药，且可从皮肤吸收，如与手接触，应立即用清水冲洗，忌用碱性肥皂，因敌百虫在碱性条件下会变成毒性作用更强的敌敌畏。

2. 给药前擦干唾液和尿粪，利于实验观察。

3. 剪去眼睫毛，以防测量瞳孔直径时引起眨眼。

4. 因瞳孔大小受光线的影响，所以在整个实验过程中不要随便改变兔箱位置，并保持光线条件一致。

5. 本实验是为分析阿托品和碘解磷定的解毒机制而设计的。临床实际应用中，需将阿托品与碘解磷定配合应用才能获得最佳的解毒效果。因此，在实验结束后，可以再加一药品，观察两药合用的作用。

【方法评价】

有机磷药物的中毒及解救实验是胆碱能神经生理、药理知识的系统复习，不仅能观察到由于体内乙酰胆碱的大量积聚而引起的 M、N 样症状，而且可以通过不同性质的解毒药物进一步认识 M 和 N 样作用以及解毒药性质的分析，此实验增加了测定全血胆碱酯酶活力项目，使该实验成为整体描述胆碱能神经系统效应较好的实验之一。

实验 4.6　普鲁卡因和丁卡因表面麻醉作用的比较

【目的】

学习筛选表面麻醉用药的方法，了解普鲁卡因和丁卡因作用的区别。

【原理】

角膜为一单纯均一膜，仅有无髓鞘神经纤维而无其他感觉细胞及血管。常用角膜反射指标测试局麻药的穿透性能、麻醉强度及作用持续时间。

【材料】

家兔 1 只，体重 2.0~2.5kg，雌雄不限。

兔固定箱、剪刀、滴管。

盐酸普鲁卡因溶液（5mg/ml）、盐酸丁卡因溶液（6mg/ml）。

【方法与步骤】

取家兔 1 只，检查两眼情况（无眼疾），放入固定箱内，剪去两眼睫毛。须以大致均等的力量轻触角膜，试验正常的角膜反射。触及部位可按 1，2，3，4，2，5 的顺序（图 4-2），刺激 6 个位点。全部阳性（6 次都不眨眼）时记 6/6，全部阴性（6 次都眨眼）时记 0/6，余类推。

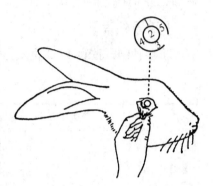

图 4-2　拉开家兔眼睑滴加药液的方法与测试角膜反射时的刺激位点顺序

然后用拇指和示指将家兔眼睑拉成杯状，中指压住鼻泪管，分别在两眼滴药。左眼：盐酸普鲁卡因溶液 2 滴，右眼：盐酸丁卡因溶液 2 滴，轻轻揉眼睑，使药液与角膜充分接触，并在眼眶中存留 1min，然后放手任其自溢。滴药后每隔 5min 测试角膜反射 1 次，到 30min 为止，同时观察有无结膜充血等反应。记录并比较两药作用。

【结果处理】

将两眼的角膜反射的记分按各时间的情况填入表 4-3。

表 4-3　普鲁卡因和丁卡因表面麻醉作用的比较

兔眼	滴入药物	滴药前角膜反射	滴药后角膜反射					
			5min	10min	15min	20min	25min	30min
左	盐酸普鲁卡因（5mg/ml）							
右	盐酸丁卡因（6mg/ml）							

【注意事项】

1. 滴药时必须压住鼻泪管。以免药液流入鼻腔，经鼻黏膜吸收而致中毒，并影响实验结果。

2. 用以刺激角膜的兔须宜软硬适中，实验中应使用同一根兔须，以保证触力均等。

3. 兔的眼睫毛应在用药前剪短，否则即使角膜已被麻醉，触及睫毛仍可引起眨眼反射，易得出错误结论。

【方法评价】

研究局麻药作用的指标常有：局麻作用强度（最小有效浓度表示），药物弥散进入神经纤维的效力和对黏膜表面的穿透力（以作用开始时间和黏膜麻醉效力表示），麻醉作用过程（以麻醉出现时间及持续时间表示）。因此研究方法也很多，如角膜麻醉法、皮丘法、神经肌肉制备法、离体神经动作电位观测法等，这些方法都是从各个方面出发评价局麻药的特点。角膜麻醉法只能提供药物对表层组织穿透力方面的资料，若要得到较全面的资料，需要用多种方法进行。

第五章　内脏系统药物实验

内脏系统是胸腔、腹腔和盆腔内各脏器系统的统称，主要包括心血管、呼吸、消化、泌尿和生殖等系统。作用于血液系统的药物一般也归入这部分。而作用于生殖系统的药物主要为性激素类，常放在"激素类药物"中讨论。由于每一系统脏器各具其生理、病理特点，作用于内脏系统的药物也就种类繁多，相应的药理学实验方法也各不相同。

心血管系统药物包括治疗心功能不全、抗心肌缺血、抗高血压，抗心律失常和防治动脉粥样硬化等药物。心血管系统药理实验主要测试药物对心肌收缩性、电生理特性、心肌代谢及血管舒缩性的影响。另外，还可制备实验性心律失常、高血压、心力衰竭、动脉粥样硬化和心肌梗死等各种动物病理模型，观察药物的实验性治疗效果。

呼吸系统药物包括镇咳、平喘和祛痰药物。镇咳药的药效可用动物咳嗽模型进行评价，引起咳嗽的方法有化学物质刺激、机械刺激和电刺激等。猫的咳嗽反射非常敏感，适用于评价镇咳药。平喘药是呼吸系统的重要药物，大都具有松弛支气管平滑肌的作用，可采用离体气管和整体肺溢流实验来观察药物对平滑肌的舒张作用。实验性病理模型一般用生物活性物质或致敏物质喷雾，引起动物"哮喘"。对平喘药最敏感的动物是豚鼠。祛痰药主要作用是促进呼吸道上皮运动，稀释或裂解痰液，使痰易于咳出。可采用呼吸道分泌液排出量来评价祛痰药。

消化系统药物主要包括抗溃疡药、止吐药、泻药、止泻药和利胆药等。抗溃疡药物的药效评价主要采用制备动物消化道溃疡模型，进行实验治疗及观察药物对胃酸分泌的影响，实验性消化道溃疡制备有外科手术法、药物法、应激法及消化道黏膜人工损伤法等。泻药和止泻药除了观察它们对动物大便形状、排便量及排便次数的影响外，还可观察药物对胃肠道平滑肌运动功能及消化道输送功能的影响。

泌尿系统药物主要是利尿药。评价利尿药药效不但要观察药物对尿量的影响，而且要研究其对尿液中电解质排泄的影响，利尿作用部位的研究对了解药物作用机制具有重要意义。肾清除率检查则是了解肾功能的一个重要方法。

血液系统药物包括促进造血细胞生长的药物和影响凝血过程的药物。血液的细胞学检查和凝血时间测定不但是血液系统药物的基础实验，而且是毒理学实验的一个重要组成部分，对新药开发具有重要意义。抗血栓药物是防治心脑血管疾病的一类重要药物，其相应的实验方法是血小板功能实验和血液流变学实验。对血小板上受体、活性物质及其功能的研究是一个很活跃的领域。

一、治疗心功能不全药物实验

心功能不全是心脏泵血功能相对不足，流经组织器官的血流量不能满足组织代谢需要的一种综合征。心脏的泵血功能不但取决于心肌的收缩性能，而且也受前、后负荷及心率的影响。

心肌收缩性能是指心肌纤维的内在收缩力，由心肌的收缩成分（肌动蛋白、肌球蛋白）

与 Ca^{2+} 的相互作用所决定。心肌周边纤维平均缩短速度是评价心肌收缩性能的合理指标，但整体实验测量条件要求较高，故较少应用。由于心室内压可反映室壁张力，而等容收缩相对心肌的收缩为等长收缩，因而在实际工作中常用等容收缩相的压力上升速率指标（dp/dt_{max}，Vpm，$Vmax$）来反映心肌收缩性能。等容收缩相指标个体差异大，因而不宜用来评价心肌收缩性能的基础水平。在整体实验中，心肌收缩力受到前后负荷的影响，而离体实验，如离体乳头肌实验可控制前后负荷，能正确地评价药物的变力性作用。

心率加快在一定范围内可增加心输出量，但同时也增加心肌耗氧量。若心率过快，超过 160～180 次/分，则由于舒张期太短，回心血量不足，心输出量反而降低。治疗心功能不全的药物最好不加快或尽可能少加快心率，以减少心肌耗氧量。

前负荷指心肌在收缩前所承受的张力，在整体实验中，可用心室舒张末期压（如左室舒张末期压）代表。

后负荷指心肌收缩时所承受的负荷，可用平均动脉血压或总外周血管阻力来代表。血管的舒缩状态对后负荷影响很大，动脉阻力血管舒张，使心脏射血阻力减小，心脏搏出量增加。

治疗心功能不全的药物，以往多用强心苷增强心肌收缩力以提高心脏泵血功能。但必须指出，心输出量较多地取决于外周因素及这些因素对前后负荷的影响，较小程度取决于心肌收缩性能的实际水平。充血性心功能不全在失代偿时，由于神经、体液因素的作用，外周血管收缩，前后负荷增加，已经衰竭的心脏负担进一步加重，这时最重要的措施是减轻心脏的前后负荷。

综上所述，评价治疗心功能不全的药物作用，应考虑以下三个方面：①对心肌收缩性能的影响；②对心脏泵血功能的影响；③对血流动力学的影响（包括心率、血压、心电图及左心室功能的各项指标）。由于心脏的舒张功能对心脏泵血也有重要的影响，而且在疾病过程中心脏的舒张功能往往比收缩功能更易受损，所以现在很重视药物对心脏舒张功能的影响。药物对心脏收缩和舒张功能的影响都可通过血流动力学和离体乳头肌实验来进行评价。另外，评价治疗心功能不全的药物不但要在正常动物身上进行，更重要的是要观察其在动物心衰模型上的作用。

实验 5.1　强心苷对离体心脏的作用

【目的】

学习八木 – Hartung 离体蛙心灌注方法。观察药物对离体蛙心收缩幅度、频率、节律和心输出量的影响。

【原理】

两栖类动物由于能生活在水中，故其心脏较能耐受缺氧的环境，在给予合适的营养液的情况下，其心脏能较长时间地存活并维持心肌收缩。将药物加入到灌流液中可观察药物对心脏的直接作用。采用低钙任氏液造成心衰模型，可较明显地显示药物的强心作用。

【材料】

蛙或蟾蜍 2 只，体重 70g 以上，雌雄不限。

手术器械、毁髓针、蛙板、八木 – Hartung 蛙心插管、蛙心夹、张力换能器和生理信号采集记录系统、烧杯、注射器、滴管。

5%洋地黄、任氏液、低钙任氏液（Ca^{2+}含量为正常任氏液的1/4）。

【方法与步骤】

1. 取蛙或蟾蜍1只，用毁髓针捣毁脑及脊髓，仰位固定在蛙板上。依次剪开胸前区皮肤、胸骨和心包膜，充分暴露心脏（图5-1）。

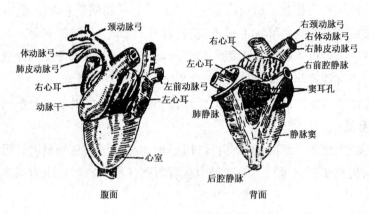

图5-1 蛙心解剖图

2. 在左右主动脉下穿二线，然后将心尖翻向头侧；暴露出静脉窦和后腔静脉。小心分离两侧肝脏与肝间的韧带，游离后腔静脉后，在其下面穿一线，在穿线处的下方剪一小口，把盛有任氏液的静脉插管从此口插入，用线结扎固定，立即用任氏液从静脉插管冲洗心脏，洗净余血。

3. 翻正心脏，在左主动脉远端剪口，向心脏方向插入动脉插管，如灌流液从动脉插管流出通畅，则用预置的一根线连同右主动脉一起将动脉插管扎紧。用剪刀将心脏从周围组织中游离出来，调整好方向、角度，将动、静脉插管固定在一起。用主动脉下另一丝线结扎除主动脉和后腔静脉以外的所有血管。制成蛙心标本（图5-2）。

4. 用任氏液反复冲洗心脏，直至动脉流出液无色为止。调节静脉插管液面1.5~2cm，在整个实验过程中液面高度应保持不变。用蛙心夹夹住心尖，通过张力换能器与生理信号采集记录系统相连。

5. 描记一段正常曲线，观察心脏收缩幅度、心率、心输出量（滴/分）。然后按下列步骤实验。

（1）换入低钙任氏液，待收缩明显减弱后描记曲线，观察上述指标。

（2）向静脉管内加5%洋地黄1~2滴，作用明显后，观察记录各项指标。

6. 比较给药前后心脏收缩强度、频率、节律以及从动脉管中搏出液体的流速（滴/分）。

【结果处理】

1. 剪贴或复制心脏收缩曲线，并作注明。

2. 给出用药前后心输出量。

【注意事项】

1. 在手术和实验过程中不可损伤静脉窦，并要防

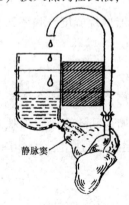

图5-2 八木-Hartung 离体蛙心制备

止标本漏液。

2. 动脉插管位置应离动脉球远些，以保证动脉流出通畅。

3. 每次换药前后，静脉插管中液面高度应尽可能一致。

4. 加洋地黄时，应逐滴加入，以免药量过大造成中毒。

5. 离体心脏要经常保持湿润。

【方法评价】

1. 本实验为一经典方法，取材容易，仪器设备简单，对实验要求低，成功率高。

2. 可同时评价药物对离体心脏的收缩幅度、心输出量和心率的影响。

3. 由于冷血动物心脏对药物的反应与温血动物有许多差异，在实验研究中使用较少，但在教学中却是一较简易明了的示教实验。

【思考题】

1. 在本实验中，若逐步提高任氏液中钙浓度会出现什么结果，为什么？

2. 洋地黄对离体蛙心有何作用？

3. 此实验能否观察药物对心脏前后负荷的影响？为什么？

实验 5.2　药物对离体乳头肌收缩、舒张性能的影响

【目的】

学习离体乳头肌的制备方法以及用其测定药物对心肌收缩和舒张性能的影响。

【原理】

乳头肌是心脏的一种特殊结构，具有心肌的各种特性。其肌纤维排列一致，在离体情况下不受心率因素干扰，用于测定心肌的张力变化、张力发展速度（dT/dt）及舒张性能等，较之完整的心脏更具独特优点，是确定正性肌力作用或负性肌力作用药物的重要实验。在适宜的温度、供氧、合适的营养液中，用电刺激驱动乳头肌可使其保持良好的舒缩活动达几小时。

【材料】

猫 1 只，体重 2~3kg，雌雄不限。

超级恒温水浴箱、浴管、铁支架、氧气瓶（充于 95% O_2 和 5% CO_2 的混合气体）。药理生理多用仪、刺激电极、生理信号采集记录系统、微分器、张力换能器、手术器械、注射器、烧杯、平皿。

改良 Tyrode 溶液（mmol/L）：NaCl 137，KCl 5.4，$MgCl_2$ 1.05，NaH_2PO_4 0.43，$CaCl_2$ 1.8，$NaHCO_3$ 12，葡萄糖 10。一般先将除 $NaHCO_3$ 和葡萄糖以外的各成分配成浓缩 10 倍的母液，用时将母液稀释 10 倍，再缓缓加入 $NaHCO_3$ 和葡萄糖。刚配制好的溶液 pH 一般在 8.1~8.4，用前通混合气体后 pH 降至 7.35~7.45。营养液也可用 K–H 液。

10^{-5} 异丙肾上腺素、10^{-4} 哇巴因、乙醚。

【方法与步骤】

1. 将猫用乙醚麻醉后，颈动脉放血处死，迅速剖开胸腔后将心脏取出，立即置于混合气体饱和的营养液中洗去余血，然后移入盛有营养液的平皿中，沿右室左缘将右心室剪开，

充分暴露乳头肌，选用细长形者为好。适当游离乳头肌基底部，用丝线连同少量心室肌结扎，用丝线结扎乳头肌腱索后，剪下腱索端及基底端。乳头肌一端固定于刺激电极上的固定钩上，迅速移入浴管中（20ml 营养液），另一端通过丝线与张力换能器相连。标本静息负荷 0.5 ~ 1g，电刺激（频率 0.5Hz，波宽 3ms，120% 阈电压，方波）驱动下稳定 30min，稳定期间换液 3 ~ 4 次。稳定后调整负荷使收缩幅度最大。

2. 收缩性能指标测定以 100 ~ 200mm/s 纸速记录单次收缩曲线及其微分曲线，从中测取①张力峰值（PT，mg）；②收缩张力达峰时间（TPT，ms）；③张力上升最大速度（dT/dt_{max}，g/s）；④张力上升达最大速度时间（$t - dT/dt_{max}$，ms）；⑤PT 下降 50% 的时间（1/2PT，ms）；⑥张力下降最大速度（$-dT/dt_{max}$，g/s）。参数测定方法见图 5 - 3。

3. 记录给药前收缩曲线后，加入 10^{-5} 异丙肾上腺素 0.2ml，作用明显后测定用药后的收缩曲线。用营养液冲洗标本 3 次以上。

4. 待收缩幅度基本恢复后，记录收缩曲线。加入 10^{-4} 哇巴因 0.2ml，作用明显后，记录用药后收缩曲线。

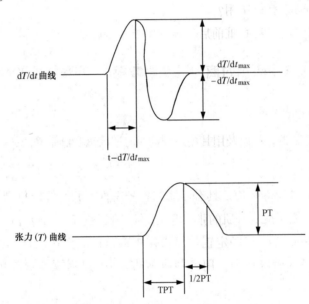

图 5 - 3　离体乳头肌收缩性能参数测定方法

【结果处理】

由于各个乳头肌大小不一，各标本间的数值可能会有较大差距，这时可测量乳头肌基部的直径，计算出乳头肌的横截面积，将所记录的 PT、$+(-)dT/dt_{max}$ 等按截面积进行校正。也可直接计算这些参数的百分比，使各标本间的结果更具可比性。药物浓度要以浴管中终浓度为准。

【注意事项】

1. 在制备乳头肌标本的过程中要细心，动作轻柔，避免过度牵拉和撕伤标本。

2. 为保持乳头肌收缩幅度稳定，营养液的 pH 应在 7.4 左右；刺激频率不能过高，一般采用 0.5Hz 或 1Hz；温度也不宜过高，应维持在 30℃ 左右。

3. 根据乳头肌的大小调节前负荷，使收缩幅度最大。

4. 注意记录仪基线零点的调节。

5. 因心房肌和心室肌对药物的反应可能有所不同，故在了解药物对心肌的收缩性能时，最好将心房及乳头肌同时进行。

6. 加药量的体积不要超过营养液体积的 5%，计算药物浓度时可忽略不计。

【方法评价】

1. 用本方法研究药物对心肌基本特性的影响，对于阐明药物对心肌作用的本质具重要意义。如配合血流动力学等整体动物试验，可对药物的心血管药理作用获得较全面的了解。

2. 标本缺乏内源性自律性，因而可用于心肌的兴奋性、不应性和自律性等指标的观察测定（有效不应期测定参见心房肌实验）。

3. 乳头肌肌纤维呈线性排列，这对测定分析心肌收缩性能的改变较完整心脏更简便。

4. 离体标本不受心率、冠脉血管舒缩等因素的影响，适合观察药物对心肌的直接作用。

5. 引入 $\pm dT/dt_{max}$、TPT、$t-dT/dt_{max}$、1/2PT 等力学指标，有利于研究药物对心肌收缩性能的影响。

6. 标本制备简单，可供实验时间较长，稳定性好，但技术要求比离体心房肌高。

【思考题】

1. 离体乳头肌测定药物对心肌收缩、舒张功能的影响比整体实验有什么优点？它能否代替整体实验？

2. 用本实验能否同时测定药物对心肌兴奋性和不应期的影响？

实验 5.3　药物对大鼠左心功能与血流动力学的影响

【目的】

学习血流动力学实验方法和大鼠左心室插管技术。了解各种血流动力学参数及其评价药物对心功能影响的作用。

【原理】

整体试验中的心脏泵血功能（每搏量、每搏功、射血分数、心脏指数等）都是心肌收缩性能、前负荷、后负荷三者综合作用的表现。在药理实验中，常需评定药物对在体心肌收缩性能的影响。血流动力学方法是研究药物对心血管功能影响的一种常用方法，其指标包括心脏泵血功能、血流量、心内压力、压力变化速率、心腔容积、血压、血管阻力及心率等。根据心室内压，压力变化速率的改变，特别是等容收缩期和等容舒张期的指标，可推测心肌收缩功能和舒张功能的变化。

本实验的主要指标及意义如下。

1. 左心室压力（LVPp）代表等容收缩期左心室内压力的变化，当前后负荷升高或心肌收缩力加强时 LVP 上升。

2. 左室等容期压力最大变化速率（$\pm dp/dt_{max}$）一定程度上反映室壁张力的变化速率，$+dp/dt_{max}$ 用于评价收缩功能，$-dp/dt_{max}$ 反映心肌舒张时收缩成分延长的最大速度，用于评价舒张功能。

3. 左室开始收缩至左室内压上升速率峰值时间（$t-dp/dt_{max}$）在变力因素作用下 $+dp/dt_{max}$ 与 $t-dp/dt_{max}$ 变化方向相反，而负荷状态改变时变化方向相同。

4. 左室压力对数值变化速率 $[(dp/dt)\,p_{max}^{-1}]$ 也属反映心肌收缩性能的指标，较 dp/dt_{max} 受负荷影响较小，但灵敏度较差。

5. 左室舒张末期压（LVEDP）代表左室前负荷,是分析心功能的重要参数,一般在 ±1.3kPa 以内。

6. T 值（等容舒张期左室压下降的时间常数）为等容舒张期中间压力对数对时间作图的直线斜率,反映心肌的舒张性能。

7. 血压（BP）包括收缩压（SAP）、舒张压（DAP）和平均动脉压（MAP）。

8. 心率（HR）。

9. 心肌力－速向量环［LVP－(dp/dt) p^{-1}环]将 LVP 和（dp/dt）p^{-1}两路信号分别输入双线示波器的 x、y 轴而得。主要用于测量 Vmax。该环正向上升支的顶端至零线高度即为 Vpm［相当于（dp/dt）p^{-1}的峰值],沿环正向曲线初降支经 Vpm 向 y 轴作切线,该切线与 y 轴之交点读取 Vmax 即零负荷时心肌缩短最大速率。

＋dp/dt_{max}是评价心肌收缩性能的常用指标,对各种变力性干预十分敏感,但在一定程度上受心率及前后负荷的影响,并与其呈正相关。当心率、前后负荷不变或降低时,＋dp/dt_{max}上升或不变则表示心肌收缩性能增强。前后负荷升高时可结合 t－dp/dt_{max}进行判断,＋dp/dt_{max}上升同时伴 t－dp/dt_{max}缩短（即两者变化相反）,提示心肌收缩性能加强。（dp/dt）p$_{max}^{-1}$和 Vmax 等 VCE 类指标受负荷的影响较小,特别是 Vmax 认为它已排除了后负荷的影响,生理状态下的前负荷对它的影响也很小,但对变力性干预敏感性较低。目前认为：根据＋dp/dt_{max}、（dp/dt）p$_{max}^{-1}$、t－dp/dt_{max}及 Vmax 等指标来综合判断心肌收缩性能变化较为全面。

－dp/dt_{max}是评价心室舒张功能改变的敏感指标,但易受左室压（LVSP）、收缩末期容积（ESV）、后负荷和心率的影响。采用－dp/dt_{max}·LVSP^{-1}可以校正 LVSP 对－dp/dt_{max}的影响。T 值是反映心脏舒张功能较敏感的指标,它不受后负荷的影响,但受 LVEDP 的影响。LVEDP 亦可间接反映左室功能,左室舒张不全或回心血量增加时 LVEDP 可升高,反之左室舒张加强或回心血量减少则 LVEDP 降低。

当 BP 下降时,DAP 下降大于 SAP 下降表明降压主要是由外周阻力下降所致。此外,t－dp/dt_{max}与外周阻力呈正关。

【材料】

雄性大鼠 1 只,体重 200～250g。

多道生理记录仪（4～8 道）、双线示波器（带照相装置）、压力换能器、直流放大器、PE－50 聚乙烯管（也可用塑料管加热拉制成内径 0.5mm,外径 1mm 的导管）、手术器械、烧杯、注射器（注：如用微型计算机联机适时分析系统,则只需二路压力换能放大装置和一路微分装置,可不用多道生理仪和示波器）。

0.4% 戊巴比妥钠,0.5% 肝素生理盐水、0.001% 异丙肾上腺素、0.002% 硝苯啶。

【方法与步骤】

1. 大鼠称重,用 0.4% 戊巴比妥钠 40mg/kg 腹腔注射麻醉,背位固定,剪去颈部被毛。将动脉插管充满 0.5% 肝素生理盐水。

2. 颈部正中切开皮肤,分离左、右颈总动脉,从右颈总动脉插管进入左心室,用压力换能器测取左室压力,并经微分器和压力处理器获得 ±dp/dt 和（dp/dt）p^{-1}信号。插管时根据荧光屏上血压波是否变为典型的室力压波来确定是否插入心室。左侧颈总动脉插管连接另一压力换能器记录动脉血压。一侧颈外静脉插管,准备给药用。

3. 调整好定标值（详见后），动物稳定 15min 后记录给药前的各项指标。

4. 从静脉插管中注入药物，记录给药后 1min，3min，5min，10min，20min 时的各项指标。

5. 待各项指标基本恢复后给下一个药物，记录给药后不同时间的各项指标。

按以下顺序给药：①0.001% 异丙肾上腺素 0.01mg/kg，静脉注射；②0.002% 硝苯啶 0.02mg/kg，静脉注射。

6. 定标及各项指标的测取：

（1）LVP 曲线　LVP 定标敏度 2.7mm/13.3kPa。由于 LVP 的最低点可接近于零，这时 $(dp/dt)\ p^{-1}$ 将趋向于无穷大，结果无法处理。如在放大 LVP 的载波放大器调零完成后再旋动载波放大器使基线抬高 4mm（即相当于预先输入 $\Delta p = 2.7$kPa 的压力），这样可保证在整个心动周期中的 LVP 信号都大于零。一般 LVEDP + Δp = （1.1~1.3）kPa 为宜，如用微型计算机适时分析则可直接计算 Vpm 和 Vmax，不需 $(dp/dt)\ p^{-1}$ 信号，也不需输入 Δp 调整 LVP 输出信号。从 LVP 曲线上可得到 LVSP 和 LVDP、LVP 信号，经直流放大器放大 10 倍后再记录下来，可从中读取 LVEDP。

（2）dp/dt 曲线　微分器时间常数 1.0ms，高频滤波 50Hz 调整微分器的标准三角波定标压力的信号幅度等同于 LVP13.3kPa 的幅度（三角波从最低点到最高点时间为 0.1s），这时微分器输出的矩形波定标信号为 ±133.3kPa/s（266.7kPa/s）调整矩形波幅度为 5mm、10mm。从该曲线上可测定 +dp/dt_{max}（最大值），-dp/dt_{max}（最小值），t-dp/dt_{max}（曲线正向上升支起点至 +dp/dt_{max} 的时间）。

（3）$(dp/dt)\ p^{-1}$ 曲线　将压力处理器开关拨向 $(dp/dt)\ p^{-1}$ 档，其输出定标信号为反向双曲线。按上述调整其标准三角波幅度，这时双曲线幅度为 ±10s^{-1}，调整双曲线幅度为 2mm，即 10mm/100s^{-1}。曲线的最高点即实测左室肌最大缩短速度 Vpm（亦称生理最大速度）。由于为避免出现 $(dp/dt)\ p^{-1}$ 出现无穷大数值而输入 Δp，因此，实际曲线数值是 $(dp/dt)\ /\ (p + \Delta p)$，这时可将实测值乘以 $(1 + \Delta p/p)$ 进行修正。若 $\Delta p \ll p$，也可不作校正。

（4）LVP - $(dp/dt)\ p^{-1}$ 环　LVP 和 $(dp/dt)\ p^{-1}$ 电信号分别输入 SBR - 1 型双线示波器的 x 轴和 y 轴以获取该环并摄影记录。定标：将定标三角波输入示波器 x 轴，$(dp/dt)\ p^{-1}$ 双曲线输入至 y 轴作直流放大，调 x 轴增益使图形宽度为 2.5cm，调 y 轴增益使定标图形右端垂直部分为 1cm，此时 y 轴刻度即为 20s^{-1}/cm，然后将 y 轴增益衰减至 1/4（即 80s^{-1}/cm）。零负荷时的收缩成分最大缩短速度（Vmax）为环的正向降支之切线与 y 轴交点之读数。

（5）T 值测取和计算　从 -dp/dt_{max} 后 20ms 处开始的 40ms 时间内在对应时间的 LVP 曲线上读取 LVP，并将其值取自然对数（ln$p$），以 x 轴为 ln$p$，y 轴为对应的时间 t 进行直线回归，这时的斜率即为 T 值。

【结果处理】

根据上述方法测取，计算各给药前后的参数，进行分析、评价。

【注意事项】

1. 记录压力的管道系统不能留有任何气泡，否则记录就会失真而出现正弦波样波形。同时管道系统也不能有渗漏和凝血现象，否则波形将变小、失真。

2. 左心室插管不能太长（应为 2～15cm），否则将因插管内阻力大而使压力波失真。

3. 在左心室插管插入颈总动脉后，应在荧光屏监视压力波的情况下缓缓向左室推进。如出现低平波或波动消失，表明前端受阻，应将插管稍后退，恢复波动后再推进，千万不能在波动消失后继续往前插管，以免插破血管或心脏。

4. 在进行插管时一定要把插管前端的血管拉直，以使插管能顺利推进。

5. 左室插管在主动脉瓣口不易进入左室时（这时从插管可感到心脏跳动），可将插管稍退出，改变角度和方向或抖动插管向前推进，这样往往可顺利插入左心室。

【方法评价】

1. 血流动力学和整体心功能评价是开发心血管药物的重要一环，所有的心血管药物都要进行这方面的评价，因此，这方面的实验是心血管药物开发必不可少的。通过药物的血流动力学研究，可了解药物对心脏功能和外周血管的影响。

2. 大鼠动物小，耐受力良好，手术操作简便，经济实惠。改进实验方法，还可进行清醒大鼠血流动力学参数的测定。

3. 该方法未测量心输出量，因而无法获得泵功能和外周阻力变化等一系列重要血流动力学参数。

4. 实验数据的获取需记录、摄片、测量、计算等，要花费不少时间和人力，如采用计算机联机实验则可免去这些步骤，并可省去示波器、照相机甚至多道生理记录仪。

5. 等容收缩期指标很适宜于评价给药前后的心肌收缩性能变化，但其正常值范围广，故不宜用来评定收缩性能的基础水平，而应用射血相指标。

【思考题】

1. 评价药物对心肌收缩性能的影响在此实验中应主要选用哪些指标？评价对心肌舒张功能的影响应选哪些指标？

2. 如一药物使 dp/dt_{max}、$t-dp/dt_{max}$、动脉血压都明显升高，而 Vpm，$Vmax$ 无明显改变说明药物的主要作用是什么？

二、抗心律失常药物实验

按心率的快慢，心律失常可分为快速性心律失常和缓慢性心律失常，但目前常用的抗心律失常药物主要是用于治疗快速性心律失常，研究方法也主要是针对快速性心律失常。抗心律失常药物的研究方法主要分为两大类：一类是观察药物对心肌电生理特性的影响，如心肌的兴奋性、自律性、传导性等。还可用玻璃微电极记录跨膜动作电位或接触电极记录单向动作电位，研究药物对动作电位各时相的影响，并推测药物对离子通道的影响。这类方法可用于研究药物的抗心律失常作用机理或筛选具有某些电生理特点的抗心律失常药。另一类是利用动物造成心律失常模型，直接观察药物的抗心律失常作用。制造动物心律失常模型的常用方法有：①药物诱发法；②电刺激法；③结扎冠状动脉法三类。

尽管诱发动物心律失常的方法和模型很多，但没有一种与临床的相关性很好而具有决定性意义。因此，在实际工作中都是用多种动物模型来评价新药的抗心律失常作用。根据药物可能的作用机理可先选用相应的模型，如Ⅰ类药可选强心苷和乌头碱诱发心律失常的模型；Ⅱ类药可选肾上腺素、三氯甲烷引起的心律失常模型，抗纤颤药可用电致室颤模型；研究Ⅲ类药及了解药物电生理特性则先用心肌动作电位分析，然后再用心律失常模型。从动物方面来讲，冷血动物诱发的心律失常与温血动物不同，现很少采用。大鼠对强心苷不敏感，故不宜用哇巴因诱发心律失常。小动物心脏（大鼠、豚鼠、兔和猫）的心室纤颤有自发性恢复的可能，可反复测定室颤阈。豚鼠和兔的心脏适合作离体标本。猫体格健壮，耐受性较好。犬、猪等大动物的室颤很难自然恢复，必须用除颤器。犬对引起心律失常的刺激很敏感，比人更易发展成室颤。猪的冠状血管系统与人的很相似，适宜结扎冠状动脉引起心律失常。

实验 5.4　奎尼丁拮抗乌头碱诱发大鼠心律失常的作用

【目的】

学习乌头碱诱发大鼠心律失常模型的制备方法，观察药物对此种心律失常的保护作用。

【原理】

乌头碱主要通过直接兴奋心肌，促使心肌自律性亢进而诱发心律失常。使用乌头碱后，能促使钠通道开放，加速 Na^+ 内流，使细胞膜去极化，提高心房传导组织和房室束 – 浦氏纤维系统等快反应细胞的自律性，形成一源性或多源性异位节律。乌头碱可引起室性早搏、室上性早搏和室性心动过速、室颤等。

【材料】

大鼠 1 只，体重 180～250g，雌雄不限。

心电图机、心电示波器、手术台、手术器械、注射器、静脉插管。

20% 乌拉坦、0.001% 乌头碱、0.5% 奎尼丁、生理盐水。

【方法与步骤】

1. 取大鼠称体重，用 20% 乌拉坦（1g/kg）腹腔注射麻醉，仰位固定在手术台上。

2. 颈部切开皮肤，分离一侧颈外静脉，行静脉插管（也可从股静脉插头皮针代替颈外静脉插管）。

3. 连接心电图导联线和心电示波器，记录给药前的 II 导联心电图。然后从静脉插管快速（5s 左右）注入 0.001% 乌头碱（25μg/kg），观察并记录出现的心律失常。

4. 出现心律失常稳定 5min 后，静脉 0.5% 奎尼丁 10mg/kg，观察心律失常的变化，记录转为窦性心率，再次出现室性早搏、室速、室颤，直至死亡的时间（观察时间以 60min 为限）。对照组用等量生理盐水代替奎尼丁。

【结果处理】

以给奎尼丁到室速转为窦性心律的时间为药物潜伏期，以窦性心律持续时间及转成窦性心律到出现室颤的时间作为药效持续期。剪贴心电图，与对照组对比，评价药物的抗心律失常作用。

【注意事项】

乌头碱的注射速度要控制好，一般在 5～10s 内注射完毕。

注意动物保温。乌头碱配成溶液后，不宜冷藏过久，一般不超过 2 周。

【方法评价】

1. 乌头碱诱发的心律失常可以持续 1h 以上，一般不能自行转为窦性心律，实验方法简单，结果可靠。由于心律失常持续时间长，可预防给药，也可治疗给药。对于未知药物，还可多次给药，测定最小有效量。

2. 乌头碱还可直接用在心房表面形成持续性的房性心动过速，房扑和房颤。

【思考题】

乌头碱诱发心律失常模型与哇巴因诱发心律失常模型的主要异同点何在？

实验 5.5　药物对家兔电刺激致室颤阈的影响

【目的】

学习整体动物电刺激诱发室颤的方法。了解电刺激心脏诱发心律失常在抗心律失常药物研究中的作用。

【原理】

在心肌除极后的复极过程中，有一段易损期，它位于心电图的 T 波处，约在动作电位的相对不应期。这个时间心肌的复极程度不均匀，当足够强度的刺激落在易损期时，就可引起折返活动而致室颤。采用串刺激可增加心肌复极的不均一，使刺激容易落在易损期上产生室颤。

小动物（如大鼠、兔和猫）产生的室颤，在停止刺激后，大多能自然中止并恢复窦性节律，而大动物（如犬和猴）一旦产生室颤则不能自然恢复，需用除颤器。

【材料】

兔 1 只，体重 2～3kg，雌雄不限。

药理生理多用仪、心电示波仪或心电图机、刺激电极、兔手术台、手术器械、注射器。

3% 戊巴比妥钠、1% 利多卡因、生理盐水。

【方法与步骤】

1. 取兔 1 只，称体重，用 3% 戊巴比妥钠（30mg/kg）耳缘静脉麻醉，背位固定，剪去胸前兔毛。

2. 胸前正中切开皮肤，沿胸骨左缘剪断第三、四肋软骨，可见心包膜下跳动的心脏。

3. 剪破心包膜，并将其固定于胸壁上，以使心脏抬高。将电极负极固定于心尖部，正极固定于左右室交界近房室交界处。两电极相距约 2cm。

4. 休息 15min 左右，开始测定给药前的心室纤颤阈（VFT）。刺激参数：方波宽度 0.3～0.5ms，频率 50Hz；电压从 1V 开始，刺激持续时间每次 10s，每隔 1min 刺激一次，逐渐增加刺激强度（每次增加 0.5V）直至室颤出现，这时的电压值即为 VFT。如用心电图机，在刺激时不能描记，刺激一停，则马上记录。休息 5min 后，重复一次，以两次平均值作为给药前 VFT。

5. 休息 5min 后从耳缘静脉缓慢注射 1% 利多卡因（10mg/kg），测定给药后 1min、5min、10min、15min、20min、25min、30min 的 VFT。

【结果处理】

以给药前 VFT 为基准，计算给药后各不同时间的 VFT 升高值，即 ΔVFT。对 ΔVFT 的上升相和下降相（如可能的话）进行线性回归，算出上升速率和下降速率，以表示药效上升和下降的速率。按三角形或梯形公式计算 ΔVFT 面积。如分组较多，50% 动物用作对照组，最后将给药组和生理盐水组结果对比，进行统计学检验。

【注意事项】

1. 家兔胸前区胸膜与心包膜易分开，所以如手术时注意，可不破胸膜即可进行心脏手术。由于不用呼吸机，要求手术中从中间剪开心包膜，用拉钩牵拉胸壁，不要用力过大，以保护胸膜完整。

2. 剪断肋软骨时，必须紧靠胸骨下剪开，以免剪破乳内动脉引起大出血。

3. 心包膜固定在胸壁上形成心包摇床，抬高心脏有利于手术操作。兔子心包膜较脆弱，易撕裂，用力要适当。

4. 心脏电极固定可用缝线固定，也可用小金属夹固定，但要注意两电极不能短路。

5. 电压增加幅度一次不要太大，以免引起严重室颤不易恢复。如室颤在数十秒内不能恢复，可进行胸外心脏按压和人工呼吸以助恢复。

【方法评价】

1. 此方法简便易行，为常用的电刺激引起心律失常的模型之一。

2. 实验结果稳定，重复性好，可对药物提高 VFT 的幅度和时程进行评价。

3. 如果用程控电刺激器可测量易损期，或在起搏情况下用单个期外刺激引起室速，室颤，测定 VFT，其实验结果更有价值。

4. 家兔、猫和大鼠等小动物的室颤容易自然恢复窦性，不需使用除颤器。

5. 由于刺激时有刺激干扰，而刺激一停，室颤又很快消失，故有时难于判断结果。如同时用动脉插管测量血压，对判断是否出现室颤很有帮助。

6. 心率改变可影响 VFT，如有条件，应用电起搏装置控制心率。

【思考题】

1. 复习心肌电活动中兴奋性的周期性变化。

2. 了解心肌复极程度与动作电位传导、折返形成之间的关系。

实验 5.6　利多卡因对氯化钡诱发心律失常的治疗作用

【目的】

学习用氯化钡诱发大鼠心律失常的方法，观察利多卡因的抗心律失常作用。

【原理】

氯化钡能促使浦氏纤维的钠离子内流，提高舒张期的除极速率，从而诱发室性心律失常，可表现为室性早搏、二联律、室性心动过速、心室纤颤等，也是一种筛选抗心律失常药物的模型。奎尼丁、利多卡因、β 受体阻滞药等对之有效。

【材料】

大鼠 2 只。

心电图机、心电图示波器、手术剪、眼科剪、大鼠固定台、注射器、头皮静脉注射针头、棉球。

10% 水合氯醛溶液、0.4% 氯化钡溶液、0.5% 利多卡因溶液、生理盐水。

【方法与步骤】

取大鼠1只，称其体重，用水合氯醛0.3g/kg腹腔麻醉，背位固定于手术台上。颈外静脉插管，以备给药。

将心电图机的针形电极插入大鼠四肢皮下，作描记心电图的准备。选用Ⅱ导联、振幅1mV＝10mm、纸速50mm/s。描记一段正常心电图后，静脉注射氯化钡4mg/kg，立即描记心电图20s，以后每隔1min再描记心电图一小段，或连续用示波器监视，直至恢复窦性节律。记录心律失常的持续时间。

取另一大鼠，用水合氯醛麻醉后以同样方法诱发心律失常的心电图后，立即由股静脉注射盐酸利多卡因5mg/kg，按上述要求描记心电图或示波器监视。以能否立即制止心律失常或心律失常的持续时间有无缩短为指标，评价利多卡因对氯化钡诱发心律失常的治疗作用。

【结果处理】

报告两只大白鼠前后所用药物，出现的心电图变化以及心律失常的持续时间（表5－1）。剪贴或复制有代表性的心电图段落。初步评价利多卡因对氯化钡诱发心律失常的拮抗作用。

表5－1　利多卡因对氯化钡引起的心律失常的对抗作用

药物＼组别	1	2	3	4	5	6	7	8	$\bar{x} \pm SD$
生理盐水组									
利多卡因									

【注意事项】

1. 本实验中的麻醉药水合氯醛不能以戊巴比妥钠等替代，否则就不易引起较恒定的心律失常。用利多卡因拮抗氯化钡诱发的心律失常作用，奏效极快。因而在推注利多卡因期间即可开始描记心电图，以便观察其转变过程。

大鼠氯化钡中毒后的心电图变化见图5－4。

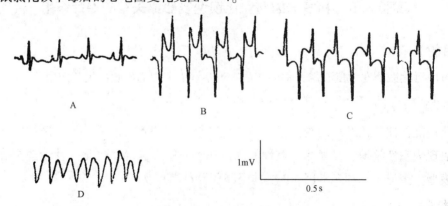

图5－4　大鼠氯化钡中毒后的心电图变化

注：A. 给药前；B. C. 分别为给药后3min与5min，出现室性早搏，呈二联律；D. 给药后7min出现室颤。均为Ⅱ导联，纸速50mm/s

2. 小鼠、大鼠、豚鼠等小动物即使发生室颤，也常有自然恢复之可能。而犬、猴等大

动物则不然，发生室颤后多以死亡告终。

实验 5.7 利多卡因对哇巴因诱发心律失常的对抗作用

【目的】

学习哇巴因诱发心律失常模型的制备，观察利多卡因对哇巴因诱发心律失常的治疗作用。了解哇巴因诱发心律失常的机制。

【原理】

强心苷中毒一方面可抑制心肌细胞膜上的 $Na^+ - K^+ - ATP$ 酶，使细胞内 K^+ 减少，导致最大舒张电位减小；细胞内 Na^+ 增加，通过 $Na^+ - Ca^{2+}$ 交换使细胞内 Ca^{2+} 增加，导致振荡性后电位及触发活动而使自律性增高。另一方面强心苷直接抑制心脏传导系统，最大舒张电位减小，动作电位幅度降低，使传导减慢易导致折返形成。

强心苷中毒可产生各种心律失常，最常见的是多源性室性早搏、室速和室颤以及传导阻滞。

【材料】

豚鼠 1 只，体重 300～400g，雌雄不限。

心电图机、心电示波器、手术台、手术器械、注射器、静脉插管。

20% 乌拉坦、0.01% 哇巴因、0.5% 利多卡因、生理盐水。

【方法与步骤】

1. 豚鼠称体重后，用 20% 乌拉坦（1.2g/kg）腹腔注射麻醉，仰位固定于手术台上，剪去颈部被毛。

2. 沿颈部正中切开皮肤，分离一侧颈外静脉，将充满生理盐水的静脉插管插入 1～2cm 深并用丝线固定。

3. 连接心电图导联线，记录给药前的 II 导联心电图。

4. 在心电示波器监视下，静脉注射 0.01% 哇巴因，首次 90μg/kg，以后每 5min 静注 20μg/kg，直到持续性室速出现为止。记录心电图。

5. 从静脉插管注射 0.5% 利多卡因（5mg/kg），观察并记录从室速转为窦性心律、室速再次出现、室速转为室颤（如出现的话）的时间和相应的心电图，给利多卡因后观察时间以 1h 为限。对照组注射等量生理盐水。

【结果处理】

以给抗心律失常药到室速转为窦性心律的时间作为药物起效时间，以窦性心律持续时间及转成窦性心律到出现室颤的时间作为药效持续时间。剪贴心电图，与对照组对比，评价药物的抗心律失常作用。

【注意事项】

1. 出现室性早搏后仍要给哇巴因，直到典型的室速出现后，才能给利多卡因。

2. 静脉插管时可不必把静脉完全游离，只需把静脉上面的脂肪、结缔组织分离干净，在静脉充有血液的情况下剪口插管，这样易于插入。

3. 注意动物保温。

【方法评价】

1. 强心苷诱发心律失常模型是一常用方法，方法稳定，结果可靠。

2. 豚鼠对心血管药物的反应与人相近，且对强心苷敏感，价格较便宜，很适宜于该模型，可用于新药筛选。另一常用的动物是犬。大鼠对强心苷不敏感，不能用于该模型。

3. 该实验为治疗给药，必要时，也可采用预防给药，即在给抗心律失常药后再静脉恒速灌注哇巴因，计算引起室性早搏、室速、室颤和死亡时的哇巴因用量。

【思考题】

哪些药物治疗哇巴因诱发的心律失常效果较好？为什么？

实验 5.8　药物抑制大鼠缺血 - 再灌注心律失常的作用

【目的】

学习结扎大鼠冠状动脉引起心律失常的方法。观察大鼠缺血 - 再灌注心律失常的特点，了解缺血 - 再灌注心律失常发生的机理。

【原理】

结扎动物的冠状动脉后，由于心肌缺血，代谢产物积聚，心肌细胞膜对离子的通透性发生改变，缺血区和非缺血区心肌电生理特性不均一，功能紊乱导致心律失常。冠脉结扎后数分钟内即可发生室性早搏、室性心动过速，甚至室颤。与急性心肌梗死患者发病早期发生心律失常的过程相似。缺血心肌再灌注时，由于氧自由基的生成，钙离子的内流加重心肌损伤和电生理紊乱，更易发生室速、室颤等严重室性心律失常。

【材料】

大鼠 1 只，体重 180 ~ 250g，雄性。

心电图机、小动物人工呼吸机、气管插管、手术器械、小动脉夹、小段硅胶管（内径 2 ~ 3mm）、注射器。

0.5% 美西律、1.5% 戊巴比妥钠、生理盐水。

【方法与步骤】

1. 取大鼠 1 只，称体重，用 1.5% 戊巴比妥钠（45mg/kg）腹腔注射麻醉。仰卧位固定于手术台上。

2. 颈部正中切开皮肤，作气管插管接呼吸机进行正压人工呼吸（频率 50 次/分，潮气量每分钟 1000ml/kg），颈外静脉插管准备给药用。

3. 连接心电图机，记录标准 Ⅱ 导联心电图。

4. 从左胸第 4、5 肋间开胸，暴露心脏，用左手挤压胸廓或用环形镊将心脏提出胸外，用无损伤缝合线（5/0）在距左冠脉根部 2 ~ 3mm 处围绕冠脉穿线，迅速将心脏放回胸腔。将缝线头穿过一小段硅胶管后引出，用于阻断冠脉。

5. 稳定 10 ~ 15min 后，拉紧缝线，并用小动脉夹固定，使硅胶管压迫冠脉，完全阻断其血流。观察记录心电图，是否有明显的心肌缺血表现（J 点抬高）及有无心律失常，如有及时记录。

6. 缺血 10min 后放开结扎线，造成缺血心肌复灌，并观察记录 0 ~ 30s、1min、1.5min、

2min、3min、4min、5min 的心电图。一般在再灌后 1min 内最易发生室速，室颤等心律失常，如 5min 内未出现心律失常，则以后很少再出现心律失常。

将整个实验分二组进行，一组在冠脉阻断前给美西律（5mg/kg），另一组给同量生理盐水作为对照组。

【结果处理】

根据心电图结果计算室速（VT），室颤（VF）的发生率和持续时间以及死亡率。再灌注 30s 内室性早搏次数。还可采用等级记分法测定室性心律失常的严重程度分数。等级划分可参考下列标准：

0 级：无室性心律失常；

1 级：偶发室性早搏（<5%）；

2 级：频发室性早搏，二联律，三联律；

3 级：短时阵发室性心动过速；

4 级：持续室性心动过速；

5 级：室扑，室颤；

6 级：死亡。

心律失常分数的组间显著性检验不能用参数统计，可用 Ridit 检验或等级序值法。最后根据整理的结果对药物的抗心律失常作用进行评价。

【注意事项】

1. 阻断冠脉后，心电图应有明显的缺血改变，否则很可能没扎住冠脉。

2. 再灌注心律失常必须一次缺血再灌注成功，多次缺血后一般不再出现心律失常。

3. 温度可明显影响动物的心律失常发生率，所以在温度较低时要采取保温措施。

4. 血液 pH 对心律失常发生也有明显影响，要严格按体重调整潮气量。

5. 阻断冠脉时缝线拉得不能太松，也不能太紧，以免勒断冠脉不能进行再灌注。

6. 再灌注前的缺血时间对再灌注心律失常的发生率有显著影响。麻醉大鼠缺血 5～10min 后再灌注的室颤发生率最高。

7. 冠脉结扎位置对心律失常的发生有很大影响，要求结扎部位保持一致。

【方法评价】

1. 大鼠冠脉结扎 – 再灌注心律失常方法可靠，重复性好，与临床的发病机理相近，是研究抗心律失常药物的常用方法之一。

2. 冠脉结扎要求位置准，动作快，因而操作者要经过一段时间的操作训练才能做好。

3. 麻醉大鼠缺血 – 再灌注心律失常的发生率比清醒大鼠低，但后者实验难度更高。

【思考题】

1. 缺血性和再灌注心律失常的产生机制。

2. 比较早期缺血性和再灌注心律失常和冠脉二期结扎形成的心律失常（Harris）。

3. 美西律抗心律失常的作用机制是什么？

实验5.9　药物对离体心房肌有效不应期和收缩力的影响

【目的】

掌握离体豚鼠心房标本的制备方法，学习用刺激法测量心肌有效不应期和用离体心房标本研究药物对心肌收缩性的影响。

【原理】

离体豚鼠心房在保持一定温度、pH和氧供充足的营养液中，在固定的电刺激驱动下，能存活并保持稳定的收缩幅度达几小时。根据用药前后心房收缩幅度的变化可反应药物对心肌收缩性能的影响。采用较短间隔的成对方波刺激，当其间隔小于有效不应期时，心房只发生一次收缩反应；当其间隔大于有效不应期时，心肌可产生二次收缩反应。当两方波的间隔刚好能引起二次收缩时，这成对方波的间隔时间为这时心房的有效不应期。测定有效不应期可用于研究抗心律失常药物对心肌电生理特性的影响及其作用机制。

【材料】

豚鼠1只，体重300~400g，雌雄不限。

温血动物离体器官实验装置（超级恒温水浴、浴管、铁支架、氧气瓶等）、药理生理多用仪、生理信号采集记录系统、示波器、张力换能器、刺激电极、手术器械、注射器、烧杯、平皿。

Krebs – Henseleit（K – H）液［组成（mmol/L）：NaCl 118；KCl 4.7，$CaCl_2$ 1.25，$MgSO_4$ 1.2，KH_2PO_4 1.2，$NaHCO_3$ 25，葡萄糖11］、10^{-4} mol/L奎尼丁、5×10^{-5} mol/L异丙肾上腺素，10^{-4} mol/L氯化乙酰胆碱。

【方法与步骤】

1. 制备离体豚鼠心房。取豚鼠1只，用木槌击头致昏，迅速剪开胸腔，取出心脏，立即置入预先加温的通入混合气体（95% O_2，5% CO_2）的K – H液中，此时心脏自动收缩把血液泵出。在房室交界处剪下心房，换入干净的K – H液，分离修整左心房，将其一端固定在刺激电极上，另一端用丝线扎住，置入浴管后与张力换能器相连。调节静息负荷为1.0g左右，浴管内K – H液体积为20ml，温度30℃±0.5℃，不断通入混合气体。电刺激驱动心房收缩（刺激参数：波宽2~4ms，频率1Hz，电压为阈值的120%）。标本在浴管中稳定30min后，开始进行实验。稳定过程中换营养液2~3次。

【附】豚鼠左右心房区别：左房较大、边缘较整齐，呈贝壳形；右房较小，边缘不规则，一端尖细，因与窦房结相连，有较高的自律性。

2. 记录给药前的收缩幅度和有效不应期。在基础频率刺激下，在生理信号系统记录仪上记录一段正常心房收缩曲线。然后用不同间隔时间（从200ms起）的成对方波刺激，在示波器上以心房收缩波形为指标，测定给药前的有效不应期。示波器采用刺激触发扫描，以使收缩波显示同步。当成对刺激的间隔不足有效不应期时，示波器上显示的收缩波与单次刺激产生的收缩波相同。当刺激间隔超过有效不应期时，心房产生的收缩波比单次刺激时高或可分成两个波。刚刚能使心房收缩波变化的成对刺激的间隔时间即为有效不应期。要求连续两次测量的有效不应期基本不变，两次测量的间隔约10s。

3. 加入被试药物10min后，按步骤2记录给药后的心房收缩幅度和有效不应期。20min

时再测量一次，然后用 K – H 液洗去药物。

按以下顺序给药：10^{-4} mol/L 乙酰胆碱 0.2ml，5×10^{-5} mol/L 异丙肾上腺素 0.2ml，10^{-4} mol/L 奎尼丁 0.2ml。

4. 用 K – H 液冲洗标本 3 ~ 5 次，待收缩曲线和有效不应期基本恢复后加另一被试药物，重复步骤 3，记录收缩幅度和不应期。

【结果处理】

剪贴记录的收缩幅度曲线，将收缩幅度按定标值换算成张力（g 或 mg）与有效不应期（ms），按相应的药物和时间记录下来，分析讨论结果。在实际工作中，如各标本在给药前的收缩张力相差较大，则可将给药前张力作为百分之百，给药后的张力换算成给药前的百分数，然后各组间进行统计学检验。

【注意事项】

1. 制备标本操作要迅速，尽量在 2 ~ 3min 内完成。

2. 温度控制在 30℃ ±1℃ 以内，太高收缩幅度容易自然衰减，过低则兴奋性不好。

3. 实验时间如超过 4h 或用了多种药物，最好要检查标本的反应性，以免因标本反应性不好而得出虚假结果。

4. 根据心肌收缩波形测定不应期时，最好用示波器观察，也可用二道生理记录仪记录，但不能用平衡记录仪。后者频响太低。

5. 加入到浴管中的药液体积应小于其中营养液的 5%，这样加入药液的体积影响可忽略不计。

【方法评价】

1. 离体豚鼠心房标本制作容易，实验结果稳定，方法易于掌握。采用快速走纸记录单次收缩波后，可对心肌的收缩速度和舒张速度等进行分析（具体方法参见离体乳头肌实验）。另外，离体豚鼠右心房在 37℃ 左右时可自发收缩跳动，频率可稳定 1h 以上，可用于观察药物对窦性心率的直接影响。

2. 由于标本为心房肌，肌纤维走向不一致，评价药物对心室肌作用价值不如离体乳头肌。后者可同步记录心肌收缩和动作电位，但实验技术和条件要求较高。

【思考题】

1. 维持温血动物离体心房持续跳动需哪些基本条件？

2. 如以动作电位为指标应怎样确定有效不应期？

3. 乙酰胆碱、异丙肾上腺素和奎尼丁使有效不应期改变的主要机理。

三、抗心肌缺血药物实验

抗心肌缺血药作用的主要途径有：保护缺血心肌，减小心肌梗死范围及损伤程度；改善冠脉循环；调节心肌代谢；调节心脏功能和血流动力学及引起血液流变学改变，如血凝状态、血小板聚集、血脂代谢等等。根据这些药物作用途径就产生了相应的多种实验方法。近年来，抗心肌缺血药在理论及新药研制方面均有很大进展，其实验方法也有较大进展。心肌缺血或梗死一定时间后再供给血液，常导致再灌注损伤，加重原有的缺血或梗死心肌损伤。心肌缺血与再灌注损伤的模型可通过整体动物结扎冠脉、离体心脏缺氧或结扎冠脉及体外心肌细胞培养缺氧等进行。

结扎冠脉引起心肌缺血和梗死可产生形态学、酶学和电生理学上的改变。用光镜作组织学切片检测心肌缺血和梗死范围是直接可靠的方法，而酶学和电生理方法所得结果均应以形态学方法为标准，与之比较才能确定其可靠程度。冠脉流量不但受冠脉血管收缩程度和血压的影响，而且还受心肌收缩力的影响，因此，在测定冠脉流量时要注意血压和心肌收缩力的变化。另外，在测定冠脉流量时，最好还要测定冠状动静脉氧分压差的改变，以了解是否增加心肌氧耗引起冠脉扩张。传统的动物耐缺氧实验筛选抗心肌缺血药的方法，由于特异性差已渐淘汰。

实验 5.10　结扎兔冠状动脉引起的心肌梗死

【目的】

学习结扎冠状动脉，建立心肌梗死模型的方法。了解估计心肌缺血和梗死范围的方法和心肌梗死发展的过程。

【原理】

临床上心肌梗死的常见原因是冠心病。当冠状动脉粥样硬化导致动脉严重狭窄或闭塞时，产生心肌缺血或心肌梗死。结扎冠状动脉后可使心肌长时间缺血引起心肌梗死。结扎冠脉后产生的血流动力学、心肌代谢改变及心律失常等，与冠心病产生的心肌梗死时的改变有相似之处。冠状动脉结扎后梗死发展快，缺血范围大致固定，可进行组织切片染色、心电图 ST 段标测和血清酶学检查等指标测定，从而确定心肌缺血/梗死范围和损伤程度。测定药物对这些指标的影响可评价药物抗心肌缺血和缩小梗死范围的作用。家兔心前区心包膜与胸膜容易分开，因此可在不破胸膜的情况下剪开心包膜，结扎冠脉。

【材料】

家兔 1 只，体重 2 ~ 3kg，雌雄不限。

兔手术台、心电图机、手术器械、小开胸器。

3% 戊巴比妥钠、2% 碘酊、75% 乙醇、龙胆紫、庆大霉素针剂。

【方法与步骤】

1. 取家兔 1 只，称体重，仰位固定，用 3% 戊巴比妥钠 30 ~ 45mg/kg 静脉麻醉，手术前去毛。局部用 2% 碘酊消毒，75% 乙醇脱碘。

2. 心电图标测　以胸骨左缘旁开 1cm 第 4 肋间为中心，上下左右各 1cm 范围，用龙胆紫标记 9 个点，记录结扎前这 9 个点的胸前导联心电图。

3. 从胸骨中线切开皮肤，暴露胸骨，沿胸骨左缘剪断第 1 ~ 3 肋软骨，用小开胸器轻轻撑开胸腔切口，可见心包及跳动的心脏。

4. 提起心包膜，用眼科剪小心将心包膜前部剪开，注意不要弄破胸膜。用止血钳将左心耳轻轻提起，用持针器持无损伤缝针在冠状动脉前降支根部下约 1cm 处穿线结扎。为减少侧支循环，增大心肌梗死范围，可在结扎线下约 0.5cm 处再穿线进行冠脉结扎。

5. 关胸后，再次记录胸前 9 个标测点的心电图，观察 ST 段的变化，注射庆大霉素 4 万单位，预防感染。

6. 一天后，再次记录 9 个标测点的心电图。处死动物，取出心脏进行 NBT 染色估计梗死范围。

7. 如要测定血清肌酸激酶或其 M 型同工酶的变化，则应在手术前及梗死后分别取血清进行酶活力测定。

【结果处理】

1. **心电图 ST 段和 Q 波标测** 胸前多导联标测的心电图 ST 段一般在结扎后 2h 明显抬高，1 天达高峰，3 天内持续抬高，3 天后逐渐自发缓解。胸前任一导联的 ST 段变化不能定量反应心肌梗死的范围，但一般认为胸前多导联的 ST 段抬高总 mV（∑ST）可以定量代表心肌梗死范围。ST 段异常抬高或降低的导联数（NST）和平均每导联 ST 段移位的 mV 值（即 ∑ST 除以全部标测点）也可作为表示梗死范围的参考指标。此外，Q 波深度的总 mV 即 ∑Q 与出现 Q 波的导联数（NQ）也可作为反映心肌梗死范围的指标。

2. **硝基四氮唑蓝（NBT）大体标本染色** 参见硝基四氮唑蓝染色法测量心肌梗死范围。

3. **CK 或 LDH 的测定** 以结扎前和结扎后 1h、3h、6h 和 24h 做比较（参见有关书籍）。

【注意事项】

1. 开胸和结扎冠状动脉时要注意保持胸膜的完整，这样可不用人工呼吸。

2. 剪开肋软骨时，要靠着胸骨边缘下剪，以免剪破乳内动脉，引起大出血。

3. 家兔冠脉前降支结扎部位应深一些，并双重结扎以减少侧支循环，形成较大的梗死范围以便观察药效。

4. 此法产生的心肌梗死范围在 3 天内较稳定，3 天后有自发缓解的趋势，实验时应加以注意。

5. 如果家兔的前降支变异大，长度不到 1.5cm，则此兔结扎前降支后造成的梗死范围过小，应弃之不用。

【方法评价】

1. 家兔不破胸膜结扎冠状动脉，方法简便，而且家兔耐受力较犬强，冠脉结扎后较少发生致命性心律失常，成功率较高。

2. 家兔冠状动脉前降支配范围较小，如不采用双重结扎则梗死范围太小不利于药效评价。采用双重结扎后可阻断侧支循环，增大梗死范围，便于观察药效，但动物死亡率也有所提高。

3. 兔大小适中，不但可用大体标本染色或组织切片和酶学检查来估计梗死范围，还可进行心电图标测。其价格也比犬便宜。

【思考题】

1. 心肌缺血后出现心肌梗死、心电图改变、血清酶活力改变的时间顺序如何？为什么？

2. 为什么心肌梗死范围太小不利于药效评价？

3. 心肌梗死后测定梗死区心肌的肌酸激酶和乳酸脱氢酶将会有什么改变？

实验 5.11 药物对离体豚鼠心脏心肌收缩力和冠脉流量的影响

【目的】

学习 Langendorff 心脏制备方法，观察药物对离体心脏收缩力和冠脉流量的影响，了解怎样评价药物对离体心脏冠脉流量的影响。

【原理】

温血动物心脏在供氧、保温、有一定离子浓度和供能物质的情况下，能自动收缩，存活一段时间。通过完整的离体心脏，可观察药物直接对冠脉流量、心肌收缩力和心率的影响。

【材料】

豚鼠 1 只，体重 350～450g，雌雄不限。

恒温、恒压离体器官灌流装置（灌流瓶、蛇形管、超级恒温水浴锅），心脏保温套管，主动脉插管，供氧装置，定滑轮，蛙心夹，张力换能器，生理信号采集记录系统，手术器械，小量筒，烧杯，注射器。

1% 肝素、10^{-5}mol/L 肾上腺素、10^{-5}mol/L 异丙肾上腺素、2.5% 氨茶碱、3% 戊巴比妥钠、Krebs - Henselit9（K - H）液。

【方法与步骤】

1. 豚鼠称体重，3% 戊巴比妥钠 30～45mg/kg（1～1.5ml）腹腔注射麻醉，颈外静脉注射 1% 肝素 10mg/kg 抗凝，1min 后开胸取出心脏，置预通混合气体的冷 K - H 液中，轻轻挤出余血。

2. 在营养液下，将主动脉插管插入主动脉内并用丝线结扎固定。

3. 将连着心脏的主动脉插管连接到灌流装置的出口，用 37℃、充以混合气体、50～60cm 水柱压力的 K - H 液灌流心脏。灌流装置内应预先排出气泡，不能让气泡灌入心脏内。

4. 用蛙心夹夹住心尖部，通过丝线经滑轮转换方向后与张力换能器连接，并连接于生理信号采集记录系统上，给心脏罩上保温套管保温。用量筒在心脏下面收集流出液，测定冠脉流量。

5. 待心脏收缩稳定后，连续测定 2 个 3min 的冠脉流量，若数值相近，则计算平均每分钟流量作为给药前的对照值，并记录心肌收缩幅度和心率。

6. 从主动脉插管上方将药物注入到灌流液中，然后记录给药后 1min、3min、5min、10min 的冠脉流量，心肌收缩幅度和心率。待冠脉流量和收缩幅度基本恢复后给下一个药物。

给药顺序为：10^{-5}mol/L 肾上腺素 0.5ml，10^{-5}mol/L 异丙肾上腺素 0.5ml，2.5% 氨茶碱 0.5ml。

【结果处理】

根据生理信号采集记录系统上的心脏收缩曲线，计算出心肌收缩力和心率。计算给药后的冠脉流量、心肌收缩力和心率的绝对变化值和相对变化值（百分变化）。列表，评价分析药物对这些指标的影响。

【注意事项】

1. 营养液要求新鲜配制。用 K - H 液需充以混合气体，用任 - 洛氏液可直接充纯氧。

2. 心脏的离体，插管等操作必须迅速。从取出心脏到开始灌流最好在 2min 之内完成，以免因心肌缺血、缺氧造成心肌损伤。

3. 插管需在液面下进行，切勿让空气进入冠脉内造成栓塞。注射肝素为防止微血管内凝血之用，如操作熟练迅速可以不用。

4. 制备离体心脏时，主动脉插管不宜插入过深，以免堵塞冠脉口，并不要损伤窦房结。

【方法评价】

1. 本实验为一经典方法，所需设备简单，操作简便，可同时观察心脏收缩功能、心率、冠脉流量及测定组织和灌流液中的生化指标。方法稍加改变，还可造成离体心律失常模型、心肌缺血模型，观察药物的抗心律失常作用或抗心肌缺血作用。

2. 冠脉流量不但受冠脉舒缩程度的影响，而且在很大程度上受心肌收缩力的影响，因此在分析药物对冠脉流量的影响时要考虑心肌收缩力的变化。必要时可电刺激致室颤，消除心肌收缩的影响。

3. 在整体条件下，心脏的能量来源主要为血液中的脂肪酸，而离体心脏的能量来源为灌流液中的葡萄糖，故离体心脏收缩维持时间不能太长，实验操作必须在较短的时间内完成。

4. Langendorff 离体心脏排除了神经体液的调控作用，但不能同时控制前负荷、后负荷及心率。离体工作心脏的左心室充盈压（前负荷）及主动脉柱高（后负荷）可以保持恒定，心率亦可通过电起搏装置加以控制。因此，可根据需要将三者同时控制，观察药物对心肌收缩性能的影响，或控制其中任两项，观察心肌收缩性能与另一项的关系。

【思考题】

1. 温血动物心脏的实验条件与蛙心（冷血动物心脏）实验条件有何不同？

2. 本实验是否为评价药物对心肌收缩性能影响的好方法？为什么？

实验 5.12　硝基四氮唑蓝染色法测量心肌梗死范围

形态学方法测量心肌缺血范围有两种方法：一是组织学方法，一是大体标本染色法。组织学切片法定量准确可靠，但要作一系列切片才能准确定量，费时费力，且一般要在心肌梗死 24h 后才能获得较满意的结果。现常用大体标本活体染色法测量心肌梗死范围，可采用硝基四氮唑蓝（Nitro – blue tetrazolium，NBT）或氯化三苯基四氮唑（Tripheny tetrazolium chloride，TTC）染色法。

【目的】

学习 NBT 染色法测量心肌梗死范围。

【原理】

正常心肌细胞含有脱氢酶，在 NADH 存在的条件下，能将无色的氧化型染料 NBT 还原成还原型的蓝色 NBT，而使活体心肌染色。心肌梗死一定时间后，细胞中脱氢酶因细胞损伤而释放丢失，不能再使 NBT 还原染色，故梗死的心肌不被染色。因此可把不被染色的梗死区与染色正常的心肌分离，用称重法或用平面切片的面积求积法估计心肌梗死范围。

【材料】

兔梗死心脏（参见结扎总冠状动脉引起心肌梗死法）。

恒温水浴箱、烧杯、平皿、手术刀。

生理盐水、0.5% NBT 溶液。

【附】0.5% NBT 溶液的配制：称取 NBT 250mg，加 80ml 磷酸钾缓冲液（pH = 7.4），摇匀后加蒸馏水至 500ml，即得 0.5% 的 NBT 溶液。

磷酸钾缓冲液的配制：称取磷酸二氢钾 4.08g，加 0.1mol/L 的 NaOH 溶液 237ml，溶解后再加蒸馏水稀释至 600ml。

【方法与步骤】

1. 将实验后心脏取下，用盐水冲洗，除去血污，剔除血管脂肪等非心肌组织，用吸水纸吸去水分，称全心湿重。

2. 沿冠状沟切除心房，留下心室称重，顺房室沟从心尖到心基部平行将兔心室切成 0.3 ~ 0.5cm 厚的心肌片，用生理盐水冲洗干净。

3. 将心肌片放在 0.5% 的 NBT 溶液中，在 37℃ 温孵 10 ~ 15min 染色，染色进程中不时摇动或搅拌染色液使之与心肌有充分的接触机会。

4. 染色后立即用水洗去多余的染料，梗死区不着色，非梗死区被 NBT 染为蓝色。

5. 剪去各心肌片被染色的非梗死区心肌；把未染色的梗死心肌称重。

【结果处理】

按下式计算梗死范围。

心室梗死范围百分率 = 梗死心肌重量/心室重量 ×100%

全心梗死范围百分率 = 梗死心肌重量/全心重量 ×100%

左心室梗死范围百分率 = 梗死心肌重量/左心室重量 ×100%

【注意事项】

1. 心肌染色应在取下心脏后立即进行，或将心肌冰冻后染色，否则非梗死区脱氢酶继续释放而影响染色结果。对冰冻的心脏，不需完全融化即可染色。

2. NBT 染料溶液应用磷酸钾缓冲液新鲜配制并调 pH 到 7.4 ~ 7.8。

3. 心肌切片应被染料溶液盖过，并不时摇动，使染料与心肌充分接触，染色时间不宜过长或过短，以免染得太深或太浅，影响观察。

4. 心肌切片不宜过厚。

【方法评价】

1. 用活体染色法测定心肌梗死范围是简便、快速易行、准确实用的方法，适用于心脏较大的动物如犬、猫、猪、家兔等。对大鼠等较小动物的心脏，此法误差较大，用切片求积方法可提高其精确度。

2. 结扎冠脉后 3 ~ 6h，NBT 染色法即可测梗死范围，此时光镜和电镜检查仅有糖原丢失而未表现出心肌坏死，故该法可比镜检更早发现梗死，现已成为国际常用并公认的心肌梗死范围定量方法。其缺点是残留有脱氢酶而染色的细胞不一定是活细胞，故此法常比组织学切片法低估梗死范围。

【思考题】

1. 影响 NBT 染色法测量心肌梗死范围的实验因素有哪些？如何控制？

2. NBT 染色法测量心肌梗死范围的同时，可测定哪些生化指标？

实验 5.13　丹参注射液对垂体后叶素致兔心肌缺血的作用

【目的】

学习用垂体后叶素引起心肌缺血的实验方法。观察药物抗心肌缺血的作用。

【原理】

垂体后叶素可使包括冠脉在内的全身血管收缩。利用这一作用，静脉注射垂体后叶素可使动物产生急性心肌缺血状态。凡可以对抗垂体后叶素收缩冠脉血管这一作用的药物，均可使缺血性心电图得到改善。以心电图 ST 段及 T 波产生的变化为指标，观察给予药物后的对抗作用。

【材料】

家兔 2 只。

电子秤、兔手术台、线绳、10ml 注射器、1ml 注射器、心电图机、秒表。

垂体后叶素注射液、丹参注射液、3% 戊巴比妥钠、生理盐水。

【方法与步骤】

挑选心电图正常的家兔 2 只，以 3% 戊巴比妥钠耳缘静脉注射（24mg/kg）麻醉动物，固定于手术台上，记录 Ⅱ 导联心电图（1mV = 10，纸速 50mm/s）。给家兔耳缘静脉注射垂体后叶素 2.5u/kg（体重）（用生理盐水稀释到 3ml）30s 注射完，并立即于注射后 30s、1min、3min、5min、7min、10min、15min、30min 记录心电图的变化。待心电图恢复正常后，给动物静脉注射丹参注射液 2ml/kg（体重）。5min 后再给同量的垂体后叶素，观察上述同样时间内心电图的变化。对照组给予等容量的生理盐水，实验方法同上。综合全实验室的结果进行比较。

【结果处理】

填入表 5 – 2。

表 5 – 2　丹参注射液对垂体后叶素所致兔心肌缺血的对抗作用

组别	R – R 间期（s）		T 波（mV）		ST 段（mV）		心率（次/min）	
	给药前	给药后	给药前	给药后	给药前	给药后	给药前	给药后
生理盐水								
丹参注射液								

【注意事项】

1. 第 1 次给予垂体后叶素后，如果家兔心电图未出现缺血性改变（尤其是 ST 段和 T 波），则淘汰该动物。

2. 给予垂体后叶素的剂量可依据其效价调整。

3. 心电图的缺血性变化多发生在注射垂体后叶素后 15min 内。

4. 本实验所用家兔体重应在 2kg 左右，雄雌均可，但雌兔不得有孕。

5. 可使用大鼠代替家兔，体重 200g 左右。

6. 根据注射垂体后叶素后心电图的异常以及药物对抗的情况，选择某一时刻的数据加以比较，并在表下注明。

7. 如应用垂体后叶素剂量不大时，动物可迅速恢复正常，故可反复在同一动物进行多次实验。

【方法评价】

1. 此方法是研究抗心肌缺血药物的常用急性实验方法，简便易行，仅需心电图机及慢性注射装置即可。

2. 在脑垂体后叶素注射后 1.5min 之内，ST 段改变；在 45s 内 T 波升高；25min 至 1h，恢复正常。

【思考题】

1. 用垂体后叶素复制动物心肌缺血病理模型的原理及优点。

2. 阐述丹参抗心肌缺血的作用、作用机制以及有效成分与其功效的关系。

实验 5.14 血脂测定法

动脉粥样硬化的发病与脂质代谢紊乱有密切关系，测定血脂水平和建立动脉粥样硬化病理模型，是研究抗动脉粥样硬化药的重要手段。

【目的】

学习血清总胆固醇和甘油三酯的测定方法，了解动脉粥样硬化与高脂血症的关系。

（一）血清总胆固醇（TC）的定量测定法——高铁-醋酸-硫酸显色法

血清中的胆固醇（CH）有 25%～30% 为游离胆固醇（FC），70%～75% 为胆固醇酯（CE），两者总称 TC。

【原理】

用异丙醇提取血清中胆固醇并沉淀蛋白质，同时加吸附剂去除磷脂、胆红素及其他干扰胆固醇显色反应的物质。胆固醇与浓硫酸及三价铁离子反应生成稳定的紫红色物质，与同样处理的标准液对照比色，求得胆固醇含量。

【材料】

1. **仪器** 721 可见分光光度计、台式离心机、振荡器、磨口试管、吸量管。

2. **试剂** ①异丙醇（AR）、②冰醋酸（AR）。③吸附剂（氧化铝）：层析用I级中性氧化铝，用约 4 倍体积的蒸馏水洗 8～9 次，直至不易下沉的细颗粒完全被除去。滤干后在 110℃烤箱中干燥活化 10～18h，密闭或干燥器内保存。④0.1% 三氯化铁（含 $6H_2O$，AR）冰醋酸溶液，可长期保存。⑤显色剂：0.1% 三氯化铁冰醋酸溶液与浓硫酸（GR 或 AR）按 1∶1 体积混合，在室温下可稳定约 2 个月。⑥胆固醇标准液（2.0mg/ml）：精确称取干燥纯胆固醇 200mg，用异丙醇溶解并定容至 100ml，冰箱贮存备用。

【方法与步骤】

1. 取血清 0.1ml 于具塞磨口试管中，加异丙醇 2.5ml（冲入，使血清成细颗粒状），加氧化铝 0.4g，加塞混匀（置 60℃水浴中 1～2min），置振荡器上振荡 10min，2000 转/分离心 10min。标准管中用胆固醇标准液代替血清，与测定管同样处理。

2. 取试管 3 支，按下表操作。

加入物	空白管（ml）	标准管（ml）	测定管（ml）
血清上清抽提液	—	—	1.0
标准上清抽提液	—	1.0	—
异丙醇	1.0	—	—
60℃水浴预热5min			
显色剂（在水浴中沿管壁加入）	3.0	3.0	3.0
充分混匀后，60℃加温15min			

3. 置室温冷却后用721型分光光度计比色，1cm比色杯，波长530nm。

【结果处理】

按下式计算：

血清总胆固醇（mmol/L）=（测定管吸光度/标准管吸光度）×5.17

【注意事项】

1. 如需同时测定甘油三酯时，可采用此同一异丙醇抽提液，标准液也可将胆固醇和甘油三酯配在一起。

2. 测定范围可达血清总胆固醇13mmol/L（500mg/dl），超过此值时，血清标本量应减半。

【方法评价】

本法显色稳定，重复性很好，回收率接近100%。因加吸附剂去除了非特异性反应物质，可能所得结果较其他方法稍低。

（二）血清甘油三酯的定量测定——乙酰丙酮显色法

【原理】

先用异丙醇沉淀血清蛋白，抽提血清脂类，用吸附剂去除磷脂、甘油、葡萄糖和胆红素等干扰物质，再以氢氧化钾溶液将甘油三酯皂化成甘油，加偏高碘酸钠使甘油氧化成甲醛。甲醛与乙酰丙酮和氨缩合形成黄色的3,5-二乙酰-1,4-二氢二甲吡啶（Hantzsch缩合）；与同样处理的标准液比色，计算出血清中甘油三酯的含量。其反应式如下：

$$H-\overset{O}{\overset{\|}{C}}-H+2CH_3\overset{O}{\overset{\|}{C}}CH_2\overset{O}{\overset{\|}{C}}CH_3+NH_3 \xrightarrow{-3H_2O}$$

甲醛 　　　乙酰丙酮 　　　　　　3,5-二乙酰-1,4-二氢二甲吡啶

【材料】

1. 仪器　同胆固醇测定实验。

2. 试剂　①异丙醇（AR）。②吸附剂（氧化铝）。③皂化试剂：取分析纯氢氧化钾10g，溶于75ml蒸馏水中，再加异丙醇25ml，置棕色瓶中保存。④偏高碘酸钠试剂：取无水醋酸铵7.7g，溶于70ml蒸馏水中，加冰醋酸6ml，偏高碘酸钠65mg，再加蒸馏水100ml，贮棕色瓶中置室温下，至少可保存6个月。⑤乙酰丙酮试剂：准确吸取乙酰丙酮0.4ml，加异丙醇至100ml，贮棕色瓶中，在室温下可保存6个月。⑥标准贮存液：精确称取三油酸甘油酯1.000g，溶于异丙醇中，加异丙醇至100ml，置冰箱保存，至少可用两个月。⑦标准应用液（100ml/200mg）：取贮存液2.0ml，放10ml容量瓶中，用异丙醇稀释至刻度，置冰

箱保存，须每周新配。

【方法与步骤】

1. 取带塞离心管 3 支，按下表操作。

步骤	试剂	空白管	标准管	测定管
抽提	血清（ml）	—	—	0.1
	标准应用液（ml）	—	0.1	—
	蒸馏水（ml）	0.1	—	—
	异丙醇（ml）	3.0	3.0	3.0
	氧化铝（g）	0.4	0.4	0.4
充分振荡 10min，离心 5min，取上清液				
皂化	上清液（ml）	2.0	2.0	2.0
	皂化试剂（ml）	0.6	0.6	0.6
混匀，在 65℃ 水浴中放 5min				
氧化	偏高碘酸钠试剂（ml）	1.5	1.5	1.5
充分混匀				
显色	乙酰丙酮试剂（ml）	1.5	1.5	1.5

2. 混匀各管，置 65~70℃ 水浴中至少 15min，取出各管置室温中冷却后于 420nm 波长下比色，以空白管调零点，读取各管吸光度。

【结果处理】

按下式计算：

血清甘油三酯（mmol/L）＝（测定管吸光度/标准管吸光度）×2.26

【注意事项】

1. 黄疸及溶血标本对实验基本无影响，抗凝剂肝素，$Na_2 - EDTA$ 和草酸钠均无干扰，但枸橼酸在正常浓度会使结果偏低。

2. 吸光度高于 0.7 者，应用空白液稀释后比色或将血清减半操作。

【方法评价】

此法颜色稳定，显色后 1h 内色泽无明显变化。近年发展的酶试剂法测定血清总胆固醇、甘油三酯具有简便、快速、微量和精密等优点，为发展的必然趋势，但需专门的酶试剂盒。

【思考题】

1. 几种脂蛋白与动脉粥样硬化和冠心病之间的关系是什么？
2. 如何控制血清总胆固醇和甘油三酯测定过程中的影响因素？

四、抗高血压药物实验

抗高血压药物的临床前药效学研究一般分三个阶段：①在麻醉动物身上观察急性降压作用，常用猫、大鼠和犬等动物。观察药物对高血压动物的急性降压作用。②进行高血压动物的慢性实验性治疗，常用肾性高血压大鼠、自发性高血压大鼠、DOCA 盐型高血压大鼠等。③对有希望的药物进一步研究其降压作用机制。

判断药物的抗高血压作用主要靠实验性治疗，但这需要较长时间。动物高血压模型建成后，连续给药 1~2 周，最长 1 个月，如 1 个月不显效，一般就无效。停药后观察血压恢复到给药前水平为止。由于抗高血压大多长期给药，因此要求口服有效。

血压测定的方法包括直接测压法和间接测压法。直接测压法又称插管法，主要是将心导管或聚乙烯塑料管插入动脉中，以测定血压的变化，也可用动脉穿刺法直接测定血压。插管手术往往需要在全麻或局麻下进行，带有创伤性质，导管中的血液压力通过液体传递到压力感受器，能精确测定血压数值和反应波形变化，此法主要用于急性实验，若进行慢性实验，则需插慢性导管，技术要求较高，对导管质量有一定要求。每天要冲以肝素生理盐水，以保持导管通畅。因此在研究实验性高血压的病理生理过程或药物筛选时，往往采用非创伤性、可重复测定血压的间接测压法。间接测压法主要用充气加压法压迫某一动脉，使血流中断，然后减压，以容积改变或脉搏搏动出现为指标，来测定血压值。该法有大鼠尾容积测压法、大鼠尾脉搏测压法、大鼠脚测压法、犬颈动脉皮鞘法、兔耳测压法等。

1934 年 Goldblatt 等证实狭窄犬肾动脉可产生持续性高血压，开创了实验性高血压研究的新阶段。实验性高血压动物模型，如神经源型、肾型、内分泌型、饮食型等，都要经过一定的手术、药物或其他附加因素处理，与人类高血压病的临床不完全一致，但是对于筛选有效降压药及研究高血压发病机制，仍是十分重要的手段。常用动物为犬和大鼠，猴、猫来源不易，家兔血压升高不够显著，且不稳定，故应用较少。

1955 年 Smirk 报道一种血压自发升高的遗传性高血压大鼠，之后在日本和美国陆续培育出各种遗传性高血压大鼠模型，以自发性高血压大鼠（spontaneously hypertensive rat strain，SHR）、易卒中自发性高血压大鼠（SHR – stroke proce strain，SHRSP）、Dahl 盐敏感大鼠（Dahl salt – sensitive stain，DS）、米兰种高血压大鼠（Milan hypertensive strain，MHS）应用为多，特别是 SHR 和 SHRSP 已在世界各地被广泛应用，其特点如下。

1. SHR 与人类高血压病十分类似，是研究高血压病发病机理和筛选降压药物较为理想的动物模型，相似之处表现为：①遗传因素占重要地位，红细胞等细胞膜离子转运正常；②在高血压早期无明显器质性改变；③病程相似，血压随年龄增加而加剧，6 个月鼠龄时上升到最高水平；④血流动力学改变的特征一致，血管总外周阻力明显升高；⑤随着疾病发展可出现心血管病损如心脑肾合并症，用降压药物等治疗措施可预防或减轻病变的进展和合并症的发生；⑥应激和摄取过量盐等环境因素能加速高血压的发展及加重合并症。

2. SHR 与人类高血压病也有不少差异，如：①它主要通过遗传学上选择性繁殖而得，与高血压病的发生有一定的差异；②甲状腺和免疫功能存在异常。故将 SHR 研究结果推论到人类高血压时应谨慎，但 SHR 与 SHRSP 仍是目前研究高血压病的发病机理和寻找防治措施的最理想的动物模型。

抗高血压药物可作用于中枢神经系统、自主神经节、交感神经末梢、交感神经递质受体、血管平滑肌和体液调节因素及血容量等。作用于神经节的降压药因其不良反应大多已被淘汰，作用于交感神经末梢的药物也用得越来越少，作用于血管平滑肌、交感神经递质受体和体液调节因素的抗高血压药是药物开发的主要方向，如钙拮抗药、α 受体阻断药、β 受体阻断药及血管紧张素转换酶抑制剂等。根据抗高血压药作用的机理不同而设计了不同的实验方法，反过来通过相应方法的实验就可推断药物的作用机理。

实验 5.15 六烃季铵降压作用机制的分析

【目的】

学习抗高血压药急性降压实验方法，分析六烃季铵的降压作用机制。

【原理】

交感、副交感神经中的传出神经纤维要经过神经节换元至节后神经才能到达效应器起作用，两种神经节前纤维均释放乙酰胆碱。交感、副交感神经的节后神经末梢分别释放去甲肾上腺素和乙酰胆碱，兴奋心脏和血管的相应受体而引起血压的变化，外周血管的舒缩以交感神经调节为主，神经节阻断剂阻断神经节中的神经冲动传递而产生药理作用。根据用药后能否阻断刺激交感、副交感神经节前纤维及直接使用神经递质引起的血压变化，可推测该药是否阻断神经节。

【材料】

兔 1 只，2 ~ 3kg，雌雄不限。

药理生理多用仪、兔手术台、手术器械、测压装置、动脉插管、动脉夹、小儿头皮针、刺激电极、注射器等。

2.5% 溴化六烃季铵、20% 乌拉坦、0.01% 重酒石酸去甲肾上腺素、0.001% 氯化乙酰胆碱、0.2% 肝素（或 5% 枸橼酸钠）、生理盐水。

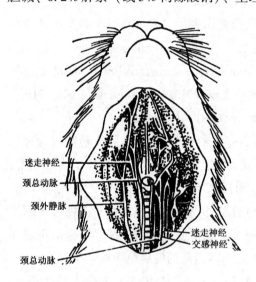

图 5 - 5 兔颈部解剖图

【方法与步骤】

1. 取兔 1 只，称体重，耳缘静脉缓慢注射 20% 乌拉坦（1g/kg）麻醉。

2. 麻醉后，将兔背位固定于手术台上，剪去颈部被毛，正中切开颈部皮肤，在胸锁乳突肌与气管之间分离出左右颈总动脉及右侧迷走神经，于右侧颈总动脉下穿一线用于阻断血流，于右侧迷走神经下穿二线靠近头端结扎，保留近心端迷走神经结扎线，以备电刺激时提起（图 5 - 5）。

3. 将充满抗凝剂的动脉插管插入左颈总动脉，与测压装置相连，以便记录血压。

4. 自一侧耳缘静脉插入充有生理盐水的小儿头皮针，用胶布固定，以备注射给药。

5. 待血压平稳后，描记一段正常血压曲线，然后按下列顺序进行实验。

（1）阻断右侧颈总动脉血流 15s，观察血压的变化。

（2）电刺激迷走神经近心端，找出引起血压反应的最低刺激强度，观察刺激引起的血压变化。电刺激参数：方波 8Hz、波宽 2ms、120% 阈电压（3 ~ 4V），刺激 15s。

（3）静脉注射 0.01% 重酒石酸去甲肾上腺素（10μg/kg），观察血压变化。

（4）静脉注射 0.001% 氯化乙酰胆碱（1μg/kg），观察血压变化。

（5）静脉注射 2.5% 溴化六烃季铵（0.1mg/kg），观察血压变化。

（6）待血压降至最低点后，迅速重复上述（1）、（2）、（3）、（4），观察血压变化。

【结果处理】

测量、计算血压变化的数值，根据实验步骤所用药物及刺激等对应记录，并分析实验结果。

【注意事项】

1. 麻醉不可过深，以免血压过度下降。

2. 注意动脉插管和静脉头皮针内不要凝血。

3. 分离迷走神经时注意不要损伤神经，实验中要使其保持湿润。

【方法评价】

兔来源容易，动物温顺，体形大小适中，适合于一般实验及进行基本操作训练。由于兔血压不够稳定，在进行降压药筛选时一般不选用它，而多选猫、犬和大鼠等动物。猫的瞬膜受颈上交感神经节后纤维支配，故也可观察瞬膜的收缩反应来了解药物对交感神经节的阻断作用。

【思考题】

1. 实验中各步骤引起血压变化的作用机制如何？

2. 如何解释六烃季铵对各实验步骤改变血压的影响？

3. 如将六烃季铵改成中枢性降压药将可能产生什么样的结果？

实验 5.16　离体兔耳血管灌流

【目的】

学习离体兔耳血管灌流法，观察药物对离体血管平滑肌的作用。

【原理】

根据血管阻力（R）与灌注压（P）成正比，与流量（Q）成反比，即 $R \propto P/Q$ 的原理，将兔耳与身体血液循环隔断后，以恒定的压力从耳动脉近心端灌入充氧、恒温的洛氏液，灌流液经耳血管灌流后从耳静脉流出。若给药后流量减少，表明阻力增大，血管收缩。观察给药前后灌流量的变化，即可反映药物对血管的作用。

【材料】

家兔1只，体重2~3kg，雌雄不限。

循环恒温水浴装置、手术器械、混合气体（95%氧气、5%二氧化碳）供气装置、兔耳动脉插管、注射器、量筒、烧杯、兔耳固定装置。

洛氏液［成分：NaCl 9.2g/L、KCl 0.42g/L、CaCl$_2$ 0.24g/L、NaHCO$_3$ 0.15g/L、葡萄糖1.0g/L］，20%乌拉坦，10^{-5}、8×10^{-5} 异丙肾上腺素。

【方法与步骤】

1. 取兔1只，称体重。股静脉缓慢注射20%乌拉坦（1~1.2g/kg）麻醉，腹位固定，剪去耳根部毛。

2. 在耳根部背面顺血管走向切开皮肤约2cm，在中央静脉下面和耳大神经间找到并分离耳后动脉，该动脉与静脉平行，但位置较深，不易触到搏动，在动脉下方预置2根丝线。

操作时，可用手术灯隔着兔耳透视，帮助确定血管位置。

3. 结扎动脉的近心端，向远心端插入动脉插管，用较快的速度向动脉内推注充氧的洛氏液，冲去血管内的血液，使兔耳静脉内呈现无色的营养液。迅速剪下兔耳，继续冲洗血管除去残存的血液，直至静脉流出液体无色。将兔耳用胶泥固定在倾斜呈 45°的玻璃或塑料板上。耳尖在上，耳根在下，以便从静脉中流出的灌流液直接沿板下角流出。动脉插管与输送 37℃的充氧洛氏液乳胶管连接，洛氏液瓶高距兔耳动脉插管口约 60cm 水柱，调节至兔耳灌流液的滴数为 30 ~ 40 滴/分。待流速稳定后，连续记录 3min 的流量，取平均值作为给药前的对照值。

4. 从连接动脉插管的乳胶管处，将待试药物直接缓慢注入灌流液中，观察并记录灌流液的流速变化。每种药物的注射速度和容量应基本相同，速度不宜超过 1ml/min。给药顺序如下：① 8×10^{-5} 异丙肾上腺素 0.5ml（30s 内注完）。② 10^{-5} 去甲肾上腺素 0.5ml（30s 内注完）。

【结果处理】

按表 5 – 3 填入数据，比较实验结果。

表 5 – 3　药物对离体兔耳灌流量的影响

药物	给药量（ml）	灌流液流出速度（ml/min）						
		给药前	给药后					
			1min	2min	3min	5min	10min	15min

血管灌流量减少百分率计算公式如下：

$$血管灌流量减少百分率（\%） = \frac{给药后均值 - 给药前均值}{给药前均值} \times 100\%$$

【注意事项】

1. 实验必须在恒温、恒压下进行。恒压灌流装置中不能有气泡，如发现气泡应随时排除，以免栓塞血管，影响结果。

2. 在剪下兔耳时，必须用灌流液将血管内血液完全冲净，以免在血管内产生凝血。剪断兔耳的剪刀需锋利，做到一剪即断，以免兔挣扎而将插入的插管挣脱或戳破血管。

3. 给药前后的动脉插管和兔耳位置要保持一致，不能移动，以免插管移动引起动脉扭曲等影响灌流速度。

4. 在注入下一种药时，要充分洗去前一种药，使流量尽可能恢复到给药前水平。

5. 实验项目应安排紧凑，尽快完成，以防兔耳出现水肿现象，影响实验结果。

【方法评价】

1. 该方法用于评价药物对血管平滑肌的直接作用，简便易行，能反映药物对中小动脉和静脉的整个血管阻力的影响。

2. 由于离体兔耳无中枢神经控制，血管张力降低，故对缩血管药敏感，对扩血管药的敏感性较差。

3. 离体兔耳血管阻力易受温度、牵拉及插管位置改变的影响，因此要控制好条件，否则结果相差较大。

4. 此法可在短时间内反复注入药液对多种药物进行测试，是观察药物对血管是否具有药理活性的常用方法。

【思考题】

1. 离体兔耳血管灌流法适用哪类药物的实验？

2. 影响离体兔耳血管灌流实验因素是什么？如何控制？

五、利尿药和脱水药实验

利尿药的动物实验方法包括急性实验和慢性实验两大类。前者一般是直接从输尿管或膀胱收集尿液，适用于犬、猫、家兔等较大的动物，实验可在较短时间内完成，受外界环境影响也较小，缺点是动物需在麻醉或手术等非生理状态下进行实验，与清醒动物并不完全相同。若欲在动物清醒状态下进行，可采用输尿管瘘或膀胱瘘法，可避免麻醉对尿液分泌的影响，但实验较复杂，筛选实验较少采用。后者一般是用代谢笼收集小动物尿液数小时，称为"代谢笼实验法"，适用于大鼠、小鼠。为了减少尿液的蒸发和粪便的污染，可用特殊的集尿装置或用滤纸吸尿液加以称重。动物在生理或接近生理状态下进行实验，所得结果较为可靠，缺点是受实验环境影响较大，实验时间较长。

在利尿药筛选实验中常用的动物为大鼠和犬，其次为家兔和小鼠。对人体有利尿作用的药物大多可在大鼠实验中获得较好的利尿效果，因此，受选动物多采用大鼠，必要时用犬做进一步的验证或深入研究。因家兔价廉易得，某些初筛实验也可用家兔代替犬进行。

各种利尿药不仅促进水的排泄，而且也都影响盐类的排泄，因此，利尿指标除观察尿量外，还需分析尿中离子（Na^+、K^+、Cl^-、HCO_3^-）量。通过尿中多种离子的测定还将药物分为若干类，如排钠-保钾利尿药等。至于药物利尿作用机制的研究，尚需配合其他分析方法，例如游离水清除率（free water clearance）实验法可衡量肾脏对尿液浓缩和稀释的能力，分析利尿药对尿浓缩和稀释功能的影响；停流法（stop-blow method）可分析肾小管各段的运转功能，对利尿药作用部位进行初步定位分析：肾小管穿刺（micropuncture）技术则可对利尿药的作用部位作出更精确、更直接的定位。

实验 5.17 呋塞米和高渗葡萄糖对家兔的利尿作用

【目的】

了解急性利尿实验的方法，观察呋塞米和高渗葡萄糖对麻醉兔的利尿作用。

【原理】

呋塞米属高效利尿药，又称呋喃苯胺酸、速尿，主要作用于髓袢升支粗段的上皮细胞，抑制此段管腔膜上 $Na^+ - K^+ - 2Cl^-$ 同向转运系统。抑制 Cl^- 的主动转运，Na^+ 的重吸收也随之减少，导致管腔内 Na^+、Cl^- 浓度增高，降低肾对尿液的稀释功能。同时，由于从髓袢升支重吸收到髓质间液 Na^+、Cl^- 的量减少，影响其高渗透压状态的形成，使肾浓缩尿的功能降低。肾小管对 Na^+、Cl^- 重吸收减少，Mg^{2+}、Ca^{2+} 等二价阳离子重吸收也减少，由于大量 Na^+ 转运到远曲小管和集合管，促进 $Na^+ - K^+$ 交换，故 K^+ 排出也增多，而 Cl^- 不受离子交换影响，因而尿中 Cl^- 多于 Na^+。因此，呋塞米通过排出大量的电解质和水分而产生强大的利尿作用。高渗葡萄糖为渗透性利尿药，近曲小管对葡萄糖的重吸收是有一定的限度的，该限度即肾糖阈，当一次大量静脉注射 50% 葡萄糖溶液，超过其重吸收的极限时，便可在管腔液中形成高渗透压，多余的葡萄糖随尿排出，同时带走大量的水分，产生利尿作用。因部分葡萄糖可从血管中扩散到组织中，且易被代谢利用，故作用弱而短。通过收集给药前后的尿量，计算单位时间内尿量增加毫升数，可分析各药的起效时间、作用强度及作用维持时间。

【材料】

家兔 1 只，体重 2~3kg，雌雄不限。

兔箱、兔手术台、兔开口器、导尿管（灌胃用）、婴儿秤、量筒、烧杯、注射器、聚乙烯管、手术刀、组织剪、眼科剪、血管钳。

20% 乌拉坦溶液、1% 呋塞米溶液、50% 葡萄糖注射液、生理盐水。

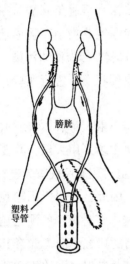

图 5-6　急性利尿实验插管及尿液收集示意图

【方法与步骤】

1. **给予水负荷**　取家兔 1 只，称重后置于兔箱中，灌胃给温水 40ml/kg。

2. **麻醉**　20min 后，耳缘静脉注射 20% 乌拉坦溶液 1.0g/kg。

3. **手术**　待动物麻醉后背位固定于兔手术台上，剪去下腹部毛，于耻骨联合上方切开皮肤 4~5cm，沿腹白线剪开腹壁及腹膜，暴露膀胱，在膀胱底两侧找出输尿管，稍加分离后在输尿管下各穿两根线，一线结扎近膀胱端，在结扎线上方用眼科剪朝肾脏方向剪一小口插入聚乙烯导管，用另一线结扎固定。将两根导管的游离端一并放入量筒内，收集记录正常尿量（ml/5min），见图 5-6。

4. **给药**　自耳缘静脉注射 50% 葡萄糖（2.5g/kg），每隔 5min 收集并记录一次尿量，连续 6 次。给予生理盐水以补充排出的尿量，待尿量恢复正常后，再静脉给予 1% 呋塞米（4mg/kg），同样每隔 5min 收集并记录一次尿量，连续 6 次。

5. **计算单位时间内尿量增加毫升数**　单位时间内尿量增加毫升数 = 给药后单位时间内尿量毫升数 - 给药前单位时间内尿量毫升数。

【结果处理】

1. 报告实验动物的种类、性别、体重、给水负荷经过及所给药物的名称、剂量和途径。

2. 收集全实验室数据，计算各单位时间内尿量增加毫升数的均数（x）和标准差（SD），以尿量增加毫升数为纵坐标，给药后不同时间为横坐标作直方图，比较呋塞米和高渗葡萄糖的作用高峰时间和作用持续时间。

【注意事项】

1. 乌拉坦静脉麻醉时需缓慢推注，边注射边观察角膜反射、呼吸和肌肉松弛情况。

2. 沿腹白线打开腹腔时，应小心，切勿损伤腹腔脏器；分离两侧输尿管时应注意避开血管进行钝性分离。

3. 家兔的输尿管较纤细脆弱，插管时动作应细致轻巧，切忌将输尿管插穿。

4. 静注高渗葡萄糖和呋塞米溶液后，一般在 1~2min 和 3min 即发挥利尿作用，如届时无尿滴出，应检查导管内是否凝血或输尿管扭曲。

5. 须等前一药物作用基本消失，尿量恢复正常后方可注入后一药物。

6. 实验过程中，应用温生理盐水纱布覆盖手术野，以保持动物腹腔温、湿度。

【方法评价】

输尿管插管法是较为理想的急性利尿实验方法之一，实验可在较短时间内完成，成功的把握性较大，受外界环境影响较小，与膀胱中余尿的量无关，结果较准确，但动物是处于麻醉状态下，与清醒动物的机体状况有所不同。与该法相类似的还有膀胱插管法，该法动物麻醉、固定、开腹方法同前，找到膀胱后，将膀胱顶上翻暴露膀胱腹面，在腹侧面避开血管作一荷包缝合，在荷包中间剪一小口，插入膀胱套管（套管内预先充满水，排掉空气），套管漏斗口需对准两输尿管，收紧荷包即可。

欲进行清醒动物的利尿实验，可采用膀胱造瘘法，即预先给动物进行膀胱造瘘手术。2周后切口愈合，再将动物固定于特殊支架上收集尿液进行实验。该法可避免麻醉药物的干扰，但实验过程较繁杂。

此外，也常采用导尿法，此法简便并可避免实验动物的手术创伤，但雌性动物易误插到子宫腔内而造成实验失败。现将其方法简要介绍如下：通常选用雄性动物，先将导尿管尖端用液状石蜡润滑，再自尿道轻而慢地插入，导尿管通过膀胱括约肌进入膀胱后即有尿液滴出，再插入 1~2cm 即可。插入总深度视动物大小而定，一般家兔 8~12cm，犬 22~26cm。最后用胶布将导尿管与动物体固定，最初 5min 滴出的尿液弃去不计，待滴数稳定后，在导尿管下接一量筒，开始收集和记录尿量。

观察尿量的方法除计毫升数外，还可连接记滴器，记录单位时间内尿液滴数。

【思考题】

1. 利尿药和脱水药的定义各是什么？本实验中能否看出两者的区别？如不能则还应补充什么实验？

2. 本实验设计的给药顺序是先给葡萄糖后给呋塞米，如果反之先给呋塞米后给葡萄糖，是否合理？为什么？

实验 5.18　氢氯噻嗪对大鼠的利尿作用

【目的】

了解慢性利尿实验方法，观察氢氯噻嗪对大鼠尿量的影响。

【原理】

氢氯噻嗪属中效利尿药，利尿的作用部位是远曲小管的前部，抑制远曲小管开始部分 Na^+-Cl^- 同向转运系统而减少对 Na^+、Cl^- 重吸收，故噻嗪类利尿药也称 Na^+-Cl^- 抑制剂。抑制 Cl^- 的主动转运使 Na^+ 的重吸收相应减少，致使管腔内渗透压增加，大量 NaCl 带着水分排出体外。因排出 Na^+ 和 Cl^- 几乎相等，故其对体液的酸碱平衡影响不大，只是排出 K^+ 较多是其缺点。

本实验采用腹腔给药后代谢笼收集尿液的慢性利尿实验方法，通过与对照组比较，观察药物的利尿作用。

【材料】

大鼠2只，180～220g，雄性。

大鼠代谢笼、大鼠灌胃器、天平、量筒、注射器。

0.5%氢氯噻嗪溶液、生理盐水。

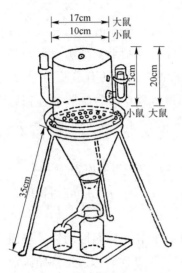

图5-7 代谢笼集尿装置

【方法与步骤】

1. **代谢笼集尿装置** 主要由圆形的笼罩、带孔的原形底盘，供饮水和摄食的装置，锥形集尿漏斗和粪尿分离器组成。粪尿分离器的侧口接一只150～200ml的量筒或烧杯收集尿液（图5-7）。动物置于圆形底盘之上，排便时可通过笼子底部的大小便分离器，将尿液与粪便分开，达到聚集尿液的目的。

2. **给予水负荷** 两鼠称重后，分别灌胃生理盐水（5ml/100g）

3. **给药** 给水负荷后30min给药，给药前先挤压大鼠下腹部，使膀胱排空。实验鼠腹腔给予0.5%氢氯噻嗪（25mg/kg），对照鼠腹腔给予生理盐水（5ml/kg）。

4. **收集尿液** 给药完毕，将大鼠分别放入两个代谢笼，记录时间，开始收集尿液，每隔30min测量一次各鼠排泄的尿量，直至给药后120min。

【结果处理】

1. 报告实验动物的种类、性别、体重、给水负荷经过及所给药物的名称、剂量和途径。

2. 收集全实验室数据，计算两组大鼠单位时间内尿量的平均值及其标准差，并用 t 检验进行组间显著性检验，将结果填入表5-4。

表5-4 氢氯噻嗪对大鼠尿量的影响

分组	大鼠编号	体重（g）	给药（mg/kg）	给药后不同时间的尿量（ml）				$\bar{x} \pm SD$
				0～30min	30～60min	60～90min	90～120min	
生理盐水组	1							
	2							
	3							
	4							
	5							
	..							
氢氯噻嗪组	1							
	2							
	3							
	4							
	5							
	..							

3. 将对照组尿量作为100，算出给药组的尿量增加百分率，以此值作为纵坐标，给药后时间为横坐标，作图表示不同时间下利尿作用的强度（图5-8）。

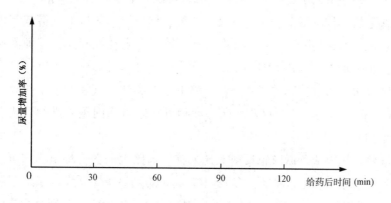

图5-8 氢氯噻嗪对大鼠的利尿作用

【注意事项】

1. 代谢笼集尿装置须保证粪尿分开，防止粪便污染尿液。此装置除支架外，均用玻璃或有机玻璃制成，便于清洗，尤其是须分析尿中金属离子时，更应避免用金属材料的代谢笼。

2. 未经水负荷的正常大鼠体液量较少，在强利尿剂作用下，容易出现脱水现象，而不能正常显示所示药物的作用。同时，由于排尿量也很少（每小时约0.5ml/100g），加上操作中的损失、尿液的蒸发、各鼠膀胱的排空不一致等，可造成较大的误差。所以实验时应先给予动物水负荷。以5%葡萄糖生理盐水作水负荷利尿效果较好。

3. 每次收集尿液前，须用手轻压大鼠下腹部，以排空膀胱的余尿。

4. 为了减少个体差异，应选用体重相近（200g左右为宜）、性别相同（雄性首选）的大鼠。实验前应使动物适应代谢笼的生活环境1～2日，观察自由饮水条件下的尿量是否稳定，再用生理盐水（2.5ml/100g）灌胃，2h内收集的尿量能达到灌入量40%以上的动物为理想的实验动物。

5. 一只大鼠尿量过少时，可将同一组2只或者3只大鼠置于同一代谢笼内。

【方法评价】

代谢笼集尿法适用于小动物（如小鼠、大鼠）的慢性利尿实验，可连续收集数小时、数天或某特定时间内的尿液，操作简便、安全，动物在生理状态下进行实验，结果可靠，但受实验环境（气温、温度）的影响较大，应尽量加以控制，室温以20℃左右为宜。

【思考题】

1. 利尿药分强效、中效和弱效三类，在临床应用中有何异同？

2. 呋塞米和氢氯噻嗪的不良反应有何异同？

六、镇咳药、祛痰药和平喘药实验

镇咳、祛痰和平喘药是支气管炎症和哮喘的对症治疗用药，其应用极其广泛。

（一）镇咳药

镇咳药分为中枢性镇咳药与末梢性镇咳药两大类。前者直接抑制延脑的咳嗽中枢，后者抑制咳嗽反射弧（咳嗽反射弧由感受器、传入神经、咳嗽中枢、传出神经和效应器五个环节组成）中的感受器或外周神经的某一环节而产生镇咳作用。引咳物不同，所致咳嗽的类型也不相同。最常用的是化学物质刺激、机械刺激和电刺激引咳实验。

1. **化学刺激法**　常用氨水、二氧化硫、硫酸、枸橼酸、醋酸的气雾或气体刺激呼吸道上皮下的感受器，引发咳嗽。本法引起的咳嗽比较接近生理性咳嗽，且刺激强度可以初步定量，缺点是同一动物不能在短时间内反复利用。

2. **机械刺激法**　通过特制的气管插管，将羽毛之类插入气管并上下拉动，可以引发咳嗽。本法简单易行，不需特殊的仪器，同一动物可在短时间内重复进行，缺点是刺激强度不易控制，无法进行定量比较。

3. **电刺激法**　用电流刺激咳嗽反射弧传入神经通路上的任何环节，均可引起咳嗽。常用的刺激部位有两处。①喉上神经：多采用猫或豚鼠；②气管黏膜：多采用豚鼠或犬。本法可在短时间内连续使用，不致"钝化"，且刺激强度可准确定量，通过测定电流的引咳阈值以评价药物的镇咳作用。如果需判断药物的镇咳作用是否属于中枢性的，可直接刺激延髓的咳嗽中枢。

在动物方面，以猫的咳嗽反射最为敏感，但猫价格较贵。豚鼠对化学刺激或机械刺激都很敏感，刺激其喉上神经亦能引起咳嗽，且一般实验室较易得到。因此，豚鼠是筛选镇咳药常用的动物。家兔对化学刺激或电刺激不敏感，很少使用。小鼠和大鼠用化学刺激也能诱发咳嗽。通常先用小鼠、大鼠或豚鼠进行初筛，然后再用猫或犬进行复筛与作用机制分析。

麻醉药能抑制咳嗽发射，影响实验结果。如果实验需要麻醉，最好选择长效的乌拉坦与氯醛酸（α-chloralose）以保证实验过程中条件的相对稳定，避免使用吸入麻醉药。

（二）祛痰药

祛痰药可通过各种方式，使呼吸道的分泌量增多，黏着于呼吸道黏膜的痰液变稀、液化而易于咳出。筛选祛痰药有直接收集气管分泌液法和测定气管的酚红排泌量法。此外，呼吸道黏膜纤毛运动对于排痰也有重要作用，因此观察纤毛运动也有助于祛痰药的研究和评价。

1. **接收集气管分泌液法**　最好用猫、犬等大动物进行。也可将大鼠进行浅麻醉，取细玻管插入气管内，使分泌液通过毛细管作用进入玻管，从收集的液体量来判断药物的祛痰作用。

2. **酚红排泌量测定法**　此法简单易行，缺点是不够精确，仅能用于初筛。

（三）平喘药

支气管平滑肌痉挛是引起哮喘的直接原因，因此，多数平喘药都作用于支气管，使平滑肌松弛。支气管平滑肌对药物反应有明显的种属差异，其中以豚鼠最为敏感，也最常用。实验可用离体气管，也可用整体动物。

1. **离体气管实验**　常用的有气管容积法、气管链法、支气管灌流法等。离体实验能直接观察药物对气管平滑肌的作用，但有其局限性，适用于初筛。

2. **整体动物实验**　给动物喷入组胺、乙酰胆碱等过敏递质的气雾，引起哮喘发作，以观察药物的保护作用。整体动物较能反映药物在临床条件的平喘作用。

由于哮喘是变态反应的一种表现，因此研究平喘药时尚需结合使用一些免疫学的实验方法。

实验 5.19 可待因对小鼠氨水引咳的镇咳作用

【目的】

学习用小鼠氨水喷雾引咳法试验药物的镇咳作用，观察可待因的镇咳作用。

【原理】

氨水为具有刺激性的化学物质，通过空气压缩机连接玻璃喷雾头，均匀地将浓氨水喷入密闭容器中，小鼠吸入氨水气雾后即可引起咳嗽。可通过计数单位时间内小鼠的咳嗽次数来分析药物的镇咳作用。

【材料】

小鼠 2 只，体重 18 ~ 22g，雌雄不限。

玻璃喷雾瓶、空气压缩机、水银检压计、玻璃三通管、秒表、注射器、玻璃钟罩（容积为 500ml）、小儿听诊器。

0.2% 磷酸可待因溶液、生理盐水、浓氨水（25% ~ 27% 氢氧化铵溶液）。

【方法与步骤】

1. 取小鼠 2 只，称重标记后置于钟罩内，观察它们的正常活动和呼吸特点。一鼠腹腔注射 0.2% 磷酸可待因（40mg/kg），另一鼠腹腔注射生理盐水（40mg/kg），以作对照。

2. 给药后 20min，将两鼠分别放入玻璃钟罩内。使空气压缩机输出管连接玻璃三通管（图 5 - 9），将气压调到 27kPa 左右。打开通向喷雾瓶的活塞，将氨水的气雾均匀地喷入玻璃钟罩内，喷雾 10s，让小鼠在钟罩内停留 2min，而后从钟罩内取出。

3. 将小鼠取出后立即置入另一钟罩内，用小儿听诊器从钟罩口上察听小鼠的咳嗽声。记录各鼠的咳嗽潜伏期（从开始喷雾到发出第一声咳嗽的时间）和 3 分钟内的咳嗽总次数。

【结果处理】

汇总全实验室结果，分别计算各组动物 3min 内咳嗽次数的平均值及标准差（$\bar{x} \pm s$），并进行组间显著性 t 检验，将结果填入表 5 - 5。

【注意事项】

1. 无特制的玻璃喷雾瓶，可用喷色层分析显色剂的瓶子代替。如无空气压缩机或喷雾装置，也可用其他简易装置代替。比如自制一水浴蒸发装置，用 1ml 浓氨水于沸水浴上蒸发，让氨水蒸气刺激小鼠 45s，而后取出观察。

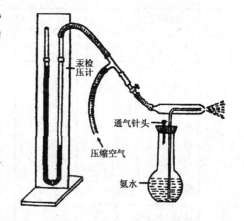

图 5 - 9 氨水引咳喷雾装置

表 5 - 5 可待因对小鼠氨水引咳的镇咳作用

小鼠编号	体重（g）	药物和剂量（mg/kg）	咳嗽潜伏期（分）	3min 内咳嗽次数

2. 若无小儿听诊器也可用肉眼观察，小鼠咳嗽时表现为腹肌收缩，同时张大嘴，观察必须细致。

3. 如需定量评价药物的镇咳作用，可以 EDT_{50}（半数小鼠喷雾致咳时间）的延长程度为指标，即逐一测定每只小鼠喷雾致咳时间，然后用序贯法（上下法）算出全组动物的 EDT_{50}。

【思考题】

常用的咳嗽模型有哪几种？各有何优缺点？

【附】 EDT_{50} 的测定：实验前预先准备好表格（表 5-6），并拟定一系列等比级数安排的喷雾时间（时间的对数间距一般采用 0.7 ~ 0.8）。相邻两个时刻的对数之差在一次实验中是固定的。

喷雾引咳装置及引咳方法同前。实验时，当前 1 只小鼠出现咳嗽反应（1min 内出现 3 次以上典型咳嗽者，算作"有咳嗽"），则后一只就用低一级的时间喷雾；相反，若前一只未出现咳嗽反应，则下一只就用高一级的时间喷雾，即按序贯法（上下法）改变喷雾时间，依次对每只小鼠进行观察，每组（给药组及对照组）均以 10 ~ 20 只小鼠为宜。测定完毕按照表中的方法求出各组的 EDT_{50}。再按下列公式算出 R 值。

$$R = \frac{给药组的\ EDT_{50}}{对照组的\ EDT_{50}} \times 100\%$$

$R > 130\%$ 判为有镇咳作用，$R > 150\%$ 则判为有明显的镇咳作用。

表 5-6　测定镇咳药的 EDT_{50} 序贯法

组别	时间 秒	lg (x)	动物 1	2	3	4	5	6	7	8	9	10	11	12	r	rx	计算
对照组	15.9	1.2															
	20.0	1.3		−											1	1.3	$n = 12\ c = \sum rx = 17.4$
	25.1	1.4	+	−		−			−		−				Z	7.0	$EDT_{50} = lg^{-1}\ (c/n)$
	31.6	1.5			+		−		+		+		+		5	7.5	$= lg^{-1}\ (17.4/12) = 28.2$
	39.8	1.6					+								1	1.6	(s)
		1.7													12		
	50.1														合计	17.4	
															↑ n	↑ c	
可待因组	20.0	1.3															
	25.1	1.4													2	3.0	$n = 12\ c = \sum rx = 19.4$
	31.6	1.5		−				−							6	9.6	$EDT_{50} = lg^{-1}\ (c/n)$
	39.8	1.6	+	−		−	+	−		−					Z	6.8	$= lg^{-1}\ (19.4/12) = 41.4$
	50.1	1.7			+		+				+		+		4		(s)
		1.8													12		
	63.1														合计	19.4	
															↑ n	↑ c	

注："+" ——咳嗽；"−" ——不咳嗽；"x" ——时间的对数；"r" ——每喷雾时间组反应动物的总和（阴性、阳性反应均包括）对照组的 EDT_{50} 一般在 25 ~ 25s

本例的 $R = \dfrac{41.4}{28.2} \times 100\% = 147\%$　结论：可待因具有镇咳作用。

实验 5.20　可待因对电刺激猫喉上神经引咳的镇咳作用

【目的】

学习用电刺激猫喉上神经引咳法试验药物镇咳作用的方法，观察可待因的镇咳作用。

【原理】

喉部的感觉神经末梢由喉上神经所支配，喉上神经是咳嗽反射弧中的重要传入神经之一。用电流刺激喉上神经可引起咳嗽，且通过测定电流的引咳阈值，可以定量评价药物的镇咳作用。

【材料】

猫 1 只，体重 2kg 左右，雌雄不限。

手术台、粗剪、手术剪、手术刀、止血钳、张力换能器、生理信号采集记录系统、药理生理实验多用仪、秒表、保护电极、静脉输液装置、纱布、棉花、丝线、缝针、注射器。

0.3% 磷酸可待因溶液、3% 戊巴比妥钠溶液、液状石蜡。

【方法与步骤】

1. **麻醉**　取猫 1 只，称重后腹腔注射 3% 戊巴比妥钠（30mg/kg）。

2. **手术**　麻醉后，将猫背位固定于手术台上，剪去颈毛，沿颈正中线切开皮肤，分离皮下组织，暴露出甲状软骨，在其附近分离出一侧迷走神经。沿迷走神经向头端分离至膨大处，此即迷走神经结状节。于该处可见神经节分出一分支斜向甲状软骨方向，与肌纤维的走向近似垂直，此即喉上神经（图 5–10）。仔细游离该神经，挂上保护电极。为了避免神经干燥，并保证神经与电极良好接触，在神经与电极的接触部位滴上少量液状石蜡。用湿纱布覆盖手术野。

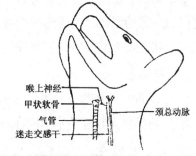

图 5–10　猫的喉上神经（左侧）位置示意图

在上腹部剑突下方皮肤上缝一丝线，丝线的另一端与肌张力换能器连接，后者又与生理信号采集记录系统相连。猫咳嗽时，由于膈肌收缩牵动腹壁，记录仪上可描记出咳嗽的次数和幅度。

再分离出一侧股静脉，插入静脉输液装置，以备给药。

3. **测试引咳阈值**　手术完毕，开始刺激喉上神经，找出引起咳嗽的阈值。将药理生理实验多用仪的刺激方式调至"连续 B"、频率 10Hz、波宽 10ms、刺激时间 5s，两次刺激之间相隔 5min。电压强度从 0.5V 起逐步递增直至出现咳嗽，一般不超过 5V。此引起咳嗽的最小电压值即为该动物的引咳阈值。连测 3 次，取其平均数作为给药前的对照值。

4. **给药**　由股静脉注入 0.3% 磷酸可待因（3mg/kg）。用药后每隔 5min 按原阈值刺激喉上神经一次，观察咳嗽次数和强度的变化。若无咳嗽，则逐步加大电压直至出现咳嗽，找出给药后的引咳阈值。记录磷酸可待因的起效时间、阈值提高最大倍数及其维持时间。

【结果处理】

按表 5 –7 做好记录。

表 5 –7　可待因对电刺激猫喉上神经引咳的镇咳作用

动物编号	药物及剂量	给药前引咳阈值（V）				给药后引咳阈值（V）					
		第1次	第2次	第3次	平均	15min	30min	45min	60min	90min	120min

【注意事项】

1. 麻醉的深度对引咳效果影响很大，麻醉过深能明显抑制咳嗽反应。有条件时最好采用氯醛糖进行麻醉（氯醛糖以丙烯甘油溶解，按 80mg/kg 腹腔注射），该药对咳嗽反射几无影响。实验过程中，若需补加麻醉药，应待动物稳定后再重新测定阈值。

2. 猫难以得到时，也可用豚鼠代替。腹腔注射乌拉坦 1g/kg 使之麻醉。切开颈部皮肤，分离出迷走神经，将其剪断，刺激向中端，可引发咳嗽。

3. 本实验除用磷酸可待因作为阳性药外，也可用盐酸吗啡和枸橼酸咳必清进行实验，前者为 0.6mg/kg 静脉注射，后者为 10mg/kg 静脉注射。

【方法评价】

猫电刺激引咳法，目前最常用的是电刺激喉上神经引咳。用一定的刺激频率和刺激强度可引起可靠的咳嗽，用药前后可进行定量的比较，方法准确可靠是寻找镇咳药的重要方法之一。缺点是咳嗽性质与生理性咳嗽有所差异，手术需要一定的条件和技能。

【思考题】

1. 镇咳药有哪些筛选方法？常选用什么动物？各种方法分别具有哪些优缺点？

2. 实验操作尤其是手术中应注意哪些问题？

实验 5.21　远志煎剂对小鼠气管酚红排泌量的影响

【目的】

学习用酚红呼吸道排泌试验筛试祛痰药的方法，观察远志煎剂对小鼠呼吸道酚红排泌量的影响。

【原理】

指示剂酚红给小鼠腹腔注射后，可部分地由支气管排泌。有祛痰作用的药物在使支气管分泌液增加的同时，也使呼吸道黏膜的酚红排泌量增加，因而可从供试品对气管内酚红排泌量的影响来间接推断药物的祛痰作用。酚红在碱性溶液中呈红色，用碳酸氢钠溶液将呼吸道内的酚红洗出后，可通过比色法来定量。

【材料】

小鼠 2 只，体重 24 ~ 28g，雌雄不限。

注射器、小鼠灌胃器、手术剪、眼科镊、小试管、721 分光光度计、大头针、棉线。

100% 远志煎剂（取远志切片 200g，加乙醇 300ml，水浴回流 2h，冷却后过滤，滤液蒸去乙醇，加蒸馏水至 200ml 即得）生理盐水、5% 碳酸氢钠溶液、0.25% 酚红溶液（准确称取酚红 0.25g，用 1mol/L 氢氧化钠溶液 2.5ml 溶解，加生理盐水至 100ml，摇匀即得）。

【方法与步骤】

1. 取小鼠 2 只，称重后标记。实验前禁食 8 ~ 12h。一只用 100% 远志煎剂灌胃，每公斤体重给药剂量相当于 25g 生药材，另一只给同量生理盐水。

2. 30min 后，每只小鼠腹腔注射 0.25% 酚红溶液 0.25ml。再隔 30min，将小鼠脱颈椎处死。将小鼠仰卧位用大头针固定于木板上，将颈部拉直，切开颈正中皮肤，分离出气管，在气管下穿一线，以备固定针头。

3. 用 1ml 注射器抽取 5% 碳酸氢钠溶液 0.5ml，接上磨钝的 7 号针头，从甲状软骨处插入气管内 0.3 ~ 0.5cm，用线结扎固定，避免针头滑脱。来回抽洗 3 次，取下注射器，将冲洗液注入小试管内，重新吸取 5% 碳酸氢钠溶液 0.5ml，按上法抽洗，重复 2 次。将 3 次冲洗液混合后，在 721 分光光度计上于波长 558nm 处比色。

【结果处理】

收集全班实验数据，分别算出给药组和对照组的平均数和标准差，并进行组间显著性 t 检验，将结果填入表 5 – 8。

表 5 – 8　远志煎剂对小鼠气管酚红排泌量的影响

分组	鼠号	体重	剂量	A 值	显著性 t 检验
给药组	1 2 3 4 M $\bar{x} \pm S$				
对照组	1 2 3 4 M $\bar{x} \pm S$				

【注意事项】

1. 剥离气管时操作要轻柔，勿损伤甲状腺及周围血管，以免出血后将血液带进冲洗液而影响比色。

2. 将针头插入气管时勿用力过度，以致刺破气管。用线结扎固定针头时，也勿用力过大，以免将气管绞断。

3. 用 5% 碳酸氢钠溶液抽洗气管时，用量要准确，速度宜慢，以免胀破气管。要尽可能将液体抽尽，同时避免将空气注入气管内。

【思考题】

祛痰药通过哪几方面的作用使痰液易于咳出？祛痰药是否具有镇咳作用？

实验5.22 氨茶碱对豚鼠组胺－乙酰胆碱引喘的平喘作用

【目的】

学习用乙酰胆碱和组胺喷雾引起豚鼠哮喘的方法。观察氨茶碱的平喘作用。

【原理】

乙酰胆碱和组胺等药物，以气雾法给药，可引起豚鼠支气管痉挛、窒息，导致其抽搐而跌倒。这种动物模型可用于观察支气管平滑肌松弛药的平喘作用。

【材料】

豚鼠2只，体重150~200g，雌雄不限。

喷雾装置、空气压缩机、玻璃钟罩（容积为2L）、注射器、秒表。

2%氯化乙酰胆碱溶液、0.4%磷酸组胺溶液、12.5%氨茶碱溶液、生理盐水。

【方法与步骤】

1. 实验前一天，将豚鼠分别放入玻璃钟罩内，以53~67kPa的压力恒压喷入2%氯化乙酰胆碱和0.4%磷酸组胺混合液（2∶1）8~15s，密切观察动物的反应，气雾引喘装置见图5－11。动物一般是先呼吸加深加快，继而发生呼吸困难，最后出现抽搐和跌倒。如见到豚鼠跌倒，应立即将其取出，以免死亡，并记录引喘潜伏期（从喷雾开始到抽搐、跌倒的时间），一般不超过150s，超过150s者可以认为不敏感，不予选用。

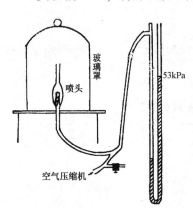

图5－11 药物气雾引喘装置

2. 次日取经过预选的豚鼠2只，一只腹腔注射12.5%氨茶碱（125mg/kg），另一只腹腔注射等容量生理盐水。30min后，将两只豚鼠分别置于玻璃钟罩内，同前法进行喷雾和测定其引喘潜伏期，若超过6min仍不出现哮喘者即取出按6min计算。

【结果处理】

按表5－9的项目做好记录。汇总全实验室结果，分别计算豚鼠给药前和给药后引喘潜伏期的平均数及标准差（$\bar{x} \pm S$）。并对给药前后引喘潜伏期进行自身对照的显著性t检验，以P值表示给药前后有无显著性差异（也可进行组间比较）。

表5－9 氨茶碱对豚鼠的平喘作用

豚鼠编号	药物	剂量及途径	引喘喷雾后反应	引喘潜伏期（s）	
				给药前	给药后
1					
2					

【注意事项】

1. 豚鼠必须选用幼鼠，体重不超过250g，且引喘潜伏期不超过150s。

2. 判断药物有无平喘作用的指标：用药后引喘潜伏期明显延长或用药后动物不会因呼

吸困难、窒息而跌倒，一般观察6min，不跌倒者引喘潜伏期以6min计算。

3. 抗组胺药无直接松弛支气管平滑肌作用，但用于这种动物模型，也能得到平喘效果。因此，在分析实验结果时，应排除这种假阳性现象。

4. 多次重复接触组胺，部分豚鼠可能出现"耐受"现象，因此在实验安排上要注意各鼠接受喷雾的机会相等。一般各鼠每天只能测定引喘潜伏期一次。

【方法评价】

喷雾引喘药是从呼吸道吸入，吸入量受呼吸量的影响；刺激性供试药由腹腔给药，若引起疼痛可能抑制呼吸，使引喘药（乙酰胆碱和组胺）吸入减少，而造成引喘潜伏期延长的假阳性。此外，还受引喘药液浓度、喷雾压力、喷雾头结构等因素的影响。喷雾颗粒直径小于5μm者能吸入肺泡，作用快而强；喷雾颗粒稍大者在支气管吸收；喷雾颗粒更大者就在气管或上呼吸道凝聚，作用慢而弱。

根据哮喘发作的表现分为Ⅰ级、Ⅱ级、Ⅲ级、Ⅳ级反应，根据反应级别来判断哮喘的轻重程度。Ⅰ级：呼吸加深加快。Ⅱ级：呼吸困难。Ⅲ级：抽搐。Ⅳ级：跌倒。但Ⅰ级、Ⅱ级、Ⅲ级之间无明显界线，观察中有时难以准确判断。有效药物多半能延缓或阻止Ⅲ级或Ⅳ级反应的出现。用药后引喘潜伏期明显延长或不出现呼吸困难、窒息、跌倒等现象。

【思考题】

常用的平喘药有哪几类？各类有何特点？临床意义如何？

实验5.23 药物对豚鼠离体气管的作用

【目的】

学习离体豚鼠气管链的制备方法，观察药物对气管平滑肌的收缩或松弛作用以及它们之间的相互关系。

【原理】

豚鼠离体气管平滑肌上主要分布有β_2受体、M受体和H_1受体。β_2受体兴奋使气管平滑肌松弛，M受体和H_1受体兴奋使平滑肌收缩。异丙肾上腺素是β_2受体激动药，可使平滑肌松弛；乙酰胆碱和组胺分别是M受体和H_1受体的激动药，可使平滑肌收缩。

【材料】

豚鼠1只，体重400~500g，雌雄不限。

麦氏浴槽、恒温水浴、温度计、张力换能器、生理信号采集记录系统、充气球胆、剪刀、眼科镊、培养皿、铁支架、双凹夹、棉线、注射器。

0.2%磷酸组胺溶液、0.05%氯化乙酰胆碱溶液、2.5%氨茶碱溶液、0.1%硫酸异丙肾上腺素溶液、0.5%硫酸阿托品溶液、克-亨氏营养液（NaCl 8.0g，$MgCl_2$ 0.42g，$CaCl_2$ 0.4g，用蒸馏水溶解并稀释至1000ml，临用前加入葡萄糖1.0g）。

【方法与步骤】

1. **调机** 接通生理信号采集记录系统，并调节基线至适当位置。加上前负荷0.5~1g，拨动量程开关调至20mV。走纸变速调到4mm分档上（4mm/min）。

2. **制备气管链** 取豚鼠1只，用木棒猛击头部致死。剖开颈部皮肤和肌层，自甲状软

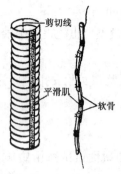

图 5 - 12　气管链的制备法

骨以下至气管分叉处剪下整条气管，置于盛有克 – 亨氏营养液的培养皿中，剪成宽度为 3 ~ 4mm 的气管圈 5 ~ 6 个，再把各个气管圈在软骨的中点剪断，制成两端连着软骨、中间为平滑肌膜的气管条片。用棉线将 5 ~ 6 个气管条片连接成一个气管链（图 5 - 12），链的长度视浴槽大小而定，容量为 30ml 的浴槽，气管链长 3 ~ 4cm，容量为 10ml 的浴槽，长 1.5 ~ 2cm。

3. **安装气管链**　将制备好的气管链放入盛有 37℃ 克 – 亨氏营养液的麦氏浴槽中，一端固定在浴槽基部，另一端挂在连有生理信号采集记录系统的换能器小钩上。插入通气管，从充气球胆缓缓放出气泡（一个接一个），以供给气管氧气。让气管链在营养液中适应 10min。描记一段正常曲线作为基线。

4. **给药**　待基线稳定后，给药观察气管链的反应（浴槽容量为 30ml）。每次给药，其作用明显后，换液洗去前一种药物，待描记基线恢复至原水平后，再给予下一种药物。

给药次序为：① 0.1% 硫酸异丙肾上腺素 0.1ml；② 2.5% 氨茶碱溶液 0.1ml；③ 0.2% 磷酸组胺溶液 0.1ml，作用达高峰后加入 0.1% 硫酸异丙肾上腺素溶液 0.1ml；④ 0.2% 磷酸组胺溶液 0.1ml，作用达高峰后加入 2.5% 氨茶碱溶液 0.1ml；⑤ 0.05% 氯化乙酰胆碱溶液 0.1ml，作用达高峰后加入 0.1% 硫酸异丙肾上腺素溶液 0.1ml；⑥ 0.05% 氯化乙酰胆碱溶液 0.1ml，作用达高峰后加入 2.5% 氨茶碱溶液 0.1ml；⑦ 0.05% 氯化乙酰胆碱溶液 0.1ml，作用达高峰后加入 0.5% 硫酸阿托品溶液 0.1ml。

【结果处理】

复制气管链的描记曲线，并在曲线下加注给药、换液等说明。

【注意事项】

1. 分离气管及用线结扎气管条时，动作要快而轻巧，避免扯伤或用镊子夹伤气管平滑肌。

2. 气管平滑肌在加药以前并无自发的节律性收缩，这点与肠管有所不同，故基线稳定后即可给药。

3. 每加入一种药物，观察 5min，待其作用明显后换液。充分洗去前一种药物（一般换液 3 次），待描记基线恢复至原水平后，再加入下一种药物。更换浴槽溶液时，应关闭记录开关，以免描笔大幅度移位。

4. 实验过程中供氧要充分。如基线升高或不易恢复到原来水平时，可充分供氧，促使其恢复。

【方法评价】

离体气管法是常用的筛选平喘药的实验方法之一，具有快速、方便、经济和节省试药的优点，并可直接观察到药物对气管平滑肌的收缩和松弛作用。常用的实验动物中，豚鼠的气管对药物反应较敏感，且接近于人的支气管，因此首选豚鼠的气管进行实验。

根据气管取下后切开的方法不同，又可分为气管环法、气管螺旋条法及本实验中所采用的气管链法。①气管环法：取下气管后，沿软骨环间横切成宽度相近的 5 ~ 6 个环，再用线将这些环结扎成一串（图 5 - 13）。这种方法制备的离体气管在应用支气管平滑肌收缩剂或松弛剂后反应的幅度不大，约为气管链法的1/3。②气管螺旋条法：可避免气管环法反应幅度小的缺陷，适用于研究支气管平滑肌收缩剂和松弛剂。制备方法为将气管由一端向另一端剪成螺旋形条状，每2~3个软骨环剪成一个螺旋条，宽2~3mm，长3~4cm（图5-14）。

另外，还可采用完整气管标本，由于气管平滑肌成环行排列（部分成斜行或纵行排列），环状肌的收缩或松弛作用可引起气管内径缩小或扩大，使气管容积相应缩小或扩大，此反应可通过连接到气管上的检压计内液面高度的改变反映出来，此即气管容积测定法。

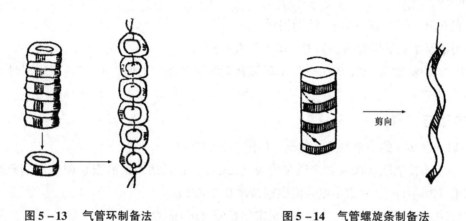

图5-13　气管环制备法　　　　　　　　图5-14　气管螺旋条制备法

【思考题】

异丙肾上腺素、氨茶碱、磷酸组胺、硫酸阿托品在豚鼠气管链上所显示作用的机理有何异同？有何临床意义？

七、消化系统药物实验

常从对胃肠道平滑肌运动的影响，对溃疡病的防治作用和利胆作用等方面研究消化系统药物。

药物对胃肠道平滑肌运动功能的影响：有离体豚鼠、家兔胃肠道平滑肌运动记录法，胃排空、肠推进运动的实验法，用压敏传感器研究消化器官运动的实验法，用生物电研究消化器官运动的实验法等。

实验性消化溃疡模型：按其疗效试验的方法可分为四类。一是外科手术法，大鼠、犬可采用结扎幽门法；二是药物法，给予阿司匹林、吲哚美辛、利血平等药物；三是应激法，可用束缚应激法和束缚水浸应激法等；四是消化管黏膜的人工损伤法，如热灼法、冰醋酸法等。这些方法就其操作的难易程度、结果的重现性、对药物的敏感性以及与病因的关系等而言，各有优点。

药物对胆汁排泄的影响：常用犬、猫、兔等动物，麻醉以后作总胆管插管引流，来观察药物对胆汁排泄的影响。还可以自总胆管向肠道方向进行灌流，以观察药物对Oddi括约肌排放活动的影响。大鼠因无胆囊，尤便于从总胆管定量收集胆汁。

实验5.24　药物对胃肠道蠕动的影响

【目的】

测定炭末在胃肠道的移动速度，观察药物对胃肠道蠕动功能的影响。

【原理】

动物小肠平滑肌由很厚的环行肌层和很薄的纵行肌层组成，在肠内容物向肛端推进运动中，环行肌的收缩起主要作用。小肠任一点受到食物刺激时，刺激点的上方发生收缩，下方发生舒张，使食团向大肠方向移动，从而形成肠蠕动。正是由于肠肌的这种规律性运动，产生了食糜由小肠向大肠的推进运动。有些药物可作用于肠道平滑肌，导致肠蠕动的增强或减弱，从而影响小肠的推进运动功能。

【材料】

小鼠 6 只，体重 20 ~ 24g，性别相同。

注射器、小鼠灌胃针头、剪刀、镊子、直尺。

0.01% 盐酸吗啡溶液、0.01% 甲基硫酸新斯的明溶液、生理盐水、5% 炭末混悬液（含阿拉伯胶 10%）。

【方法与步骤】

1. 取禁食 24h 的小鼠 6 只，称重、标记、分成三组。

2. 甲组小鼠灌服 0.01% 盐酸吗啡溶液（2mg/kg）；乙组小鼠灌服 0.01% 甲基硫酸新斯的明溶液（2mg/kg）、丙组小鼠灌服生理盐水 0.2ml/10g。

3. 15min 后，每只小鼠均灌服 5% 炭末混悬液（0.1ml/20g）。

4. 灌服炭末 20min 后，用颈椎脱臼法将动物处死，剖开腹腔。将消化管自幽门至直肠末端完整地摘出，不加牵引铺平，测其全长和炭末的前沿至幽门的距离，计算每只小鼠炭末移动的距离与胃肠道全长的百分比。

【结果处理】

按下式计算，并汇集全班结果，取平均值及标准差进行比较。

$$炭末移动距离占胃肠道全长的百分比 = \frac{炭末移动距离}{胃肠道全长距离} \times 100\%$$

【注意事项】

1. 动物必须事先禁食 1 日。

2. 灌服炭末和处死动物时间必须准确，否则对实验结果影响较大。

3. 剪取肠道要避免牵拉，否则影响测量长度的准确性。

【方法评价】

研究胃肠推进运动时，常安放一种示踪物质在肠腔内并追踪它的前进，观察一定时间内该物质在胃肠推进的距离。

这种方法简单、安全，但仅测量了物质在胃肠道中总的通过情况，不能得到有关收缩形式等细节，而且实验完成时必须处死动物。近年来，研究胃肠道平滑肌的电活动，以胃肠肌电作为平滑肌活动的指标，是比较活跃的研究方法。

【思考题】

盐酸吗啡和甲基硫酸新斯的明对胃肠道的作用有何异同？有何临床意义？

实验5.25 药物对实验性胃溃疡的防治作用

【目的】

学习结扎大鼠幽门以诱发胃溃疡的实验方法，观察药物对实验性胃溃疡的防治作用。

【原理】

将大鼠胃的幽门结扎以后，胃液在胃内停滞，对胃壁产生消化作用，可以造成溃疡。此外，手术前禁食48h，也是生成胃溃疡的重要因素。此法于1945年由Shay等首先报道，以后被广泛用于抗溃疡药物的筛选。

【材料】

大鼠6只，体重200～250g。性别相同。

铁丝鼠笼，大鼠手术板、手术刀、手术剪、镊子、外科缝针、丝线、纱布、大鼠灌胃针头、注射器、量筒、pH试纸、漏斗、显微镜。

1%氢氧化铝凝胶、2%西咪替丁、生理盐水。

【方法与步骤】

1. 大鼠6只，标记，禁食不禁水48h，然后进行手术。

2. 取大鼠用乙醚浅麻醉，仰位固定于手术板上，剪去腹部被毛，用2%碘酊及75%乙醇消毒皮肤。自剑突下切开腹壁约1.5cm，用钝头的镊子将胃引出腹腔，避开肠系膜血管，在幽门和十二指肠的交接处作结扎。将胃放回原位，缝合腹壁，将大鼠放于铁丝鼠笼内，禁食、禁水。

3. 做完手术的大鼠分为三组，每组2只，甲组每只大鼠灌服1%氢氧化铝凝胶5ml；乙组每只皮下注射2%西咪替丁6mg/100g；丙组每只灌服生理盐水5ml。

4. 于手术后18h，断头处死大鼠，剪开腹壁，在贲门部结扎，取出胃，立即泡于1%的福尔马林液中，5min后取出用滤纸吸干。在胃大弯处切一小口，将胃内容物经漏斗移入量筒内，沿胃大弯切开胃，用清水轻轻漂洗胃体，平铺于玻璃板上，在显微镜下观察并计算溃疡面积及整个腺体胃的总面积。测量胃液体积及用pH试纸测胃液的酸度。

【结果处理】

计算溃疡面积，测量胃液体积、胃液pH，汇集全班结果，将三组不同给药组的以上三个指标进行比较。

【注意事项】

1. 手术前的绝对饥饿是造成溃疡的必要条件。应将大鼠关在架空的铁丝鼠笼内，以防其吞食粪粒及铺垫物。

2. 结扎幽门时应避开血管，以免妨碍胃肠道的血液循环。

3. 用镊子夹取胃部时，动作要柔和，以免损伤组织器官。

【方法评价】

幽门结扎法诱发的胃溃疡发生率为85%～100%，常与水浸拘束法配套应用。幽门结扎法诱发的胃黏膜病损程度，与动物手术前的禁食情况和结扎后经历的时间有关。该模型还可用胃内滞积的胃液分析测定其体积、胃液酸度、总酸度以及胃蛋白酶活力，用于观察药物对以上各指标的影响作用。

【思考题】

1. 幽门结扎法造成胃溃疡的因素有哪些？

2. 氢氧化铝凝胶、西咪替丁对溃疡病有何作用？其临床效果如何？

实验 5.26　去氢胆酸对大鼠的利胆作用

【目的】

学习测定大鼠胆汁分泌量的实验方法，观察药物的利胆作用。

【原理】

本实验利用去氢胆酸能使胆红素或其他胆汁成分浓度变稀，胆汁水分大量增加而增加胆汁分泌的作用，观察催胆剂对大鼠的利胆作用。

【材料】

大鼠 2 只，体重 300g 左右，性别相同。

注射器、细塑料管（直径为 1～2mm）、手术剪、眼科镊、试管夹、止血钳、手术刀、大鼠手术台、刻度吸管（1ml）、烧杯、纱布、丝线、铁架台、量筒、眼科剪。

3% 戊巴比妥钠溶液、2.5% 去氢胆酸、生理盐水。

【方法与步骤】

1. 大鼠禁食、禁水 12h 后，称重、标记，分为两组。

2. 腹腔注射 3% 戊巴比妥钠溶液（30mg/kg）麻醉，仰位固定。腹部正中线剃毛后切开皮肤及腹膜 2cm，以幽门部为标准，翻转引出十二指肠，即可见到白色的十二指肠乳头部。从乳头部追踪总胆管。在乳头部上方 3～5mm 处，用镊子将覆盖在上面的被膜连续剥离 5～10mm，总胆管完全暴露。

3. 在经过剥离的胆管乳头侧及其上方，穿过 2 根丝线备用。将靠近乳头部的线牢固结扎。用眼科剪在胆管上作一切口，从切口向肝脏方向插入聚乙烯塑料管，确认胆汁流出后，将预先穿过的线把套管固定，用止血钳暂时关闭腹腔。

4. 用量筒收集胆汁 1h，计量。作为给药前胆汁分泌的正常值。

5. 甲组由十二指肠注入生理盐水 4ml/kg，乙组由十二指肠注入 2.5% 去氢胆酸（100mg/kg）。分别收集给药后第 1h 及第 2h 的胆汁流出量，与给药前作自身对照比较后第 1h 及第 2h 的胆汁流出量，与给药前作自身对照比较。

【结果处理】

汇集全班结果，进行比较。

胆汁增加量 = 用药后 1h 内胆汁分泌量 – 用药前 1h 内的分泌量

将将二组的数据进行配对比较。

【注意事项】

1. 手术时，创口要小并切勿损伤肝脏及十二指肠。

2. 动物要注意保温，尤其在冬季更应注意。药物要预热到 38℃，方可给药。

【方法评价】

利胆剂的效果随动物的种属不同而异，因此只有通过临床结果对它们评价最为理想。

但在临床试验中必须在患者身上采集胆汁，在方法上是相当困难的，所以，常需利用动物实验结果作为评价的参考依据。

对利胆剂特别是催胆剂进行评价的时候，必须记录实验动物的种类、胆汁采集的方法、是否麻醉及麻醉种类、利胆剂的用量和给药方式、胆汁采集时间，附带记录水分、胆红素、胆汁酸、胆固醇在胆汁内的浓度和一定时间内这些物质的排泄量，而且也需记录胆汁的外观、黏稠度和沉淀的变化等，这些资料对统一评价药物效果是必不可少的。

【思考题】

1. 本实验是否可用其他动物作为实验对象？其方法上有何不同点？

2. 去氢胆酸有何临床作用？常用于何种病症？

八、促凝血药和抗凝血药实验

在生理状态下，血液在血管中循环流动，既不溢出血管之外导致出血，也不会在血管中凝固形成血栓，这主要是由于体内存在着复杂的凝血系统和抗凝纤溶系统，而且二者维持动态平衡，一旦这种平衡遭到破坏，则可能发生出血性或血栓性疾患。

血液由流动状态转变为凝胶状态称为血液凝固，参与凝血过程的有关因子统称为凝血因子。按国际凝血因子命名委员会规定，依其发现年代从罗马字码顺编，已编号 12 个凝血因子，这些因子转变为活化型的凝血因子时，在其右下角加标一个"a"。还有激肽释放酶原（PK）、激肽释放酶（Ka）、高分子激肽原（HMWK）、血小板磷脂（PL 或 PF_3）、纤溶酶原、纤溶酶等也参与凝血与纤溶的连锁反应。

凝血与纤溶大致可分为 4 个步骤。

1. 凝血酶原激活物的形成 根据血液凝固的瀑布学说，认为血液凝固过程是由内源性途径（所有参与成分都存在于血液之中）、外源性途径（除血中成分以外，还要有内皮下细胞膜蛋白即组织因子参与）和共同途径组成，通过多种酶原被相继激活而得到加强和放大的一种连锁反应。在内源性途径中，首先是血浆中的接触因子，即因子Ⅻ、激肽释放酶和高分子激肽原暴露在带负电荷的表面，使因子Ⅻ活化为因子Ⅻa，因子Ⅻa又导致因子Ⅺ活化。然后因子Ⅺa激活因子Ⅸ，因子Ⅸa又在辅因子Ⅷa、磷脂和钙存在下，组成 X 酶复合物，激活因子 X。而外源性途径则从血浆因子Ⅶ暴露于组织因子开始，二者形成复合物后直接激活因子 X。当凝血过程通过这两种途径发展到因子 X 被激活的阶段时，两途径汇合在一起，使因子 X 被激活为 Xa，并与因子 V 通过 Ca^{2+} 连接于磷脂表面，形成复合物，此复合物即为凝血酶原激活物。

2. 凝血酶的形成 凝血酶原在凝血酶原激活物的作用下转化为凝血酶。

3. 纤维蛋白的形成 在凝血酶的作用下，使溶胶状态的纤维蛋白原转化为凝胶状态的纤维蛋白（血凝块）。

4. 纤维蛋白的溶解 纤维蛋白在纤维蛋白溶解酶（纤溶酶）的作用下液化溶解转化为可溶性纤维蛋白降解物。

促凝血药是一些通过加速血液凝固过程或者阻止纤维蛋白溶解作用而达到止血效果的物质；抗凝血药则是一些延缓血液凝固或加速纤维蛋白溶解的物质，这类物质是能预防和治疗血栓形成的重要物质。

体外法是在体外观察药物对凝血时间和纤溶时间的影响，操作简单，无需特殊设备，可用于药物的初筛。

病理模型法是在实验动物身上造成类似人体出血或凝血等病理状态，然后用促凝血药或抗凝血药进行实验性治疗，用以观察和分析药物的作用或筛选新药。这类病理模型较易形成，如给小鼠灌服双香豆素形成低凝血症的病理模型。

实验5.27　药物的体外抗凝血作用

【目的】

学习体外试管法观察枸橼酸钠与肝素的体外抗凝血作用。

【原理】

肝素在体内外均有强大而迅速的抗凝血作用，作用机制主要是作为抗凝血酶Ⅲ（AT-Ⅲ）的辅助因子，与AT-Ⅲ结合后，加速与凝血酶和因子Ⅸa、Ⅹa、Ⅺa、Ⅻa结合而使之失活。肝素对凝血酶及凝血因子Ⅹ的抑制作用最强，而这二者是内源性和外源性凝血途径必需的因子，加上其对凝血因子Ⅸ、Ⅺ、Ⅻ的抑制作用，肝素对凝血过程的每一步骤几乎均有抑制作用，从而产生强大的抗凝血作用。

枸橼酸钠可降低血中钙离子含量而使血液凝固过程受阻，常用作体外抗凝剂。

【材料】

家兔1只，体重2~3kg，雌雄不限。

试管（内径8mm）、试管架、刻度吸管、注射器、秒表、恒温水浴、小玻棒。

4%枸橼酸钠溶液、生理盐水、4U/ml的肝素溶液、3%氯化钙溶液。

【方法与步骤】

1. 取试管5支，编号。1支滴加生理盐水0.1ml，2支加4%枸橼酸钠溶液0.1ml，另两支各加4U/ml的肝素溶液0.1ml（表5-11）。

2. 从家兔心脏用9号注射针头穿刺取血约5ml，迅速向每支试管中加入兔血0.9ml，充分混匀后，放入37℃±0.5℃恒温水浴中。

3. 每隔30s将试管轻轻倾斜，观察一次血液的流动性，直至将试管缓慢倒置血流不动为止，比较5支试管的凝血时间。

4. 如果后4支试管不出现凝血现象，则可在第2、4两支试管中各加入3%氯化钙溶液2~3滴，混匀，再次观察是否出现凝血，并比较凝血时间。

【结果处理】

观察各试管出现凝血的情况，记录并比较不同的凝血时间（表5-10）。

表5-10　药物对凝血时间的影响

药物	试管编号				
	1	2	3	4	5
生理盐水（ml）	0.1	-	-	-	-
4%枸橼酸钠溶液（ml）	-	0.1	-	0.1	-
4U/ml肝素溶液（ml）	-	-	0.1	-	0.1
兔血（ml）	0.9	0.9	0.9	0.9	0.9

续表

药物	试管编号				
	1	2	3	4	5
	恒温水浴 37℃ ±0.5℃				
凝血时间					
3% 氯化钙	–	2～3 滴	–	2～3 滴	–
凝血时间					

【注意事项】

1. 试管口径大小须均匀适当，一般来说，血液在小口径试管中凝血时间短、管径大、凝血时间长。

2. 家兔心脏穿刺采血要迅速、准确，避免血液在注射器内凝固，并尽量减少组织液和气泡混入。

3. 兔血加入后须立即用小玻棒将血液与试管内的药液搅拌均匀，否则将影响测定的准确性。搅拌时注意避免产生气泡。

4. 自动物取血到试管放入恒温水浴的时间间隔不得超过 1min。

5. 恒温水浴温度要控制好，过高或过低均可使凝血时间延长。

6. 在倾斜试管时，动作要轻，倾斜度尽量小（＜30°），以减少血液与管壁的接触。

7. 注射器及试管用保持干燥、洁净，否则会加速凝血或发生溶血。

【方法评价】

本法为在体外试管内观察药物对血凝时间的影响，其操作简便，无需特殊设备，可用于药物的初筛。但影响因素较多，易影响测定结果的准确性，故用于药物初筛时，应注意各对照组与治疗组平行操作，使影响因素尽可能保持一致。

体外试管法也可用于评价志愿者或患者的凝血情况。凝血时间延长一般见于如下情况：①较显著的因子Ⅷ、Ⅸ、Ⅺ减少，如甲、乙、丙型血友病；②严重的凝血酶原减少，如肝病、阻塞性黄疸、新生儿出血病等；③严重的纤维蛋白原减少，如低（无）纤维蛋白原血症、严重肝病等；④应用抗凝药物如肝素等；⑤纤溶亢进，如弥散性血管内凝血（DIC）的后期及原发性纤维或有大量纤维蛋白降解产物（FDP）存在时。凝血时间缩短见于：①血液呈高凝状态，DIC 早期；②高血糖及高脂血症。

用类似的方法还可以测定活化凝血时间（ACT）、血浆复钙时间（RT）、血清凝血酶原时间（SPT）、活化部分凝血活酶时间（APTT）等。

【思考题】

1. 请比较枸橼酸钠和肝素抗凝血作用的异同点？

2. 鱼精蛋白对肝素的抗凝血作用有何影响？其相互作用的机理是什么？有何临床意义？

实验 5.28　药物的促凝血作用

【目的】

学习低凝血症动物模型的建立方法，观察药物的促凝血作用。

【原理】

利用口服抗凝药双香豆素的作用造成低凝血症的病理动物模型，观察维生素 K_1 的促凝血作用。

【材料】

小鼠 3 只，体重 18～22g，性别相同。

注射器、毛细玻管（内径 1mm、长 10cm）、载玻片、秒表。

蒸馏水、生理盐水、0.25% 双香豆素混悬液、1% 维生素 K_1 溶液。

【方法与步骤】

1. 取小鼠 3 只，称重，标记。

2. 甲鼠灌胃给予蒸馏水 20ml/kg，乙、丙鼠各灌胃给予 0.25% 双香豆素混悬液 50mg/kg。

3. 16h 后，甲、乙鼠各腹腔注射生理盐水 20ml/kg，丙鼠腹腔注射 1% 维生素 K_1 200mg/kg。

4. 从双香豆素灌胃给药时算起，24h 后采用毛细玻管法或玻片法测定凝血时间。

5. 凝血时间测定法

（1）毛细玻管法 用内径 1mm 玻璃毛细管插入小鼠眼内肌球后静脉丛，深 4～5mm，轻轻转动再缩回。自血液流入管内开始用秒表计时，血液注满后取出毛细管平放于桌上，每隔 30s 折断两端毛细管 3～5mm，并缓慢向左右拉开，观察折断处是否有血凝丝，至血凝丝出现为止，计算从毛细玻管采血至出现凝血丝的时间，即为凝血时间，毛细玻管两端数据的平均值即为该鼠的凝血时间。

（2）玻片法 用眼科弯镊迅速摘去小鼠一侧眼球，即有血液流出，于载玻片两端各滴一滴血，血滴直径约 5mm，立即用秒表计时，每隔 30s 用清洁大头针自血滴边缘向里轻轻挑动一次，并观察有无血丝挑起。从采血开始至挑起血丝起止，所用时间即为凝血时间，另一端血滴供复验。取两端平均值为该鼠凝血时间。

【结果处理】

汇集全实验室结果，计算 3 组小鼠的平均凝血时间，并做平均数之间差异的显著性 t 检验，从而判断药物对凝血时间的影响。

【注意事项】

1. 凝血时间可受室温影响，温度愈低，凝血时间就愈长。本实验室温最好在 15℃ 左右。

2. 灌胃前 2h，小鼠应禁食。吸取双香豆素混悬液时要充分摇匀，以免浓度不一。

3. 毛细玻管法中所用玻管内径最好为 1mm，并均匀一致，毛细玻管采血后不宜长时间拿在手中，以免体温影响凝血时间。

4. 玻片法中每次挑血滴时，不应以各个方向多次挑动，以免影响纤维蛋白的形成时间。

【方法评价】

本法是在实验动物体内造成类似人体凝血障碍的病理状态，然后用促凝血药进行实验性治疗，用以观察和分析药物的作用或筛选新药。该模型较易形成，用小鼠为实验对象操作简便、经济，可用于药物的筛选。

给药多长时间后测定凝血时间可根据不同药物和途径而定，注射给药可于给药后 30min 起，设立几个时间测定，观察药物的时效关系。

【思考题】

1. 促凝血药和抗凝血药筛选方法有哪些？
2. 双香豆素和维生素 K_1 各对凝血时间有何影响？作用机理如何？临床用途有哪些？

九、抗血小板药实验

在正常条件下，血小板以分散状态在血管内运行，但当血管损伤、血流改变或受到化学物质刺激时，血小板则发生彼此相关的变化，即形态改变、黏附、聚集和释放。

血小板数量减少、黏附、聚集或释放能力降低可导致出血。血小板数量过多，聚集功能过强可增强血液凝固性，形成血栓。血小板的黏附、聚集和释放反应是血小板的生理条件下止血功能的基本条件，也是血小板病理情况下形成血栓的主要因素。

当血管受损后，血小板与破损内皮所暴露的胶原纤维等接触，并互相聚集，形成牢固的，不能解聚的血小板血栓。血小板聚集后，释放凝血因子，加之血管壁受损均可激活凝血系统，促进纤维蛋白的形成，进一步形成血小板纤维蛋白血栓。

调节血小板功能的因素很多，主要有花生四烯酸（AA）系统，环核苷酸系统，包括环磷酸腺苷（cAMP）和环磷酸鸟苷（cGMP）系统，磷脂酰肌醇（PI）系统和 Ca^{2+} 等。随着生物科学和医学的发展，人们对血小板的生理功能及在病理状态下的作用进行了深入探讨，研究血小板的方法也得到迅速发展。

抗血小板药是一类新型的药物，目前其临床应用多限于心血管系统疾病方面，如缺血性心脏病和血栓性疾病等。现从药物对血小板黏附性、聚集性和反应产物释放的影响等方面来介绍抗血小板药实验。

实验 5.29　血小板黏附性测定法

【目的】

学习血小板黏附性实验原理和操作。

【原理】

血小板能黏附于损伤血管表面或异物表面的特性，称为血小板黏附性。正常情况下，血小板表面与血管内皮细胞表面都带有负电荷，由于同性相斥，血小板不会黏附在血管内皮上。当血管内皮受损时，内皮下胶原暴露，则带负电荷的血小板与带正电荷的胶原黏附。

根据血小板有黏附性，当血液和异物接触适当时间后，由于血小板黏附在异物表面，使血液中血小板数目减少，测定接触异物前后血液中血小板数目之差，即为黏附于异物表面的血小板数，由此可计算出血小板黏附率。下面主要介绍两种改良旋转玻球法。

【材料】

家兔 1 只，3kg 左右，雄性。

血小板黏附仪，硅化注射器，硅化刻度试管，1ml 硅化刻度吸管，玻璃球瓶，血球计数板，尖滴管，显微镜。

3.8% 枸橼酸钠液，1% 乙醚 – 甲基硅油溶液（1ml 硅油，乙醚加至 100ml）。

【方法与步骤】

1. 取家兔 1 只，用硅化注射器自心脏取血。

2. 血小板黏附性测定方法。

（1）A 法　取兔血 2.7ml，置于含有 0.3ml 3.8% 枸橼酸钠的硅化试管中，轻轻摇匀。随后取 1.5ml 抗凝血，加入 12ml 的玻璃球瓶内。将玻璃球瓶固定在血小板黏附仪的转动装置上，以 3r/min 转速旋转 15min，使血液与瓶壁充分接触。旋转后从玻璃球瓶（黏附后）中及试管（黏附前）中各取 1ml 血液，分别加入到盛有 3.8% 枸橼酸钠溶液 19ml 的硅化试管中，以塑料膜覆盖试管口，反复清道 3 次，使其均匀，在室温下静置 2h，待红细胞部分下沉后，取试管上层液体作血小板计数，测得黏附前后的血小板数，每一被测标本均做双份测定，取其均值。

（2）B 法　取兔血 1.8ml，加入含有 0.2ml 3.8% 枸橼酸钠的硅化试管中，混匀。用 1ml 硅化刻度吸管吸 1ml 抗凝血，加入容量为 8ml 的玻璃球瓶中，将玻璃球瓶放入血小板黏附仪转动装置上，恒温 37℃，以 3.7r/min 转速旋转 15min，分别测定黏附前后的血小板数，计数两次，取平均值。

【处理结果】按下式计算血小板黏附率：

$$血小板黏附率（\%）=\frac{黏附前血小板数 - 黏附后血小板数}{黏附前血小板数} \times 100\%$$

【注意事项】

1. 除玻璃球瓶外，实验所用的玻璃器皿及注射针头均需用 1% 乙醚 – 甲基硅油溶液冲涂，进行硅化处理。

2. 实验选用的玻璃球瓶容量应相同，以减少接触面积变化对血小板黏附率的影响。

3. 适当选用抗凝剂，以枸橼酸钠、EDTA 为宜，且应注意抗凝剂与血液的比例尽量准确。

4. 从静脉或心脏采血不应有气泡或血凝块。采血后应于 15～25min 内测定完毕，血液不宜久置。

5. 血小板计数要力求准确。

【方法评价】

测定血小板黏附性的方法很多，但基本原理均相似。国外主张用灌注小室法，即将血液泵入盛有去除内皮层的兔主动脉壁的小室中，根据血小板与内皮黏附的多少，判断血小板的黏附性。优点是接近体内的生理或病理条件，但每次需用 50ml 血，操作比较复杂。国内常用的有旋转玻球法、玻璃纤维法、玻璃滤器法以及玻璃球法等。本文介绍的改良旋转玻球法操作简单、用血量不多，但血小板计数不易准确，影响结果。

【思考题】

1. 为什么要将实验中所用之玻璃器皿进行硅化？

2. 测定血小板黏附性方法的基本原理是什么？

实验 5.30　血小板聚集性测定法

【目的】

学习血小板聚集性实验原理和操作。

【原理】

血小板与血小板之间相互黏附、聚集成团，即为血小板聚集。在体外，血小板一般需在诱导剂刺激下才发生聚集。已知可诱导血小板聚集的诱导剂有许多，如 ADP、胶原、凝血酶、肾上腺素及花生四烯酸等。当血小板活化程度增高时，也可能发生自发性聚集。血小板聚集有两种时相，第一相聚集代表血小板聚集物的形成；第二相聚集代表释放反应。

测定血小板聚集性的方法有多种，如比值法、比浊法和血栓法等，其中比浊法最为常用，其基本原理如下。

富血小板血浆（PRP）是一种胶体溶液，血小板呈分散状态、轻度混浊，其浓度高低与所含血小板数目相关。若在搅拌的条件下，加入引起血小板聚集的诱导剂（ADP、胶原、肾上腺素等），血小板即发生聚集，致散在的血小板数减少、浓度下降、透光率增高。因此，可以 PRP 的浓度变化来表示血小板的聚集程度。利用血小板聚集仪中光电系统将 PRP 的浓度变化转换为电讯号变化，并用记录仪进行描记。通过描记的曲线求出血小板聚集的程度。

【材料】

大鼠 1 只，体重 250～300g，雄性。

大鼠手术台及器械，血小板聚集仪，钢芯或铜芯玻璃搅拌棒，离心机，硅化注射器和刻度离心管等。

二磷酸腺苷（ADP）：用 ADP 钠盐以 0.1mol/L 磷酸盐缓冲液（pH 7.2）配成 1mol/L ADP 贮存液，冰箱冷冻保存。3.8% 枸橼酸钠溶液，3% 戊巴比妥钠溶液。

【方法与步骤】

1. 将大鼠称重，用 3% 戊巴比妥钠（30mg/kg）麻醉，仰位固定，分离腹主动脉。用硅化的注射器（9 号针头）从腹主动脉取 4.5ml 血，加入装有 0.5ml 3.8% 枸橼酸钠溶液的试管中，轻轻倒置混合后，以 1000r/min 离心 5min，吸出上层米黄色悬液约 1ml 即为 PRP，余下的血浆再以 4000r/min 离心 10min，吸取上清液，制得贫血小板血浆（PPP）。

2. 计算 PRP 中血小板数目，若血小板计数过高，可用 PPP 稀释。

3. 实验开始前，聚集仪预热 15min，分别取一定量的 PRP 和 PPP 于比浊管中，将含 PPP 比浊管放入聚集仪的测定孔中，使透光度调节到 10，反复调节几次，直至基线稳定。PRP 管中应加入搅拌棒，否则血小板不会聚集。药液或对照液可加入 PRP 管中。

4. 描记一段基线后，加诱导剂 ADP 于 PRP 管中，观察 PRP 在 5min 内的最大聚集程度，计算聚集百分率或药物抑制的百分率。

【结果处理】

按下式计算药物抑制聚集百分率：

$$血小板聚集抑制率 = \frac{对照管血小板聚集百分率 - 给药管血小板聚集百分率}{对照管血小板聚集百分率} \times 100\%$$

【注意事项】

1. **采血** 受试患者或志愿者在取血前两周内避免服用阿司匹林等血小板功能抑制剂，取血当天应禁饮牛奶、豆浆等可能影响 PRP 透光度的食物。取血要迅速准确，避免反复穿刺，以免将组织液混入血液，激活血小板。大鼠以腹主动脉采血，家兔以心脏采血为好。

采血与试验的时间间隔不宜过长，以采血后 1~2h 为宜，不应超过 4h，否则将影响血小板的反应性。

2. 硅化 所有与血液接触的玻璃器皿均需硅化，包括注射器、试管、比浊管及搅拌棒等。

3. 抗凝剂 常用抗凝剂有枸橼酸钠、肝素和 EDTA，但不同抗凝剂对血小板聚集影响不同。与枸橼酸钠抗凝相比，肝素抗凝分离的 PRP 对 ADP 或肾上腺素诱导聚集的第一相反应较大。相反，肝素化 PRP 对肾上腺素诱导的第二相反应和胶原诱导的聚集却较枸橼酸钠化 PRP 弱，这可能是肝素抑制了释放机制。EDTA 由于具有较强的螯合作用，如达到抗凝浓度则将结合血浆中所有的钙和镁离子，除瑞斯托霉素（Ristocetin）可引起 EDTA 化 PRP 聚集外，如不另加钙，其他诱导剂均不能引起血小板聚集。

4. 温度 采血后标本应置于 15~25℃ 室温下，血小板在低温条件下将发生自发性聚集。在测定聚集时，聚集仪的温度应严格控制在 37℃±0.1℃。若低于 30℃，ADP 或肾上腺素都不能引起第二相聚集，即释放反应。

5. pH 一般以 7.5 左右为宜，在 6.8~8.5 反应较好。以 ADP 为例，若 pH 低于 6.4 或高于 10.0，虽有形态改变，但不能引起聚集。因此，在检测药物对血小板聚集影响时，应注意药物是否对 pH 有改变。

6. 血小板计数 血小板计数的高低影响聚集性，血小板计数愈低，聚集速率愈慢，最大聚集程度也愈低。以 PRP 为例，人、兔和大鼠的血小板计数范围分别以 $(200~250)×10^9/L$、$(400~450)×10^9/L$ 和 $(600~750)×10^9/L$ 为宜。

7. 诱导剂 ADP 配置成溶液后宜在 -20℃ 贮存，以防止其自行分解。胶原溶液宜保存在 4℃，肾上腺素、去甲肾上腺素和 5-羟色胺均能诱导人血小板聚集，但不引起动物（大白鼠、兔、豚鼠和犬）血小板聚集。血小板聚集诱导剂的作用机理不尽相同，因此宜采用两种以上的诱导剂。

8. 药物颜色 研究中草药抑制剂时，为排除药物颜色对浊度的影响，应加相应量的药液至空白管中作空白对照。

【方法评价】

血小板聚集性是血小板的重要功能，许多遗传性疾病都伴有血小板聚集性异常。血小板聚集性增高也可作为诊断高凝状态的参考指标。比值法能定量地测定血小板的聚集功能，操作较简便。但该法为体外实验方法，不能完全反映机体内血小板的聚集状态，而且影响因素较多，特别是"正常人群"对诱导剂的反应程度存在很大的差异。一般而言，血小板聚集性减低对诊断某些疾病有意义，但血小板聚集性增高仅具有临床参考价值。

该法如作体外药物试验，先将药物或对照液于 37℃ 与 PRP 孵育一定时间；如体内给药或观察疾病状态下血小板聚集性的改变，则可直接进行试验。

【思考题】

1. 根据实验原理，是否可用其他仪器代替血小板聚集仪？

2. 在分离 PRP 时，如吸入红细胞会有何影响？

实验 5.31　动静脉旁路血栓形成实验

【目的】

学习动静脉旁路血栓形成实验方法，掌握动静脉插管操作。

【原理】

利用大鼠体外颈总动脉 – 颈外静脉血流旁路法形成血小板血栓。以聚乙烯管连接动静脉，形成旁路血液循环，动脉血流中的血小板，当接触丝线的粗糙面时黏附于线上，血小板聚集物环绕线的表面形成血小板血栓。当血小板的黏附、聚集功能受到抑制时，形成血栓的重量就较轻。因此，从血栓重量可测知血小板的黏附、聚集功能。

【材料】

大鼠 1 只，体重 250 ~ 350g，雄性。

大鼠手术台和器械，动脉夹，聚乙烯管，4 号手术丝线。

3% 戊巴比妥钠，50U/ml 的肝素生理盐水。

【方法与步骤】

1. 取大鼠，称重。腹腔注射 3% 戊巴比妥钠（30 ~ 40mg/kg），仰卧位固定，分离气管，插入一塑料套管（气管分泌物多时可通过此套管吸出），并分离右颈总动脉和左颈外静脉，用动脉夹夹闭右颈总动脉。

2. 剪一根长 7cm 的 4 号手术丝线，称重后放入三段式聚乙烯管中段，使接触血液的丝线长 6cm，剩下的 1cm 从靠近动脉端的接头处露出来，以 50U/ml 的肝素生理盐水充满整个聚乙烯管。

3. 将静脉端插入左颈外静脉后，从静脉端准确注入 50U/ml 的肝素生理盐水（1ml/kg）抗凝，然后将动脉端插入右颈总动脉。

4. 打开动脉夹，计时，血液从右颈总动脉流至聚乙烯管内，返回左颈外静脉，15min 后中断血流，迅速取出丝线称重。

【结果处理】

比较对照动物和给药动物血栓湿重。

$$血栓湿重 = 总重量 - 丝线重量$$

按下列公式计算抑制率：

$$抑制率（\%） = \frac{对照组血栓湿重 - 给药组血栓湿重}{对照组血栓湿重} \times 100\%$$

【注意事项】

1. 对照组和给药组动物体重要严格配对。

2. 聚乙烯管口径大小要求一致，三段式管中间接头处要求严密，以防漏血。

3. 各动物麻醉深度尽可能一致。

4. 手术过程要求迅速，操作熟练，在 15min 内完成。

5. 注意及时吸出器官分泌物，保持呼吸道畅通。

6. 丝线上血栓比较疏松，从管内取出时不能碰到管壁。

【方法评价】

本法反映整体动物血流中血小板的黏附、聚集功能，血栓结构类似动脉中的白色血栓，故与生理病理情况比较接近。方法简便，可用于多种动物（如大鼠、家兔等），能反映药物对血小板聚集的抑制作用。如果在开放血流 15min 待血栓形成后静脉给药，还可观察药物的溶栓作用。

本法血小板血栓的形成与血流速度、血小板数目密切相关，在分析药物作用时注意。此外，本方法所形成的血栓为混合血栓，除抗血小板药外，抗凝药亦可抑制血栓形成。

【思考题】

为什么对照组和给药组动物体重要严格配对？为何麻醉条件要尽可能一致？

实验 5.32　苯海拉明对组胺的竞争性拮抗作用及 pA_2 值

【目的】

学习离体豚鼠回肠标本的制备方法，观察组胺对组胺受体的亲和力及苯海拉明对组胺的竞争性拮抗作用，了解测定 pA_2 值的方法和意义。

【原理】

拮抗剂指能与受体可逆性结合，但无内在活性的化合物。竞争性拮抗剂能使激动剂的量–效反应曲线平行右移，但最大效应 E_{max} 保持不变。组胺作用于 H_1 受体，引起豚鼠回肠收缩。当加入 H_1 受体拮抗剂苯海拉明后，若提高组胺浓度，仍能达到未加拮抗剂前的收缩高度，则表示苯海拉明对组胺呈竞争性拮抗。

pA_2 是一种拮抗参数，表示竞争性拮抗剂的作用强度。在实验系统中加入一定量的拮抗剂，使加倍浓度的激动剂只能引起原浓度激动剂的反应水平，此时该拮抗剂的摩尔浓度的负对数值即为 pA_2。

pA_2 是表示竞争性拮抗剂对相应激动剂拮抗强度的指标，其数值不因实验动物种属或实验器官差异而改变。pA_2 值越大，表示拮抗剂与相应受体的亲和力越大，对相应激动剂的拮抗力越强。不同亚型的受体其 pA_2 值不尽相同。故 pA_2 也是研究受体分型的手段之一。

假设激动剂浓度为 $[A]$，拮抗剂浓度为 $[B]$，则反应到平衡时存在下列方程：

K_A 和 K_B 分别为激动剂和拮抗剂的平均解离常数。

$$[R] + [A] \xleftarrow{\quad K_A \quad} [AR]$$

$$K_A = \frac{[A] \cdot [R]}{[AR]} \tag{1}$$

$$[R] + [B] \xleftarrow{\quad K_B \quad} [BR]$$

$$K_B = \frac{[B] \cdot [R]}{[BR]} \tag{2}$$

此时受体总数目 $R_T = [AR] + [BR] + [R]$

$$\frac{R_T}{[AR]} = 1 + \frac{[BR]}{[AR]} + \frac{[R]}{[AR]} \tag{3}$$

从式（1）和（2）得：

$$\frac{[BR]}{[AR]} = \frac{K_A}{K_B}\frac{[B]}{[A]}$$

$$\frac{[R]}{[AR]} = \frac{K_A}{[A]}$$

代入式（3）得：

$$\frac{E}{E_{max}} = \frac{[AR]}{R_T} = \frac{K_B[A]_B}{K_AK_B + K_A[B] + K_B[A]_B} \tag{4}$$

假设药物的效应与其占领的受体数目成正比，则：

$$\frac{[AR]}{R_T} = \frac{K_B[A]_B}{K_AK_B + K_A[B] + K_B[A]_B}$$

$[A]_B$为在有拮抗剂 B 存在时的激动剂浓度，如果不存在拮抗剂时，即 $[B] = 0$

$$\frac{E}{E_{max}} = \frac{[A]_0}{K_A[A]_0} \tag{5}$$

若在无拮抗剂和有拮抗剂情况下，加入不同浓度的激动剂并产生相同效应时，则存在下列等式：

$$\frac{[A]_0}{[A]_0 + K_A} = \frac{K_B[A]_B}{K_AK_B + K_A[B] + K_B[A]_B}$$

经整理得：

$$\frac{[A]_B}{[A]_0} - 1 = \frac{[B]}{K_B}$$

令 $\frac{[A]_B}{[A]_0} = dr$（Dose Ratio，剂量比）$= 2$，则 $1 = \frac{[B]}{K_B}$，即 $[B] = K_B$

$$pA_2 = -lg[B] = -lg K_B$$

【材料】

豚鼠 1 只，体重 250～300g，雌雄不限。

麦氏浴槽、换能器、记录仪、10ml 量筒、恒温水浴、剪刀、眼科镊、注射器、烧杯、培养皿等。

台氏液、$3×10^{-6}$mol/L 磷酸组胺溶液、$3×10^{-5}$mol/L 磷酸组胺溶液、$6.85×10^{-5}$mol/L 盐酸苯海拉明溶液。

【方法与步骤】

1. 猛击头部将豚鼠处死，迅速打开腹腔，取出回肠，放入通有氧气的盛台氏液的培养皿内。取豚鼠回肠 1.5～2cm，在肠段两端从里向外各穿一线，将肠段固定在浴槽中，负荷约 0.5g。

2. 在浴槽中加入 10ml 台氏液，标记液面高度，浴槽恒温至 37℃±0.5℃，插入通气管，通入以细碎气泡、不影响记录为宜，稳定 10min，其间换台氏液 3 次。

3. 累计计量法加入 $3×10^{-6}$mol/L 磷酸组胺溶液，每次加 0.1ml，直至达到最大收缩反应。

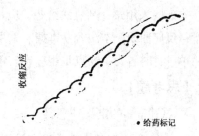

图 5-15 离体肠管累积给药法反应曲线

4. 冲洗数次，待基线稳定后加入 6.85×10^{-5} mol/L 盐酸苯海拉明 0.02ml，保温 5min，再加入 3×10^{-5} mol/L 磷酸组胺溶液重复上述实验（图 5-15）。

每次加药后一旦肠管收缩将达高峰，立即累加下次药物，因加药与肠管收缩之间有时间滞后，故应在肠管收缩至次高点时加入。

【结果处理】

1. 量出肠管收缩幅度（mm），E/E_{max} 及组胺浓度，填入下表。

表 5-11 药物对豚鼠离体回肠的作用

苯海拉明（0）				苯海拉明（1.37×10^{-7} mol/L）			
组胺		效应		组胺		效应	
C	$\lg C$	E	E/E_{max}	C	$\lg C$	E	E/E_{max}

2. 在坐标纸上以 $E/E_{max}\%$ 对 $\lg[A]$ 作图，比较两条曲线的平行程度及最大反应，并取 25%~75% 内的点回归求直线方程，K 值。

3. 用"三点法"计算 pA_2 值。

（1）存在拮抗剂的剂量-反应曲线上（左边曲线）取 25%~75% 内的二点 r_1、r_2，对应激动剂剂量为 a_1、a_2。

（2）在加入拮抗剂的剂量-反应曲线上取介于 r_1、r_2 之间的一点 R，对应剂量为 A_B。在无拮抗剂存在下引起相同反应的激动剂浓度为 A_0。

$$\frac{R - r_1}{r_2 - r_1} = \frac{\lg A_0 - \lg a_1}{\lg a_2 - \lg a_1} = \frac{\lg A_0/a_1}{\lg a_2/a_1}$$

$$\lg \frac{A_0}{a_1} = \frac{R - r_1}{r_2 - r_1} \cdot \lg \frac{a_2}{a_1}$$

$$A_0 = a_1 \left[anti\, \lg \left(\frac{R - r_1}{r_2 - r_1} \cdot \lg \frac{a_2}{a_1} \right) \right]$$

$$pA_2 = -\lg K_B = \lg \left(\frac{[A]_B}{[A]_0} - 1 \right) - \lg[B]$$

【注意事项】

1. 整个实验过程中，必须保持麦氏浴槽内液面等高（同体积营养液）。

2. 滴加药液时一旦肠管收缩，曲线趋于平坦，立即追加药液，直至达到最大收缩反应。

【方法评价】

本实验采用累计剂量法给药，应从低剂量开始，逐渐增加剂量，此法可在短时间内得到剂量-反应曲线。本法容易掌握。采用"三点法"计算 pA_2，只需两条剂量-反应曲线，计算简单、省时省力，缺点是相应比较粗，精确度较差，但此法仍是非常适用的 pA_2 估算方法。

【思考题】

1. 试述 pA_2 的定义和意义。

2. 麦氏浴槽中台氏液量的改变对 pA_2 值有何影响？

第六章　抗炎药物实验

炎症是常见的临床症状。药理研究中，常通过对实验动物人为地实施某种干扰（如给予物理性、化学性和生物性等刺激）来模拟人类炎性疾病的发生、发展和处理。但炎症过程是一个相当复杂的病理、生理过程，要制备比较完善的动物模型是相当困难的。当前，对某种药物的抗炎药理研究，主要是依据该药物在多种炎症模型中所表现的功效来综合地加以观察、分析和评价。

实验性炎症模型制作时，需从实验要求出发考虑多种因素，诸如动物的选择、致炎因子的选择、指标的选择和观察、环境因素的控制等。一般来讲，实验性炎症模型常用哺乳类动物，并根据模型差异而用不同种属的动物，如足跖肿胀模型以大鼠为宜、过敏性炎症多用豚鼠。

致炎因子种类繁多，作用机制也各不相同，但大致可归结为物理性、化学性、生物性等。理想的致炎因子应可精确定量、作用恒定、可靠、对动物个体差异小、作用持续时间长。指标的选择应是客观的，适于统计处理等，主要有肿胀度、毛细血管通透性、白细胞游走、肉芽增殖等。本章将从初步药效研究、一般机制探讨和分子机制解释等方面，简要介绍抗炎药物实验的常用方法。

实验6.1　氢化可的松对小鼠腹腔毛细血管通透性的影响

【目的】

观察糖皮质激素对腹腔毛细血管通透性的影响。

【原理】

药理剂量的糖皮质激素具有抗炎、抗毒、抗休克及抗免疫等作用。为观察其抗炎作用，可选择合适的致炎因子，在动物背部或腹部皮肤、耳郭或腹腔内造成局部炎症，然后静脉注射伊文蓝溶液（Even's blue），观察上述部位在糖皮质激素作用下，染料渗出被抑制情况，染料渗出量可通过比色法进行定量。

【材料】

小鼠10只，体重18~22g，雌雄不限。

离心机、分光光度计。

0.5%伊文蓝溶液（Even's blue用生理盐水配制）、0.5%氢化可的松、0.6%冰醋酸溶液、生理盐水。

【方法与步骤】

1. 取小鼠10只，称重后随机分为2组。甲组皮下注射0.5%氢化可的松20mg/kg，乙组皮下注射等量生理盐水。

2. 半小时后，两组小鼠均由尾静脉注射0.5%伊文蓝溶液（10ml/kg），继而腹腔内注射0.6%冰醋酸溶液（每只0.2ml）。

3. 半小时后，将小鼠脱颈椎处死，剪开腹腔。用适量生理盐水反复冲洗腹腔，合并洗涤液，使冲洗液总量达 5ml，然后 3000r/min 离心 5min。

4. 取上清液于分光光度计 590nm 波长处比色，在标准曲线上查出每只小鼠腹腔内洗涤液中的伊文蓝量（μg/ml）。按照统计要求，得出各组的均值，进行 t 检验，并以对照组（乙组）小鼠染料的渗出量为 100%，计算给药组（甲组）小鼠腹腔渗出的抑制率。

【结果处理】

按下式计算抑制率，并填写表 6 – 1 的内容。

$$抑制率 = \frac{对照组渗出量 - 给药组渗出量}{对照组渗出量} \times 100\%$$

表 6 – 1　氢化可的松对毛细血管通透性的影响

组别	鼠数	剂量 （mg/kg）	染料渗出量 （μg/ml）	抑制率
给药组				
对照组				

【注意事项】

1. 腹腔注射醋酸溶液的部位要力求一致，还应注意注入腹腔内，否则成假阴性。

2. 打开腹腔时避免损伤血管以免出血，否则血中染料大量进入腹腔影响结果。

3. 如洗涤液发生胶冻样混浊，则应弃去。

【方法评价】

1. 依据同样的原理，也可观察小鼠腹部或背部皮肤毛细血管的通透性，方法略繁，但意义相同。

2. 任何一种能引起组织损伤的物质都可成为致炎因子。因此，抑制剂的作用也是非特异的。

【思考题】

糖皮质激素抗炎作用的特点和机制是什么？

实验 6.2　吲哚美辛对小鼠巴豆油耳肿胀的影响

【目的】

掌握抗炎实验最基本方法。

【原理】

由于吲哚美辛对前列腺素合成酶具有强大的抑制作用，显著抑制前列腺素的合成和释放，故对多种因素引起的非特异性炎症均有良好的治疗作用。

【材料】

小鼠 4 只，体重 18～22g，雌雄不限。

8mm 打孔器、扭力天平。

0.5% 吲哚美辛、1% CMC 混悬液、2% 巴豆油合剂（由 2% 巴豆油、20% 无水乙醇、

73%乙醚和5%蒸馏水混合而成）。

【方法与步骤】

1. 取小鼠4只，称重，随机分为2组。甲组腹腔注射0.5%吲哚美辛（50mg/kg），乙组注射适量1%CMC混悬液（10ml/kg）。

2. 30min后，两组小鼠右耳郭两侧用微量进样器均匀涂布2%巴豆油合剂0.05ml致炎，左耳郭作对照。

3. 致炎后30min，将小鼠处死，沿耳郭基线取下两耳，用打孔器于同一部位各取一个耳片称重。致炎侧耳片重量减去对照侧耳片重量即为肿胀度。

【结果处理】

根据要求，汇集各组结果进行统计处理（参照实验6.1）。

【注意事项】

1. 环境温度不宜低于15℃，如果用二甲苯致炎，环境温度应更高些。

2. 取材力求部位一致。

3. 打孔器应锋利。

【方法评价】

本法不需特殊设备，简便易行；对两大类抗炎药物均敏感，适用于抗炎药的筛选。

【思考题】

1. 抗炎药分为哪两大类？

2. 吲哚美辛的作用特点是什么？

实验6.3 吲哚美辛对角叉菜胶诱发大鼠足跖肿胀的影响

【目的】

学习大鼠足跖肿胀常用的测定方法。

【原理】

局部应用角叉菜胶引起的炎症，前列腺素合成明显增加，并与血管活性胺类和激肽类一起诱发水肿。吲哚美辛对前列腺素为主要介质介导的炎性反应有良好的抑制作用。

【材料】

大鼠4只，体重120～150g，雄性。

外径千分尺。

0.2%吲哚美辛（用1%CMC混悬）、1%角叉菜胶（carrageenan用无菌生理盐水配制，冰箱过夜）。

【方法与步骤】

1. 取大鼠4只，随机分为用药组与对照组，用药组大鼠腹腔注射0.2%吲哚美辛（20mg/kg），对照组注射等量的CMC。

2. 30min后，用外径千分尺测量大鼠右后足跖的厚度，然后皮下注射1%角叉菜胶0.1ml致炎。

3. 致炎后30min、60min、120min、180min、240min，分别测定致炎足跖的厚度（图6-1）。

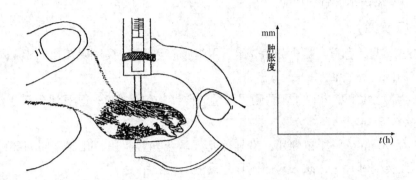

图6-1 用千分尺测量大鼠肿胀肢体厚度

【结果处理】

以致炎后减去致炎前足跖厚度为肿胀度，然后计算在某一时间的肿胀度均值与标准差，进行统计检验。以时间为横坐标，肿胀度为纵坐标，画出时程反应图。

【注意事项】

1. 1%角叉菜胶需在临用前一天配制，置4℃冰箱内贮存。

2. 测定足跖厚度的部位要一致，千分尺使用要一致。

3. 体重120~150g的大鼠对致炎剂最敏感，肿胀度高，差异性小。

【方法评价】

本法是应用最广泛的炎性水肿模型，具有差异性小、敏感和重复性高等优点，但特异性低，不少非抗炎药也有效。肿胀的测定方法除了用外径千分尺外，也有用特制软带尺测定肿胀部位周长和足跖体积。这些方法各有可取之处，目前尚无最合适的统一测定方法。用本模型所获得的某些抗炎药的效价与临床经验基本一致，故初步阳性的药物，可进一步利用本模型测定效价。

【思考题】

1. 讨论一下吲哚美辛与氢化可的松抗炎作用的区别。

2. 实验操作中应注意哪些问题？

3. 角叉菜胶诱发的水肿有双相过程，请叙述各相主要释放何物质？

实验6.4 药物对实验性胸膜炎的影响

【目的】

用在体法观察药物对白细胞游走的影响。

【原理】

当给大鼠胸腔内注射角叉菜胶后，会引起严重的胸腔内炎性渗出，大量白细胞聚集。由于胸腔渗液易于收集，且受污染少，常可用作对抗炎药物的进一步研究。

【材料】

大鼠4只，体重180~220g，雄性。

0.5%角叉菜胶、0.2%戊巴比妥钠。

【方法与步骤】

1. 取大鼠4只，随机分成用药组与对照组。

2. 抓取清醒状态下大鼠颈背部皮肤，使背部固定于掌心，胸部朝上，用75%酒精消毒右侧胸壁，在锁骨中线相当于乳房处进针，给抗炎药物（如前述的吲哚美辛或可的松）。30min后，在胸腔内注入0.5%角叉菜胶1ml致炎，然后依据药物作用的强弱及作用持续时间，决定每4h给药一次或全程只给药一次。

3. 致炎后8~12h（此时胸腔内已积聚了大量渗液），用0.2%戊巴比妥钠（40mg/kg）腹腔注射麻醉大鼠，然后剪断腹主动脉放血处死。

4. 打开胸腔，用吲哚美辛-肝素溶液湿润内壁的吸管，吸取双侧胸腔内渗液（也可直接用注射器）。

【结果处理】

准确计量内渗液后，立即作白细胞计数，渗出液涂片染色，对渗出细胞进行分类。如果将渗出液适当处理后，可进一步测定 β-葡萄糖醛酸酶活性、TXB_2 和 6-keto-PGF。

【注意事项】

1. 进针时应沿肋骨上缘刺入胸腔，进针深度以穿破胸壁肌层略深为度。

2. 遇有血性渗出物应弃去。

【方法评价】

1. 两类抗炎药对炎性渗出都有作用。

2. 甾体类抗炎药抑制细胞移行的作用较强。

3. 该法要求操作熟练、准确。

4. 该法主要适用于经初筛有效药物的进一步研究。

【思考题】

比较两类抗炎药对炎性渗出作用异同。

第七章　化学治疗药物实验

1908 年 Ehrlich 首先提出化学治疗这一概念，凡对体内、体外病原体或寄生物具有杀灭或抑制其生长繁殖的药物，皆属化学治疗这一范畴，但只有对病原体或寄生物发挥作用，而对人体无显著毒性的药物，才能在临床上作为全身性化学治疗药。

百浪多息在试管中并无抗链球菌的作用，它在体内可分解为对氨基苯磺酰胺（又称磺胺）而有抗菌活性。受此启发，一系列磺胺衍生物相继合成，使许多全身性感染得到了控制，也开辟了许多药理学新的领域。1928 年，英国细菌学家亚历山大·弗莱明在研究葡萄球菌的形态时，实验平板意外地被青霉菌污染。而青霉菌周围的葡萄球菌被溶解这一现象引起了他的兴趣和关注。这导致了青霉素的发现。由于青霉素疗效高、毒性小，许多研究工作者将注意力转移到抗生素研究上。目前，在防治感染性疾病中，抗生素占有极为重要的地位。Domagk 对磺胺的合成，Fleming 对青霉素的发现，Waksman 对链霉素的分离成功，开创了药物发展史上的黄金时期。因为他们的突出贡献，三人分别在 1939 年、1945 年、1952 年获诺贝尔奖。

恶性肿瘤是目前危害人类健康最严重的一类疾病，全世界每年死于癌症者在六百万人以上。近半个世纪以来，世界各国投入了大量人力、物力，开展抗癌药物的研究。目前研究较成熟的抗癌药物已达 310 种以上，肿瘤治疗已从姑息治疗法向根治过渡。但目前突出的问题是抗癌药物毒性太大、选择性太差，这使肿瘤依然是人类面临的最难攻克的顽症之一。征服肿瘤成为人们的共同愿望和摆在药物研究人员面前的艰巨任务。

一、抗菌药物实验

观察一种物质是否具有抗菌作用，一般先用体外法初筛，获得阳性结果后再以体内法进行复证。

（一）体外法

测定药物的抑菌能力常用的有两大类方法：琼脂渗透法与试管稀释法。

1. 琼脂渗透法　琼脂渗透法是将试验菌混入琼脂培养基，然后倾注成平板；或将试验菌涂于琼脂平板的表面，再用不同的方法将药物置于已含试验菌的琼脂平板上，利用药物能渗透至琼脂培养基的性能，经适宜温度培养后观察结果，判断药物对试验菌是否有作用，也有将药物直接混入琼脂培养基中，然后接种试验菌的。

根据加药的操作方法不同有滤纸片法、打洞法、纸条法、挖沟法、管碟法和平板稀释法。其中滤纸片法、纸条法、挖沟法用于定性测定，管碟法和平板稀释法用于定量测定，而打洞法则可根据使用的具体情况来确定是用于定性测定或定量测定。

（1）定性测定方法

1）滤纸片法：先在无菌平皿内加入已经熔化的肉汤琼脂培养基，待其凝固作为底层。再取适量已熔化的肉汤琼脂培养基，冷至 50℃左右，加入一定量的试验菌液，摇匀后取 4～5ml 铺在底层之上，即为上层，待其凝固。用无菌滤纸片沾取药液贴在培养基表面，放于适宜的温度下培养一定的时间，取出观察结果（图7-1）。

此种方法的最大特点是测定方便、迅速、样品量大，在同一个含菌平皿内同时能测定多个样品，最适用于药物的初筛。即一菌多药。

应注意选择对测定样品敏感的菌作为试验菌。在制备含菌平板时，应该控制好试验菌的浓度和琼脂的温度。

2）挖沟法和纸条法：先制备好无菌琼脂平板，然后在平板的中央挖一沟槽，将各种试验菌分别接种在沟槽的两侧，每种菌之间应间隔一定的距离，然后将待测的样品加入中央的沟槽中，放于37℃培养，18~24h后取出观察结果（图7-2）。纸条法与挖沟法相似，只是将挖沟法中的中央沟槽换成含有药液的纸条即可。

此种方法的。最大特点是能快速地检测出一种药物的抗菌谱，即一药多菌。

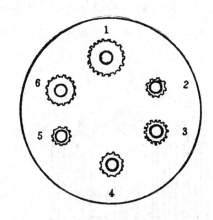

图7-1 用平皿内杯管法或挖孔法或贴纸片
法筛选抗菌药物

注：内圈为杯管或挖孔域纸片，外圈为抑菌圈

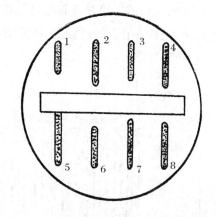

图7-2 用平皿内挖沟法或贴纸条法筛选
抗菌药物

注：中间为加药沟或加药滤纸条，两侧为以
划线法接种的8种细菌经过培养后的生长情况

（2）定量测定方法　采用平皿稀释法。将药物按倍比稀释法用无菌生理盐水稀释，即按1:2、1:4、1:8……等稀释成各种药物浓度，然后取各种稀释度的药液（每个平皿取2ml）于无菌平皿内，加入冷至50℃左右的MH培养基（每个平皿取18ml），摇匀，放置冷却备用，药物的最终稀释浓度为1:20，1:40，1:80……

试验菌液的制备：将各种试验用菌接种于定量分装的MH肉汤培养基中（特殊菌除外，如肺炎双球菌、链球菌等），于适宜的温度培养8~10h，取出按一定的比例稀释（在1:100~1:1000之间）。稀释前应该用麦氏比浊管进行比浊，菌浓度应在10^8~10^9CFU，然后再进行稀释，备用。特殊菌培养时需加少量血清（兔血清、羊血清均可）。

将各稀释好的菌液接种于含药平板上，接种量为2μl，此时活菌数最终为10^3~10^4CFU，放于37℃培养18~24h，取出观察各稀释度平皿的细菌生长情况，记录不长菌的最高稀释度即为试验药物对受试细菌的最低抑菌浓度（MIC）。

平皿稀释法所获得的结果准确性高、速度快，出现假阳性的机会少，不易出现跳管现象，能够直观反应细菌的生长情况和药物的作用效果。此法能一药多菌地进行试验，节省药物和培养基。根据目前对抗生素的报批要求，使用这种方法是非常合理而又简便的方法。因此，目前被广泛地应用在抗生素的体外抗菌活性的测定中。

目前，在化疗药物的新药审批中，要求愈来愈严格，体外抗菌活性测定的试验用菌要求必须是临床分离的菌株，并对实验菌的数量和种类都做出了明确的规定。对一类新药必须要做 1000 菌株以上，而且种类必须在 20 种以上。对二类新药必须要做 500 菌株以上，种类必须在 20 种以上。对三类及四类新药必须要做 200 菌株以上，种类必须在 20 种以上。这样，就能够显示出平皿稀释法的优越性，该方法是新药审批中药效学体外抗菌活性测定的规定方法。本法试验用菌必须是对数生长期的，因该时期的细菌对药物作用最为敏感，试验菌的浓度亦应该掌握好，否则会影响结果。

【附】MH 培养基：即为水解酪蛋白琼脂培养基，该培养基为国际通用培养基。

2. **试管稀释法** 将药物按倍比稀释法与肉汤培养基混匀成 1∶2，1∶4，1∶8……等各种浓度，取各种浓度的含药培养基 2ml 于无菌小试管中，各加入 0.1ml 经 1～1000 稀释的对数生长期敏感菌液，混匀，并以一管不加药物作为阳性对照，另一管不加菌液也不加药物作为阴性对照（目的：检查培养基是否被细菌污染）。置 37℃ 培养箱培养 24h 后取出观察结果，记录各管内细菌生长情况，以澄清不长菌的最高稀释度这一数值作为试验药物的抑菌效价（MIC）（图 7－3）。

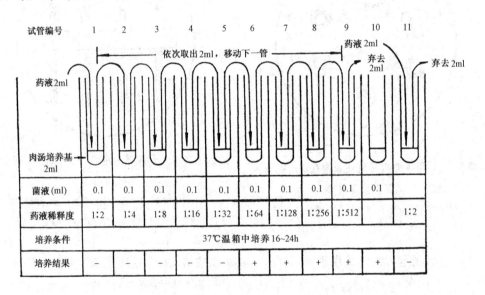

图 7－3　以试管内药液逐级稀释法测定药物的抑菌效价示例

此种方法操作较烦、工作量大、培养基多，易出现假阴性结果和跳管现象，影响结果的准确性。

【附】常用培养基的制备法

1. **肉浸液** 取新鲜牛肉，除去肌腱及脂肪，绞碎后，每 1000g 加水 3000ml，充分搅匀。在 2～10℃ 浸泡 20～24h 后，煮沸 1h，滤过，压干肉渣，补足液量，15 磅高压灭菌 20min 后冷藏备用。也可用牛肉浸膏 3g，加水 1000ml，配成溶液代替。

2. **肉汤培养基** 取蛋白胨 10g，氯化钠 5g，加入肉浸液 1000ml。微温溶解后用 0.1mol/L 氢氧化钠溶液调节 pH 为 7.6，煮沸 10min，冷却、滤过后 15 磅高压灭菌 20min。

3. **肉汤琼脂培养基** 取蛋白胨 10g，氯化钠 5g，琼脂 20g，加入肉浸液 1000ml，加热融化后滤过，调节 pH 为 7.6，15 磅高压灭菌 20min。

（二）体内法

在体外实验中呈现抗菌作用的药物可能由于毒性较大或与蛋白质结合及生物转化等原

因，在体内发挥不出抗菌效果。所以在体外实验中有效的药物须进一步了解它对感染动物是否有效。如果在体内也有效，且毒性不大，才有可能过渡到临床。

1. 菌液制备　以保存的典型菌种或临床分离的致病菌，挑选毒力强，对已知药物较敏感的菌株，移种于液体培养基，37℃培养，以供动物感染之用。

2. 动物感染　根据菌种的致病力选用实验动物。常用 20g 左右的小鼠，腹腔注射菌液进行感染。菌液的注射量应造成 90% 左右的实验小鼠死亡率。小鼠对金黄色葡萄球菌和痢疾杆菌不敏感，在这些菌液中添加适量胃黏液素可提高致病力。

3. 分组给药　将感染小鼠分成数组，除一组留作对照，其余各组均以待试药物治疗。药物的剂量应不超过小鼠的最大耐受量。一般在感染接种后 1h、6h、12h 各以灌胃法或注射法给药一次，也可在感染接种前预先给药。

4. 结果判断　通常于感染接种后 72h 清点各组死亡小鼠数，并作统计处理。如果治疗组小鼠的死亡率显著小于对照组，即说明该药有效，可考虑用其他动物进行复证并作有关的药理试验。

实验 7.1　诺氟沙星、氧氟沙星及环丙沙星的体外抗菌活性测定

【目的】

了解用平皿稀释法和纸片法试验药物抗菌作用的步骤，观察药物不同浓度对抗菌作用的影响，了解平皿稀释法的操作过程和实验结果的判断。

【原理】

诺氟沙星、氧氟沙星及环丙沙星属于第三代喹诺酮类合成抗菌药物，该类药物具有抗菌谱广、高效、不良反应少的特点，特别是对铜绿假单胞菌等厌氧菌有强大抗菌力。其主要能与 DNA 回旋酶亚基 A 结合，从而抑制了酶的切割与联结功能，阻止 DNA 的复制而呈现抗菌作用。

【材料】

已培养 16~18h 的金黄色葡萄球菌（或大肠埃希菌）菌液。

MH 琼脂培养基、无菌平皿、无菌滤纸片（直径 0.5cm）、镊子、无菌试管、无菌吸管（5ml）、微量移液器、肉汤培养基、卡尺。

80μg/ml 的诺氟沙星、氧氟沙星、环丙沙星、无菌生理盐水。

（一）纸片法

【方法与步骤】

1. 将灭菌平皿底面向上，在底面上划三条放射线，均分为 6 等分，标上 1~6 号。

2. 用无菌吸管定量吸取试验菌液 0.1ml，加于 100ml 保温于 45℃ 的琼脂培养基中，摇匀，倾注于无菌平皿中，待其冷凝后备用。

3. 无菌生理盐水将药物稀释成各种浓度，按倍比稀释的方法，稀释好备用。

4. 用镊子分别取无菌滤纸片，分别沾取不同浓度的药液，然后按划好的位置贴在含菌的平板上。

5. 将培养皿置 37℃ 培养箱中培养，24h 后观察结果。用卡尺测定每张滤纸片周围的抑菌圈的直径（mm）。

【结果处理】

按表 7 – 1 做记录。

表 7 – 1　药物的体外抗菌活性测定结果（纸片法）

纸片号码	1	2	3	4	5	6
含有药液种类及浓度						
抑菌圈直径（mm）						

【注意事项】

1. 制备含菌平板时，琼脂须保温，动作要敏捷，否则易凝块不均一。

2. 在贴放滤纸片时，纸片间必须保持一定的距离，并事先在平皿底部的适当位置上注明号码。

3. 尽量使滤纸片上的药量均匀一致，否则会给实验结果带来误差。

【方法评价】

本法最大的特点是测定方便、迅速、样品数多。在同一个含金黄色葡萄球菌平皿内，同时测定诺氟沙星、氧氟沙星和环丙沙星，甚至更多的样品，能做到一菌多药筛试。

【思考题】

1. 试验药物抗菌作用的滤纸片法适用于哪些情况？

2. 试从本次实验的结果中比较几种喹诺酮类药物的作用强弱。

（二）平皿稀释法

【方法与步骤】

1. 将经 12h 培养的菌液进行稀释（1∶100），摇匀备用。

2. 将药物按倍比稀释的方法用无菌生理盐水进行稀释：1∶1、1∶2、1∶4、1∶8……

3. 将不同浓度药物加入无菌平皿中（每个平皿 2ml），然后将冷至 50℃ 左右的 MH 培养基加入（每个平皿 18ml），摇匀，最终浓度为 1∶10、1∶20、1∶40、1∶80，待凝，备用。

4. 用微量移液器吸取各菌液 2μl 加到平板上，淌匀放置 20min 后，于 37℃ 培养箱中培养 18～24h，取出观察结果，记录不长菌的最高稀释度作为 MIC 值。

【结果处理】

按表 7 – 2 做好记录。

表 7 – 2　药物的体外抗菌活性测定结果（平皿稀释法）

药物＼浓度	1	2	3	4	5	6	7
1							
2							
3							

【注意事项】

1. 当 MH 培养基加入平皿后，必须充分摇匀，速度要快，否则会凝固，造成药物分散不均匀。

2. 使用的试验菌液必须是对数生长期的敏感菌。

3. 实验必须要做对照组。

4. 放置平皿的台面和温箱台面应校正水平。

【方法评价】

平皿稀释法目前广泛地应用在抗生素的抗菌活性的体外筛选和测定中。方法简便、合理，准确性高，速度快，假阳性少，能直观反应细菌生长情况和药物作用效果。

【思考题】

讨论一下诺氟沙星的抗菌原理。

实验 7.2　诺氟沙星对小鼠体内感染的保护性实验

【目的】

了解细菌感染实验的治疗方法的基本过程，掌握药效学体内测定的基本方法，并观察诺氟沙星对感染小鼠的疗效。

【材料】

小鼠 12 只，体重 18 ~ 20g，雌雄不限。

注射器、天平、苦味酸、菌液、鼠笼、消毒棉花。

生理盐水、诺氟沙星药液（3mg/kg）、2.5% 碘酒、70% 酒精、用 5% 胃膜素稀释的大肠埃希菌菌液。

【方法与步骤】

1. 取小鼠 12 只，标号、称重，分成 6 组，每组 2 只，5 组给药，1 组对照。

2. 药物的浓度确定：以所给药物的浓度作为中间剂量，按 1 : 0.7 的比例，向上推两个剂量，也向下推两个剂量，组成 5 个剂量组，对照组为生理盐水。给每只小鼠腹腔注射菌液 0.5ml，在给菌液后，立即灌胃给药，按体重折算，一次性给完。然后观察 72h，记录小鼠的死亡情况。

【结果处理】

算出死亡率，以统计学的方法算出 ED_{50}。

【注意事项】

1. 试验所用药的浓度必须要预试，试出恰当的浓度后再进行试验。所用试验菌必须是临床新分离的而且毒性较强的菌。

2. 试验菌必须用胃膜素进行保护，否则影响实验结果。

3. 药物浓度的确定必须严格，不应随意改变，量要给足，否则影响结果。

4. 动物的体重必须严格，否则影响实验结果。

5. 实验中带菌动物应严加管理，严禁逃逸发生。实验结束后，动物的尸体应焚化或放入置有 5% 的碳酸液缸内，活的动物应立即处死并处理掉，处理完毕必须用碘酒与酒精擦干，用肥皂洗手，以防传播疾病。所有带菌液器材均须灭菌处理。

【方法评价】

体外实验有效是体内实验的前提，体内实验有效是过渡临床的基础。一旦对感染小鼠有强大的保护作用，再用其他动物进行复证，并作进一步的药理毒理试验，证明其抗菌作用强、毒性小。这样，有可能研制出一个新的抗菌药物。因此，感染的保护性试验是关键性的一个环节。该法可靠、重复性高，能客观地反应药物的效果。

【思考题】

1. 细菌感染的实验治疗包括哪些基本步骤，应如何进行？

2. 在本实验中能否肯定诺氟沙星对小鼠大肠杆菌感染的疗效？有何根据？

二、抗肿瘤药物实验

抗肿瘤药物的筛选方法繁多，大体上分为体内法与体外法两类。每种方法各有其优缺点，用某一种方法难以肯定药物的抗癌作用。当受试样品数量少时，可先以药物对细胞系体外培养的生长抑制作用作为初筛，选用人癌细胞株作初筛可能找出对该癌有效的药物。体外实验只能用于初筛，必须经过动物体内实验才能判断药物的抗癌作用。

（一）体内法

动物移植性肿瘤实验法是最常用的方法，比自发性及诱发性动物肿瘤更易于实行。该方法可在同一时间内获得大量生长相当均匀的肿瘤，以供给药及对照之用。但移植性动物肿瘤与人癌生物学特点有较大差距，动物肿瘤恶性度高，生长迅速，对药物敏感性较人癌高得多，且该方法命中率较低。

目前常用的动物实验瘤株可分腹水癌、肉瘤及白血病三类。国内曾主张用 S_{180}（小鼠肉瘤180）、艾氏癌腹水型和 L_{615} 白血病。美国国立癌症研究所（NCI）几年前推荐采用 P_{388}（白血病）、L_{1210}（白血病）、W_{256}（大鼠瓦克癌肉瘤）、B_{16}（黑色素瘤）、C_{038}（结肠癌）、3LL（Lewis 肺癌）。

用一种模型去筛选各种不同类型的新药显然是不恰当的，各种动物移植瘤对药物的敏感性不一样。筛选烷化剂，可选用瓦克癌肉瘤258、吉田肉瘤；筛选抗代谢物时，可选用肉瘤180、L_{615} 以及 L_{1210}；从天然产物中寻找新抗肿瘤药物可选用 P_{388}、L_{615}、艾氏癌腹水型、U_{14} 等。

（二）体外法

以人或动物肿瘤细胞的短期和长期培养作为筛选系统，来观察药物的抗肿瘤作用，具有方法简便、用药量少、获得结果快、能大量筛选等优点。但体外法脱离了机体的整体性，不能反映出药效、毒性和机体代谢各方面之间的相互关系，常有假阳性和假阴性，所以体外实验必须配合体内实验。体外实验的主要方法有：

1. 接触染色法 动物的腹水癌细胞稀释液加药以后，被杀死的癌细胞因膜的通透性改变，可在37℃ 24h 内，被台盼蓝染色，而活的癌细胞则不能被染色。可在显微镜下进行鉴别计数，染色率达到50%以上者为初筛有效。

2. 亚甲蓝还原法 肿瘤细胞内含脱氢酶，该酶可使底物脱氢，将氢传递给亚甲蓝，亚甲蓝被还原而褪色。如肿瘤细胞被药物杀死，则脱氢酶活性消失，亚甲蓝就不能褪色。此法简单易行，但正常细胞也有脱氢酶，故并无特异性。

3. **呼吸抑制法** 用组织呼吸仪测定药物对肿瘤细胞需氧代谢抑制率，抑制率达到50%以上者为初筛有效。

4. **组织培养法** 将动物细胞（特别是人体肿瘤细胞人工培养后），加入一定量的药物，观察该药对细胞生长的影响、细胞的数量及形态变化。

此外，也有用精原细胞、噬菌体等非肿瘤系统来筛选抗肿瘤药物。

实验7.3 抗肿瘤药的亚甲蓝试管法初筛

【目的】

了解抗肿瘤药的一种体外初筛方法——亚甲蓝试管法。

【原理】

脱氢酶的活力与癌细胞的功能有关，抗癌药物抑制或杀灭癌细胞时，往往引起脱氢酶活力的降低或消失，可利用亚甲蓝作为指示剂而显示出来。当癌细胞处于活动状态时，其脱氢酶能把氢转给亚甲蓝，使其褪色。如果癌细胞死亡，则酶失活，亚甲蓝不能被还原，继续保持蓝色。以此可初步判定药物有无抑制癌细胞的作用。

【材料】

艾氏腹水癌（EAC）小鼠1~2只，体重、性别不限。

无菌试管、无菌吸管、恒温箱。

1%及10% 5-氟尿嘧啶（5-FU）溶液、0.05%亚甲蓝溶液，待试药物溶液。

肿瘤细胞培养液（内含0.8% NaCl，0.02% KCl，0.02% $CaCl_2$，0.01% $MgCl_2$，0.05% $NaHCO_3$，0.005% NaH_2PO_4；0.1%葡萄糖，pH 7.0~7.5），各种药液均须经过灭菌。

【方法与步骤】

1. 取接种已达8~10天的艾氏腹水癌小鼠，以无菌操作抽取腹水5ml，按1:2的比例用肿瘤细胞培养液加以稀释。

2. 取无菌试管8支，各加肿瘤细胞培养液0.75ml，1:2腹水稀释液0.25ml。然后分别加入下列物质各0.1ml：肿瘤细胞培养液2管（对照），1%及10% 5-FU溶液各2管，待试药物的溶液2管，置37℃恒温箱中保温。4h后每管再加0.05%亚甲蓝溶液0.2ml，继续37℃保温。于2h、4h、8h、12h、24h后观察各管的颜色深浅，并作记录。

【结果处理】

记录各管中先后所加物质及保温后各个时间溶液的颜色深度，根据实验结果对所试药物的作用得出结论。

【注意事项】

1. 如无艾氏腹水癌小鼠，可以任何人或动物的新鲜无菌肿瘤细胞悬液代替。

2. 检查各管的褪色程度不能振摇，以防亚甲蓝分子被氧化而出现颜色。

3. 艾氏腹水癌腹水液应呈乳白色，如已呈粉色，表明沾有许多红细胞，血性严重，不宜使用。为抽取方便，可先将无菌稀释液注入腹腔冲洗后再吸出，并可将从几只小鼠腹中抽出的悬液混合使用。

【方法评价】

1. 亚甲蓝试管法具有简便、快速等优点，但该法只能用来初步筛选，要确定药物的抗肿瘤作用须通过动物移植性肿瘤等体内实验法。

2. 本法易受氧化剂或还原剂影响而出现假阳性或假阴性的结果，因此需另设对照管。

【思考题】

1. 筛选药物如是氧化剂或还原剂应如何进行？

2. 亚甲蓝还原法与台盼蓝接触染色法有何不同，各有何优缺点？

实验 7.4　5 – Fu 对小鼠肉瘤 S_{180} 的实验治疗

【目的】

了解抗肿瘤药物的体内筛选方法，初步认识 5 – Fu（5 – 氟尿嘧啶）的抗癌活性。

【原理】

以小鼠肉瘤 S_{180} 为实验模型，给予一定剂量有抗癌活性的药物，可以抑制肿瘤的生长；以瘤重抑制率评价该药的抗癌活性。

【材料】

小鼠 20 只，体重 18 ~ 20g，接种 S_{180} 瘤源并饲养 10 ~ 12 天的小鼠 1 只。

组织匀浆器、解剖剪、眼科弯镊、培养皿、注射器、烧杯、棉球（上述器材均须灭菌）、搪瓷盘、蜡盘、小天平。

0.25% 5 – FU 溶液、灭菌生理盐水、碘酒、70% 乙醇溶液。

【方法与步骤】

1. **制备供接种用的肿瘤细胞悬液**　将已接种并饲养 10 ~ 12 天的 S_{180} 瘤源小鼠拉断脊椎处死，腹面向上固定于蜡盘上。依次以碘酒、酒精消毒肿瘤部位及其周围皮肤。于灭菌室内以无菌操作剖取肿瘤。正常肿瘤组织呈粉红色，略有弹性，含丰富血管。瘤块中心常有坏死，呈灰白色。用消毒手术剪剪取粉红色的良好肿瘤组织，用生理盐水洗去血污，移至一培养皿中称重，然后剪碎，以每克肿瘤组织 3ml 的比例加入灭菌生理盐水，于组织匀浆器中小心研磨，制成均一的细胞悬液，加盖置冰箱中保存备用。悬液颜色以乳白色略带粉色为宜，若红色较深，表示带入血液过多，质量不佳。

2. **接种小鼠**　接种时左手抓住小鼠的头背部，用碘酒、酒精消毒右前肢腋下部位皮肤后，右手持已吸取肿瘤细胞悬液的注射器，刺入腋下皮下组织（刺入后可轻轻摆动针头验证是否在皮下部位），注入悬液 0.2ml。

3. **分组给药**　接种 24h 后将小鼠编号，随机分为两组，对照组与治疗组各 10 只。治疗组腹腔注射 0.25% 5 – FU（0.25mg/10g），每天 1 次，连续 10 ~ 14 天，对照组腹腔注射生理盐水 0.1ml/10g。给药期间注意观察小鼠有无排稀便、拒食等现象，如有异常应减量给药或暂停给药，疗程结束时动物体重下降不应超过 15%。

4. **结果观察**　疗程结束后次日，小鼠逐个称重；脱颈椎处死，剖取肿瘤称重，检查肿瘤有无坏死、感染等情况。

【结果处理】

按表 7 – 3 记录实验结果，分别算出对照组与治疗组的平均瘤重，并按下式计算瘤重抑制率。

表 7 – 3　5 – FU 对小鼠肉瘤 S_{180} 的实验治疗结果

组别	接种日期	药物剂量和疗程	动物数		平均体重		平均瘤重	瘤重抑制率	平均瘤重差异的显著性
			开始	结束	开始	结束			
治疗组									
对照组									

$$瘤重抑制率 = \frac{对照组平均瘤重 - 治疗组平均瘤重}{对照组平均瘤重} \times 100\%$$

所得结果均应进行相应的统计学处理。

【注意事项】

1. 接种肿瘤的全过程应注意严密消毒及无菌操作，以免因感染而干扰肿瘤生长。

2. 剥取瘤块时，应将周围正常组织除去。

3. 对照组平均瘤块重应大于 1g。瘤重最小者亦应在 0.4g 以上，否则应弃去不计。

4. 本实验需重复三次以验证其可靠性，抑制率高于 30% 者，可考虑进一步扩大瘤谱或进行其他药理研究。

5. 接种时动作要快，整个操作应在 30min 内完成。

【方法评价】

S_{180} 肿瘤移植实验法成功率较高，较自发及诱发的动物肿瘤更易进行，假阳性及假阴性出现机会少。该方法从整体水平筛选抗癌新药，可同时观测药品的抗癌效力及动物对该药的综合反应，较体外实验更具可靠性。

【思考题】

1. 解剖荷瘤动物时，如何区分正常肿瘤组织和坏死组织？选取何种组织接种？为什么？

2. 给荷瘤动物用药期间应注意哪些问题？

3. 给小鼠接种肿瘤整个过程为什么要严密消毒？

实验 7.5　小鼠（裸鼠）肾被膜下人癌细胞移植法

【目的】

通过实验了解将人体肿瘤移植于动物体内（小鼠肾囊膜下）的方法，并利用它来筛选有效化合物。

【原理】

将人癌细胞（为抗原）移植入裸鼠体内，观察短期内（6 ~ 11 天）肿瘤生长规则。此法免受宿主免疫活性差异的影响，不致引起体液和细胞免疫反应，故接种能够成功。肾囊膜下营养丰富，适合癌细胞生长；肾被膜透明，便于镜下测量肿块大小，故人体癌细胞可以移植于小鼠肾被膜。

【材料】

裸鼠或 BDF_1、CDF_1 小鼠 12 只，体重 18 ~ 22g，雌雄不限。

人新鲜瘤组织（如肺癌、乳腺癌等瘤块）。

体视显微镜、手术刀、解剖剪、眼科镊、12 号或 18 号胸骨穿刺针、缝针缝线、烧杯。

0.2% 环磷酰胺、乙醚、碘酒、酒精。

【方法与步骤】

1. 在灭菌条件下取新鲜人瘤组织，剪去包膜及出血坏死部分，切成 1mm 小块。

2. 选用健康裸鼠或 BDF_1、CDF_1 小鼠，吸入乙醚麻醉。在其侧背部手术部位用碘酒及 70% 酒精消毒后，打开腹腔暴露左肾。

3. 将一小块瘤组织用眼科镊挟取放入 12 号或 18 号胸骨穿刺针针尖内，将穿刺针插入肾被膜下，将瘤块植入。用装有显微标尺 100 格（$0\mu m \sim 100\mu m = 1mm$）的体视显微镜观测植块的长径和短径，测毕，缝上切口。

4. 接种次日，将小鼠随机分成两组，对照组 6 只，给药组 6 只。给药组每鼠腹腔注射 0.2% 环磷酰胺 0.2ml，每天 1 次，共 5 天。第 6 天处死小鼠，切除带瘤肾脏，用体视显微镜测量瘤径大小（裸鼠给药 10 天，第 11 天处死）。

【结果处理】

$$瘤体积 = \frac{长径 \times 短径^2 （mm）}{2}$$

测得各鼠瘤体积（mm^3）和重量（g），求每组的平均瘤体积 ± 标准差，按下式计算抑制率：

$$肿瘤抑制率 = \frac{对照组平均瘤体积 - 给药组平均瘤体积}{对照组平均瘤体积} \times 100\%$$

根据瘤重计算抑制率：

$$抑制率 = \frac{治疗组平均瘤重（T）}{对照组平均瘤重（C）} \times 100\%$$

【注意事项】

1. 国内评定疗效标准仍以 T/C% ≤ 60% ~ 70% 且经 t 检验与对照组有显著差异者为阳性药，并经 3 次重复有效才能肯定疗效。

2. 严格无菌操作，瘤源应作细菌培养，有污染应立即中止实验。

3. 从手术取得的人瘤组织须在摘取后 4h 内接种完毕。

4. 植入瘤块长短径应在 9 ~ 120μm 范围内。

5. 穿刺肾被膜动作要轻，以免刺伤肾脏，小鼠出血而死。

【方法评价】

小鼠肾囊膜下移植法疗效评价客观、敏感、可靠、重复性高。移植肿块来自人体，较其他肿瘤如 S_{180} 等更能反映人体肿瘤特点，筛选的抗癌新药针对性强。本法缺点是裸鼠等动物价格昂贵，且不能长期给药用来筛选慢性抗癌药物。

【思考题】

1. 小鼠肾囊膜下移植法为什么不能长期给药筛选慢性药？

2. 为什么要以肾囊膜作为肿瘤移植部位？

第八章 避孕药物实验

实行计划生育是我国的一项国策。20世纪60年代初甾体避孕药问世，并得到了广泛应用。长期的临床实践表明，甾体避孕药的避孕效果确切，安全性较高，为其他节育方法所不及。人们把甾体避孕药的诞生称为一次重大的科学、医学和社会学上的革命。然而，人口增长依然没有得到有效控制，寻找安全、有效、方便的避孕药仍旧是药学工作者的重要目标之一。

女用避孕药的最基本筛选方法是抗生育实验，即在与雄性动物合笼期间，给雌性动物用药，观察对生育的影响。此外，还可用抗着床、抗早孕、抗排卵实验等方法，检查药物对雄性动物生育过程中各特定阶段的影响。

一、抗生育实验

1. **短效药物**　取雌性小鼠或大鼠，一般每组10只。给药组动物给药3天（化学药品）或5天（植物药制剂），然后与雄鼠合笼，每2只雌鼠配1只雄鼠，合笼期间继续给药。合笼12~14天后取出雌鼠，剖腹检查各组动物怀孕百分率，记录每只孕鼠的胚胎数，并注意有无死胎。对照组动物只给水或溶剂，其余处理均与给药组相同。结果用统计方法进行分析（图8-1）。

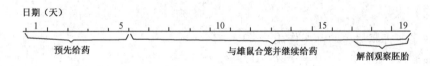

图8-1　短效女用抗生育药实验程序示意

2. **长效药物**　实验动物预先给药一次。3天后与雄鼠合笼，直到雌鼠生育。自合笼后第19天开始每天检查和记录有小鼠者及仔鼠数，计算雌鼠自合笼至生育的天数。给药组与对照组相差的天数即为避孕时间。实验结果作统计分析，抗生育实验中如对照组的生育率不及70%，结果不可靠。

在抗生育实验中需注意有无体重减轻，如体重减轻应考虑到药物的毒性作用。如初筛有效，则再降低剂量，重复实验。应每天检查阴栓（小鼠交配后，精液在雌鼠阴道中凝固为白色栓塞）。如出现阴栓，说明已交配过。检查大鼠有无交配，除观察或寻找阴栓外，尚可用浸湿了生理盐水的棉签拭阴道，涂片后在显微镜下查找精子，以了解药物对性行为的影响。

二、抗着床实验

将大鼠或小鼠合笼后，每日上午检查雌鼠有无阴栓，将出现阴栓的雌鼠取出，连续检查5~7天。将出现阴栓的雌鼠分组，一般每组10只。于出现阴栓后的1~5天期间，每日给药一次，于出现阴栓后第12天将动物剖杀，记录两例子宫内的胚胎数及怀孕的百分率。

实验结果用统计方法进行分析（图 8-2）。

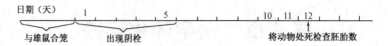

图 8-2　抗着床实验程序示意

此项实验，由于动物出现阴栓的日期不一致，因而各组动物，甚至同一组的动物，给药和处理的日期都不尽相同，只能按期分批处理。

三、抗早孕实验

方法同抗着床实验。一般于出现阴栓后第 6~9 天连续给药 4 天，第 12 天处死动物，检查胚胎数及死胎情况。如经重复实验均出现阳性结果，可减少给药天数，进行实验。如果观察长效药物，于出现阴栓后第 6 天给药 1 次即可（图 8-3）。

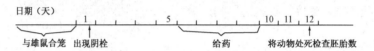

图 8-3　抗早孕实验程序示意

注：在抗生育、抗着床和抗早孕实验中最常用的动物为 28~35g 的壮年小鼠，也可用体重 200~250g 的壮年大鼠。

实验 8.1　炔诺酮的抗排卵作用 （交配法）

【目的】

观察炔诺酮抑制雌兔的排卵作用。

【原理】

家兔为诱发排卵、交配，静脉注射硫酸铜、醋酸铜或葡萄糖酸铜均可诱发排卵，以平均排卵点为效应的指标，与药物剂量之间呈指函数关系。以对照组排卵点为 100%，计算用药组排卵抑制率。求得排卵抑制率为 50% 的剂量（ED_{50}），可以定量比较药物对排卵抑制的作用强度。

【材料】

家兔，体重 2~3kg，雌雄各 2 只。

兔灌胃器、镊子、注射器、小烧杯、剪刀。

苯甲酸雌二醇注射液（1mg/ml）、炔诺酮混悬液（25μg/ml）、生理盐水。

【方法与步骤】

取预先分笼饲养 3 周的健康雌兔 2 只（经阴道涂片检查证实在动情期，即大部分为角化细胞者）。在交配前 36h 皮下注射苯甲酸雌二醇 100μg 可增加交配率。甲兔灌胃给予炔诺酮混悬液（炔诺酮 0.25mg/kg），乙兔以同法给予生理盐水，作为对照。给药 12h 后，使甲、乙两兔各与一只雄兔合笼。合笼后 24h 将 2 只雌兔处死。剖腹检查两侧卵巢有无排卵点（兔卵巢在排卵后滤泡上遗留有小突起，突起的顶端有一鲜红色小点，即排卵点。暗红色的突起或没有红点的突起都不是排卵点。正常家兔一般每次排卵 1~10 个），记录其结果。

【结果处理】

综合全实验室的结果，比较给药组与对照组排卵情况的不同。

$$抑制排卵率 = \left(1 - \frac{给药组平均排卵点}{对照组平均排卵点}\right) \times 100\%$$

【注意事项】

1. 家兔的发情交配有季节性，春季的交配率可达75%以上。将雌兔移至雄兔笼中比将雄兔移至雌兔笼中容易引起交配。

2. 如无炔诺酮纯品，可用口服避孕片1号代替，该种制剂每片含炔诺酮625μg、炔雌醇35μg，其剂量按其中含有的炔诺酮折算。

3. 兔灌胃给药时，注意勿将尿导管插入气管中，给药前导管一端放入盛有水的烧杯中，如无气泡方可注入药物。

【方法评价】

本法通过交配法观察炔诺酮的排卵作用。实验方法简便，实验结果可靠，数据重现性好。本法亦可用于避孕药物的研究。

【思考题】

1. 口服避孕药除了抑制排卵外，还可以影响其他哪些环节？
2. 试述口服避孕药的作用原理。

第九章　抗衰老药物实验

衰老是生物体内各组织、器官的退行性变化及许多病理、生理过程综合作用的结果。抗衰老药是一类从机体物质和能量代谢出发，在组织器官、细胞及分子水平上延缓各种退行性变化，提高生物活力，延长寿命的药物。迄今为止，有关衰老的学说不下数十种，类似临床衰老症状的动物模型及抗衰老药研究的实验方法也很多，本章根据一些主要的衰老学说，从物质代谢、免疫功能状态、中枢神经系统等方面介绍一些常用的抗衰老药物研究实验方法。当然这些方法仅仅反映了衰老的某一过程或某一指标，不能因为某些药物对某种衰老模型或某个指标有效就认为是抗衰老药，而要通过多种模型、多种指标进行综合评价。

一、自由基学说

衰老的自由基学说是当前衰老生化研究中极为活跃的学说。机体代谢过程中发生的氧化还原反应所形成的自由基可与核酸、蛋白质、脂质等发生反应，生成相应的氧化物或过氧化物。当组成生物膜的脂质被氧化生成过氧化物时，可使生物膜通透性改变，细胞膜发生破裂分解，造成细胞代谢和功能形态的改变，引起机体一系列衰老过程。脂质过氧化物还可经氧化酶进一步分解生成丙二醛（MDA），与蛋白质交联，最后脂褐质沉积于脑、心肌及各重要脏器，影响细胞的正常生长，加速整个机体的衰老。自由基损害的程度可用化学发光法、电子自旋波谱（ESR）直接测定自由基含量得以反映，也可测定自由基对脂质的作用产物如 MDA、LPO 的含量间接得以反映。此外超氧化物歧化酶（SOD）可催化氧自由基的歧化反应，是机体氧自由基的重要酶，故测定组织或红细胞中 SOD 活性也可作为观察氧自由基的间接指标及评价有关药物的疗效。

实验9.1　过氧化脂质的测定

【目的】

学习测定过氧化脂质的方法，观察药物的抗氧化作用。

【原理】

过氧化脂质的二级分解产物丙二醛能与硫代巴比妥酸反应生成红色产物，在 532nm 波长有最大吸收，可通过比色进行测定。又因四乙氧基丙烷与过氧化脂质在同一条件下进行化学反应均产生丙二醛，因此可用四乙氧基丙烷作为标准物质。

【材料】

大鼠 1 只，体重 250 ~ 300g，雄性。

离心机、组织匀浆机、多用振荡器、恒温振荡器、721 分光光度计、恒温箱。

三氯醋酸、硫代巴比妥酸（TBA）、四乙氧基丙烷、生理盐水、0.1mol/L 盐酸（HCL）、正丁醇。

【方法与步骤】

1. 取大鼠称重后断头处死，取出肝脏，滤纸吸去残血，剪碎称重，加生理盐水，用组织匀浆机制备1%匀浆。

2. 取1%肝匀浆0.6ml，加入20%的三氯醋酸0.3ml，沉淀蛋白，混匀静置于室温下20min，加入0.1mol/L的HCl 2ml和1% TBA 1.0ml，充分混匀。100℃沸水煮15min，冷却，加入4.0ml正丁醇提取，振摇混匀，3000r/min离心15min。

3. 取上清液4ml在532nm波长下比色测定。

4. 采用Lowry法测定肝匀浆中蛋白质含量，以四乙氧基丙烷为标准，计算每克蛋白过氧化脂质生成量。

【结果处理】

按下式计算，并列出结果（表9-1）。

$$C = \frac{A}{\text{消光系数} \times L} = \frac{A}{1.56 \times 10^{-5} \times L} \text{mol/L}$$

式中，C——丙二醛浓度；

　　　A——吸光度；

　　　L——光径（1cm）；

　　　消光系数——$1.56 \times 10^{-5} \text{m}^{-1} \text{cm}^{-1}$。

如已知被测物蛋白含量，则：

$$C = \frac{A}{0.156 \times \text{mg 蛋白质}} \text{（nmolMDA/mg pro）}$$

表9-1　药物对大鼠肝匀浆内过氧化脂质生成的影响

组别	剂量（mg/kg）	实验次数（n）	MDA（n mol/kg） （$\bar{x} \pm SD$）
对照组			
药物组			

【注意事项】

1. 制作匀浆前肝组织尽量剪碎；制作匀浆时，每次的时间和频率均应保持一致。

2. 每次取匀浆时，应摇动烧杯使所取匀浆浓度一致。

【方法评价】

此法简单易行，试剂易得。目前临床上许多具有抗衰老作用的药物都是从该实验中筛选而出。MDA含量可客观反映机体衰老的程度，指标明确。

【思考题】

说明过氧化脂质与衰老的关系。

实验9.2　超氧化物歧化酶（SOD）测定方法

【目的】

学习超氧化物歧化酶测定方法；了解超氧化酶活性与自由基浓度的关系；观察药物提

高酶活性，清除自由基的作用。

【原理】

超氧化物歧化酶是体内清除自由基的重要物质，它的作用是催化下述反应。

$$O_2^- + O_2^- + 2H^+ \xrightarrow{\text{SOD}} H_2O_2 + O_2$$

SOD 随着衰老过程而减少，故测定 SOD 活性可作为机体衰老的定量指标。

O_2^- 使 NBT 还原成甲䐶产物，在 560nm 处有吸收峰，SOD 清除 O_2^- 而抑制甲䐶产物的形成，因此测定甲䐶生成的减少，可知样品中 SOD 含量，反应式如下：

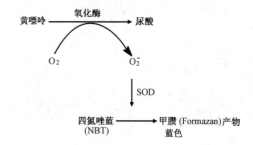

【材料】

721 分光光度计、旋涡振荡器、匀浆器。

黄嘌呤、硝基四氮唑蓝、黄嘌呤氧化酶。

黄嘌呤氧化酶：0.4u/ml，-20℃保存，同时以 pH 7.8（50mmol/L）磷酸钾缓冲液稀释，使终浓度为 0.04u/ml。

SOD 标准液：同时以 20% 乙醇配成 1mg/ml 的溶液，再稀释成 10μg/ml（58.52u/ml）。

混合底物缓冲液：A 液为 0.2mol/L 磷酸钾盐缓冲液（pH 7.8）；B 液为 0.4mol/L 的 EDTA-NaOH 缓冲液；C 液为黄嘌呤 10mmol/L，溶于 0.1mol/L 的 NaOH 内；D 液为硝基四氮唑蓝 7.5mmol/L 溶于 20% 乙醇。取 A 液 135ml、B 液 0.188ml、C 液 4.5ml、D 液 3.75ml，最后加水补足至 240ml，即为混合底物缓冲液。

【方法与步骤】

1. 在红细胞中提取 SOD。取肝素抗凝血 2ml，去血浆及白细胞，以 2~3 倍体积生理盐水洗 2 次，红细胞以冷热蒸馏水等体积稀释，充分溶血，并矫正该溶血的血红蛋白含量为 100g/L。

2. 吸取该血溶液 0.5ml，依次加蒸馏水 3.5ml，冷乙醇 1ml，三氯甲烷 0.6ml，混匀，振荡 1min，3000r/min 离心 5min，沉淀血红蛋白，上清液中含 SOD。

取小试管 3 支，每管各加混合底物缓冲液 2.4ml，于第 1 管加样品红细胞提取液 0.15ml，第 2 管加 SOD 标准液 0.15ml，第 3 管加无离子水 0.5ml，第 1、2 管亦以水补量至 0.5ml，各管于 30℃水浴中预温 5~10min，每间隙 30s 依次加入黄嘌呤氧化酶（0.04u/ml）0.3ml，反应 12min 后，用分光光度计比色计算各样品的抑制百分率与标准 SOD 抑制百分率对比，计算红细胞内 SOD 含量。

【结果处理】

按下式计算，最后计算成相当于 1gHb 含量的红细胞内 SODμg 量。

$$红细胞 \ SOD\mu g/gHb = \frac{A_3 - A_1}{A_3 - A_2} \times 1 \times \frac{5}{0.15} \times \frac{1}{0.05} = \frac{A_3 - A_1}{A_3 - A_2} \times 666.6$$

式中，A_3——未受 SOD 抑制的吸光度；

　　　A_1——测定样品的吸光度；

　　　A_2——标准 SOD 的吸光度；

　　　5——为 5ml 红细胞总体积；

　　　0.05——0.5ml 血中 100g/L 血红蛋白液中 Hb 含量；

　　　0.15ml——SOD 提取液用量。

【注意事项】

1. 血细胞及组织中 SOD 提取应在冰水浴中进行。
2. 此法形成颜色不稳定，所有比色应在 20min 内完成。

【方法评价】

1. 试剂价廉易得，一次可操作多管，但灵敏度及精确度不及邻苯三酚法。
2. 颜色不稳定，变异系数相对较大。

【思考题】

试述超氧化物歧化酶与自由基的关系。

二、对免疫功能的影响

近年来，大量实验资料表明衰老与机体免疫功能状态关系密切。人进入老年期后，胸腺激素减少，免疫功能下降或紊乱，机体抵抗外界病原体的能力明显降低，感染、肿瘤的发病率明显升高。不少扶正固本方药对机体的免疫功能具有调节作用，能改善或调整因免疫功能受损而产生的病理状态，使机体恢复健康。因此研究抗衰老药的作用时，观察其对免疫功能的影响是一个常用的指标。

实验 9.3　免疫器官重量法

【目的】

掌握免疫器官重量法，观察药物对免疫器官重量的影响。

【原理】

免疫增强剂多使免疫器官（胸腺、脾脏）增重，而免疫抑制剂则相反。用该法可观察药物对已知免疫抑制剂所至免疫器官减重的对抗作用。

【材料】

小鼠 20 只，体重 16~18g，雌雄不限。

天平。

环磷酰胺、生理盐水、待试药物。

【方法与步骤】

取小鼠 20 只，随机分成空白对照组（给生理盐水）、待试药物组、环磷酰胺组及待试药物 + 环磷酰胺组。待试药每天给药一次，连续 6 天。给予待试药物后第 4 天，一次性腹腔注射环磷酰胺 75mg/kg。末次给药后次日，摘眼球放血，剥取脾脏、胸腺。

【结果处理】

扭力天平称重，脏器重量以 mg/10g 体重表示。随后进行组间 t 检验，比较组间差异的显著性。

【注意事项】

1. 必须用年轻小鼠。

2. 胸腺和脾脏必须分离干净。

【方法评价】

1. 此法比较简单，可供中药初筛，已知许多补益中药对免疫器官有增重作用。

2. 实验结果如与其他指标所得结果平行，则比较可靠。

【思考题】

为什么本实验用环磷酰胺引起免疫功能抑制后再观察待试药的作用?

实验9.4　单核吞噬细胞功能测定法

【目的】

了解药物对小鼠单核吞噬细胞功能的影响，以便进一步探讨药物对机体免疫功能的调节作用。

【原理】

吞噬细胞具有吞噬异物，处理抗原等多种功能。一些颗粒状异物进入血循环后，迅速被单核吞噬细胞清除，其中主要为定居在肝和脾脏的巨噬细胞。若将异物量恒定，则自血流中清除速率可反映单核吞噬细胞的吞噬功能。常用的颗粒状异物为胶体碳。在一定范围内，碳颗粒的消除速率与其剂量呈指数关系，即吞噬速度与血碳浓度成正比，而与吞噬的碳粒量成反比。一些增强机体非特异性免疫功能的药物常使单核吞噬细胞的吞噬能力增加。

【材料】

小鼠15只，体重18～22g，雌雄不限。

印度墨水、秒表、721分光光度计、小吸管。

肝素、碳酸氢钠（Na_2CO_3）溶液、生理盐水。

【方法与步骤】

1. 取18～22g的健康小鼠随机分成待试药物组、阴性和阳性对照组，给药方式和途径随受试药物不同而异。

2. 按64mg/ml的浓度制备胶体碳悬液，临用前在沸水中融化、振摇并稀释至16mg/ml。

3. 于末次给药后30min，尾静脉注射印度墨水（0.05～0.1ml/10g），注射后选取不同时间（如1min、5min或2min、20min），分别从眼眶静脉丛取血20μl溶于0.1% Na_2CO_3 2ml溶液中，摇匀，在600～680nm波长下比色，测定吸光度。

4. 将小鼠处死称取肝，脾重量。

【结果处理】

1. 以不同时间测得的血中颗粒浓度之对数值为纵坐标，时间为横坐标，两者则呈线性关系。此直线斜率（K）可表示吞噬速率（或称廓清指数）。

$$K = \frac{\lg A_1 - \lg A_2}{t_2 - t_1}$$

式中，A_1，A_2——不同时间所取血样的吸光度；

　　$t_2 - t_1$——取两血样的时间差。

2. 因动物肝、脾重量可影响 K 值，故可按下式计算校正的廓清指数（α）。

$$\alpha = \sqrt[3]{K} \times 体重 / （肝重 + 脾重）$$

【注意事项】

1. 印度墨水应先用生理盐水稀释 10 倍，否则注射后可致小鼠死亡。

2. 取血时间应尽量准确。

3. 若小鼠肝、脾重量差异不大，只计算 K 值亦可。

【方法评价】

用免疫抑制剂（如环磷酰胺）引起免疫功能抑制，观察待测药的作用，所得阳性结果较可靠，且更接近临床情况。

【思考题】

1. 何谓非特异性免疫和特异性免疫？

2. 本实验属上述哪种免疫功能实验方法？

三、对应激能力的影响

所谓抗应激能力，反映了机体对不利环境的适应能力。而抗衰老药是一类提高生命活力的药物，一般都能增强机体对各种有害刺激的非特异性抵抗能力，使紊乱的功能得以恢复正常，中药上常称此种作用为适应原样作用。抗应激实验一般以小鼠为实验对象，观察各种有害刺激对小鼠生存时间的影响。

实验 9.5　小鼠耐缺氧实验

【目的】

掌握小鼠耐缺氧的实验方法，观察药物的耐缺氧作用。

【原理】

缺氧是一种紧张性刺激，可引起机体产生各种应激性反应。脑、心脏缺氧是死亡的主要原因。许多抗衰老药物可通过增加心肌供血或降低心肌耗氧，改善心肌能量代谢而延长小鼠缺氧条件下的存活时间。

【材料】

小鼠 30 只，体重 18～20g，性别相同。

150ml 广口玻璃瓶、秒表、天平、凡士林、钠石灰。

普萘洛尔。

【方法与步骤】

将小鼠随机分成 3 组，每组 10 只，分别放入容积相同（150ml）的密闭广口瓶内，瓶内装有等量钠石灰（25g）以吸收水和二氧化碳。瓶盖涂以凡士林，放入小鼠后将瓶密闭，以秒表观察小鼠呼吸停止时间。每次实验均设空白对照组和阳性药（普萘洛尔 20mg/kg，腹腔注射）对照组。

【结果处理】

计算各组小鼠死亡时间平均数（$\bar{x} \pm S$），t 检验比较组间显著性。

【注意事项】

1. 所用容器必须密封，不漏气，而且容量相等。

2. 为防止钠石灰受潮，故每次实验开启后应封口。

3. 小鼠体重、性别及室温不同，实验结果均有差异。

【方法评价】

1. 本方法简单易行，可作为初筛基本方法。

2. 本实验特异性不高，一些镇静、催眠、扩血管药及扶正固本、活血化瘀中药均呈阳性结果。

【思考题】

1. 本实验钠石灰作用是什么？

2. 为什么本实验特异性不高？

实验 9.6 小鼠耐寒实验

【目的】

学习寒冷刺激的实验方法，观察药物增强动物耐寒能力的作用。

【原理】

寒冷刺激属物理性应激原，当寒冷刺激作用于机体后，可使机体发生一系列保护反应，如皮肤血管收缩、反射性颤抖和代谢加快等，此时肾上腺皮质激素分泌大量增加，有利于机体抗应激作用。当肾上腺皮质激素储备耗竭时，许多抗衰老药能加速肾上腺皮质激素从耗竭中恢复正常，因而有利于机体提高抗应激能力。

【材料】

小鼠 30 只，体重 18～22g，性别相同。

冰箱，天平，温度计。

【方法与步骤】

调节实验用普通冰箱（冷冻室）或低温冰箱的温度，一般应达 $-5℃ \pm 1℃$。小鼠随机分组，给药 1h 后，装入鼠笼、放入冰箱，观察 50min 或 60min 的死亡率，也可观察每只小鼠存活时间，直至全部死亡。

【结果处理】

求算 50min 或 60min 小鼠平均死亡率（$\bar{x} \pm S$）或小鼠平均存活时间（$\bar{x} \pm S$），进行组间比较。

【注意事项】

小鼠性别应一致，重量宜相近，以免结果差异太大。

【方法评价】

1. 此法简单易行，但特异性不高。

2. 此法可与抗高温实验（温度 45℃ ±1℃，其他条件及操作同耐寒实验）平行进行。

【思考题】

何谓药物的适应原样作用？

实验 9.7　小鼠游泳实验

【目的】

了解小鼠游泳实验方法，观察药物的抗疲劳作用。

【原理】

以游泳时间作为检测小鼠疲劳的指标，具有抗疲劳效能的药物可使动物游泳时间延长。

【材料】

小鼠 30 只，体重 18～22g，雄性。

玻璃缸，温度计，恒温箱，胶泥（或铝块），线绳。

生理盐水、受试药物。

【方法与步骤】

取小鼠 30 只，随机分成 3 组，一组给予受试药物，一组给阳性对照药，另一组给生理盐水作为阴性对照组。给药后一定时间将小鼠投入玻璃缸进行游泳试验，水深 25cm，水温调节 30℃ ±1℃。为缩短观察时间可予小鼠尾部负重（体重的 5%），用秒表计算鼻孔沉下水面所需时间。

【结果处理】

记录每鼠游泳持续时间，计算各组小鼠游泳持续时间的平均值，进行组间显著性检验，观察药物有无抗疲劳作用。

【注意事项】

1. 严格控制水温。

2. 动物单个游泳为好，集体游泳时相互攀推会影响实验结果。

【方法评价】

1. 此法简便，但实验结果差异大。

2. 动物体重差异大会影响结果。

3. 本实验也可用冰水（称冰水游泳试验），是体力与应激反应的综合指标。

【思考题】

药物抗疲劳的可能作用机制是什么？

四、对中枢神经系统的作用

中枢神经系统与机体衰老的关系已越来越引起生物工作者的关注。衰老可引起中枢儿茶酚胺水平降低，从而导致脑的"生化损伤"，包括神经功能的退化、自主行为的改变等。Fowler 等于 1980 年发现单胺氧化酶 B（MAO－B）活性随年龄增加而升高，与衰老关系密切。许多抗衰老药通过降低 MAO－B 活性，减轻中枢儿茶酚胺水平下降所致的"生化损伤"而发挥作用。

实验9.8　单胺氧化酶-B活性测定

【目的】

学习单胺氧化酶-B（MAO-B）活性的测定方法，观察药物抑制单胺氧化酶（MAO）的作用。

【原理】

以苄胺为底物，在MAO-B的作用下生成苄醛，以环己烷提取，在242nm下测定A值，反应式如下：

$$RCH_2\!-\!NH_2 + O_2 + H_2O \xrightarrow{\text{MAO}} RC\overset{O}{\underset{H}{\diagup\!\diagdown}} + NH_3 + H_2O$$

【材料】

小鼠1只。

0.2mol/L磷酸缓冲液，8mmol/L苄胺，60%高氯酸，环己胺。

【方法与步骤】

1. 取小鼠全脑加入10倍体积预冷的0.2mol/L磷酸缓冲液（pH 7.4）制成匀浆，超声，离心5000r/min，弃去沉淀。

2. 上清液在17000r/min下离心30min，取沉淀，用磷酸缓冲液将沉淀重新悬浮，即为粗酶。

3. 取上述酶悬浮液0.5ml加入8mmol/L苄胺0.3ml，用0.2mol/L磷酸缓冲液（pH 7.4）补足至3ml，反应系统在37℃下保温3h，每15min振荡混合一次，然后加入60%高氯酸0.3ml终止反应。

4. 加环己烷3ml提取，3000r/min离心10min，取上清液在242nm下测定A值。

步骤3、4操作程序如下：

	空白管	测定管
酶液	—	0.5 ml
8mmol/L苄胺	—	0.3 ml
0.2mol/L磷酸缓冲液	3.0 ml	补足到3.0 ml
37℃下保温3h		
8mmol/L苄胺	0.3 ml	—
60%高氯酸	0.3 ml	0.3 ml
环己烷	3 ml	3 ml

【结果处理】

酶活性以每3h生成苄醛（nmol）表示，或以3h产生0.01个吸光度为一个活性单位，即每小时的u/毫克蛋白质。酶液蛋白质含量按Lowry法测定。

【注意事项】

为了消除酶液中存在的单胺底物的干扰，空白样品在保温前不加苄胺，保温后再加。

【方法评价】

样品处理较麻烦，不如同位素法灵敏、准确。

【思考题】

试述 MAO – B 活性与衰老的关系。

第十章 药物的安全性评价

一、药物的毒性试验

任何一种新药在推荐临床试用前必须进行周密、细致、认真的毒性研究，对新药的安全性作出全面的评价，以便剔除毒性大的化合物，并找出发生不良反应的靶器官和组织。此外，还要尽可能地找出这些不良反应与剂量、疗程之间的关系以及毒性作用是否可逆和如何预防。按照我国药政部门的规定，新药安全性评价的内容包括急性毒性试验、重复给药毒性试验和特殊毒性试验，后者又包括遗传毒性试验、生殖毒性试验和致癌试验。作用于中枢神经系统的新药应进行药物依赖性试验，通过皮肤给药的药物还需进行皮肤刺激性试验和皮肤过敏性试验。

（一）急性毒性试验

急性毒性试验是指机体一次或短时间内（24h）多次接受大剂量某种药物后所产生的快速而剧烈的中毒反应，包括死亡效应，是药物安全性评价的第一道关卡。其试验目的有：①测定药物的半数致死量（LD_{50}）及相关参数；②通过观察药物的急性中毒症状，揭示药物的毒性靶器官，以及对靶器官的特异性作用，提供毒性作用机制分析的资料；③为慢性毒性试验提供给药剂量设计依据。实验动物一般多用小鼠，有时也用大鼠。观察时间视毒性反应出现快慢而定，一般 1～2 周。对于拟推荐给临床的新药，按新药审批法规相关规定，要求采用两种给药途径，其中一种必须是推荐临床研究的给药途径，观察时间为14 天。

实验 10.1 普鲁卡因急性毒性试验

【目的】

通过实验了解测定药物半数致死量（LD_{50}）的方法、步骤和计算过程。

【原理】

衡量一个药物的急性毒性大小，一般是以该药物使动物致死的剂量（lethal dose）为指标。通常用半数致死量（LD_{50}）来表示，因为 LD_{50} 是剂量反应曲线上最敏感的一点。一个药物的剂量与生物反应之间有一定的关系，若以死亡率做纵坐标、剂量做横坐标，常成一长尾"S"形曲线（图 10 – 1）。这条曲线两端平缓、中间陡峭，在反应率50% 处斜率最大，右端又较左端长。这是因为一群随机取样的动物中，对于某一药物很敏感、易致死和很耐受、不易死亡的动物都较少，而大多数动物的敏感程度都是比较相近而适中的。

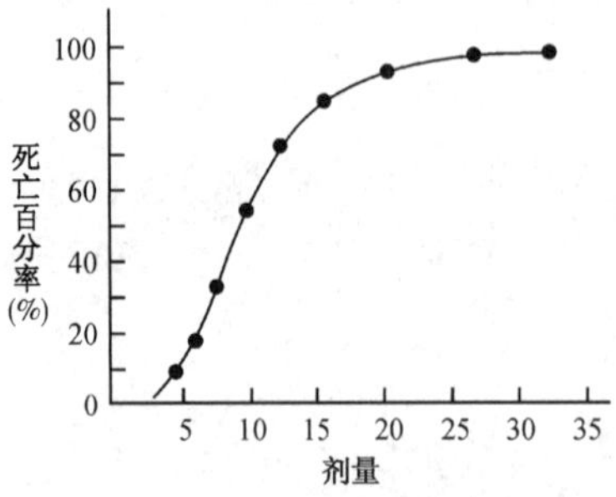

图 10 – 1 死亡率与剂量的关系

如果将剂量转换成对数剂量做横坐标，则曲线右端缩短，因而左右对称，对称点在反应率50%处（图10-2）。此处斜率最大，变化最明显，亦即剂量反应最敏感处。此时剂量也最准确，误差最小。

如果将反应率转换成一种数学函数——几率单位，则几率单位与对数剂量之间呈线性关系（图10-3）。

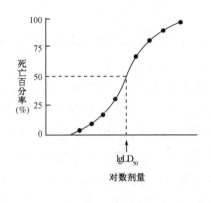

图10-2 死亡率与对数剂量的关系　　　图10-3 几率单位与对数剂量的关系

这种转换方法称为几率单位法，通过作图或公式计算可求出LD_{50}。

【材料】

小鼠50只，体重18～22g，雌雄各半。

鼠笼、天平、注射器。

1%普鲁卡因，苦味酸溶液。

【方法与步骤】

1. 将小鼠雌、雄分开。分别称重，同一体重段（如18.0～18.9g）小鼠放入同一个笼内。

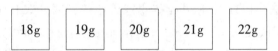

2. 雌、雄小鼠分别按体重顺序（由大→小，或由小→大），照下列方式分层随机分为5组，使不同性别和体重的小鼠能均匀分配于各组，每组10只。

组别	1#	2#	3#	4#	5#
鼠数	①	2	3	4	5
	5	①	2	3	4
	4	5	①	2	3
	3	4	5	①	2
	2	3	4	5	①

3. 按剂间比1：0.85，腹腔注射1%普鲁卡因，五组剂量分别为130mg/kg、153mg/kg、180mg/kg、212mg/kg和249mg/kg。给药后观察30min，记录各组小鼠行为反应及死亡数目。

4. 用改进寇氏法和Bliss法计算普鲁卡因的LD_{50}和95%可信区间。

【结果处理】

实验报告应包括如下内容。

1. 受试物的批号、规格、生产厂家、理化性状、溶液的浓度、实验室温度。

2. 实验动物和种系、性别、体重范围、分组情况、给药途径、剂量、给药时间、给药后的中毒症状、死亡时间和死亡率。

3. LD_{50} 的计算过程和结果（包括 LD_{50} 值的95%可信区间）。

【注意事项】

1. 实验动物应挑选体重相近（$20g \pm 2g$ 为宜）的健康小鼠，最好雌雄各半或同一性别，怀孕的雌鼠应剔除不用。

2. 精密测定 LD_{50} 前，通常先要摸索出合适剂量范围，即测出能使小鼠出现接近0%和100%死亡的剂量。若是已知药的核对试验，则可根据文献查出该药的 LD_{50}，在此剂量上、下各推两个剂量；若是新药，则可根据文献查出同类结构化合物的 LD_{50} 以供参考；若是未知药物或无文献可供参考时，则取少量小鼠，每组 $2 \sim 3$ 只，共 $3 \sim 4$ 组，按剂间比 $2:1$ 给药，找出引起0及100%死亡的剂量范围，为精密测定 LD_{50} 提供依据。

3. 在预试验所获得的0和100%死亡的剂量范围内，选用几个剂量（小鼠一般用 $4 \sim 5$ 个剂量，按等比级数增减，相邻组之间剂间比一般取 $1:0.8 \sim 1:0.7$），尽可能使半数组的死亡率在50%以上，另半数组的死亡率在50%以下。

4. 小鼠分组时应先将不同性别分开，再将不同体重分开，然后随机分配，此法称为分层随机分组法。

5. 给药时最好先从中剂量组开始，以便能从最初几组动物接受药物后的反应来判断两端的剂量是否合适，如不合适可随时进行调整。

6. 小鼠称重及给药剂量力求准确。药液的pH及渗透压应在生理范围内。

7. 动物的饥饱、实验室温度、实验时间等均会影响实验结果，应尽量保持一致。

【计算方法】

1. **孙氏改进寇氏法**　1931年 Kurber 提出寇氏原法，因算式有误，不为人重视。1952年 Finney 改正原式，得改良寇氏法。1963年孙瑞元根据点斜式直线方程，并综合寇氏法及概率单位的优点进行改进，故常称为改进寇氏法，是一种简捷且比较精确的近似计算方法。

（1）基本要求：

1）反应情况符合或接近对数正态分析。

2）相邻两剂量的比值应相等。

3）各组动物数相等或相近，一般为10只。

4）不要求死亡率必须包括0与100%，但最低与最高剂量组死亡率之和宜在80% ~ 120%范围内。

（2）计算公式：

1）当最低剂量组的死亡率为0，最高剂量组的死亡率为100%时，按下列公式计算：

$$LD_{50} = \lg^{-1} [X_m - i (\sum p - 0.5)] \tag{10-1}$$

式中，X_m——最高剂量的对数；

　　　　p——各组动物的死亡率（以小数表示）；

　　　$\sum p$——各组动物死亡率的总和（$p_1 + p_2 + p_3 \cdots$）；

　　　　i——相邻两组对数剂量的差值。

2）当最低剂量组的死亡率大于0%而又小于30%，或最高剂量组的死亡率小于100%

而又大于70%时，可按下列校正公式计算：

$$LD_{50} = lg^{-1} \left[X_m - i \left(\sum p - \frac{3 - P_m - P_n}{4} \right) \right] \qquad (10-2)$$

式中，P_m——最高剂量组的死亡率；

P_n——最低剂量组的死亡率。

3）LD_{50}的标准误按下式计算：

$$S_{lgLD_{50}} = i \cdot \sqrt{\frac{\sum p - \sum p^2}{n-1}} \qquad (10-3)$$

式中，n——每组的动物数。

4）LD_{50}的95%可信区间按下式计算：

$$lg^{-1} (lgLD_{50} \pm 1.96 S_{lgLD_{50}}) \qquad (10-4)$$

（3）例题 取体重18~22g小鼠50只，雌雄各半，随机分成5组，每组10只，按表10-1中剂量腹腔注射PAM溶液，组间剂量比为1:0.8。3天内的死亡率见表10-1，用改进寇氏法计算半数致死量、标准误和95%可信区间。

表10-1 小鼠腹腔注射PAM溶液实验结果

组别	小鼠（只）	剂量（mg/kg）	对数剂量	死亡动物（只）	死亡率（p）	p^2
1	10	300	2.48	10	1	1
2	10	240	2.38	8	0.8	0.64
3	10	192	2.28	5	0.5	0.25
4	10	154	2.18	3	0.3	0.09
5	10	123	2.08	0	0	0
					$\sum p = 2.6$	$\sum p^2 = 1.98$

按式（10-1）计算LD_{50}，现$X_m = 2.48$，$i = 0.10$，$\sum p = 2.6$

$$LD_{50} = lg^{-1} [2.48 - 0.10 (2.6 - 0.5)]$$

$$= lg^{-1} 2.27 = 186 mg/kg$$

按式（10-3）计算LD_{50}的标准误，现$n = 10$，$\sum p^2 = 1.98$

$$S_{lgLD_{50}} = 0.10 \cdot \sqrt{\frac{2.6 - 1.98}{10 - 1}} = 0.026$$

按式（10-4）计算LD_{50}的95%可信区间。

$$lg^{-1} (lg186 \pm 1.96 \times 0.026) = lg^{-1} (2.22 \sim 2.32)$$

$$= 166 \sim 209 mg/kg$$

PAM对小鼠腹腔注射的LD_{50}为186mg/kg，95%可信区间为166~209mg/kg。

2. Bliss法 此法由Bliss创建，利用对数剂量与反应百分率的转换数（即几率单位）呈线性关系而设计。在众多的LD_{50}计算方法中，其在数理上为最严谨的一种，又称之为加权几率单位法或几率单位正规法，是新药审批法中推荐使用的方法。

（1）优点 ①可求$LD_5 \sim LD_{95}$；②剂量任意，各剂量组间可以是等比级数，也可为等差或不等距的数值，只需有死亡率在50%以上及以下组出现；③计算结果精确。

（2）缺点　①计算繁琐；②须用权重表。目前由于电脑的普遍使用，开发了有关的软件，使用非常便利，完全克服了计算繁琐这一缺点。

（3）例题　取体重 18～22g 小鼠 50 只，雌雄各半，随机分成 5 组，每组 10 只，按表 10-2中剂量静脉注射三七总皂苷溶液，组间剂量比为 1∶0.85。7 天内死亡率见表 10-2，用 Bliss 法计算 LD_{50} 和 95% 可信区间、LD_5、LD_{95}。

采用 LD_{50} 计算软件，得到静脉注射三七总皂苷的小鼠 LD_{50}（95% 可信区间）、LD_5 和 LD_{95} 分别为：6.33mg/10g（95% 可信区间 5.70～7.03mg/10g）、4.44mg/10g 和 8.89mg/10g。

表 10-2　小鼠静脉注射三七总皂苷溶液实验结果

剂量 (mg/10g)	对数剂量	死亡数/动物数	死亡率 (%)	实验几率单位	预期几率单位	校算几率单位	权重系数	权重				
D	X	r/n	p	ye	Y	y	w	Nw	nwx	nwx²	nwy	nwxy
9.0	0.9542	10/10	100		6.5	7.02	0.269	2.69	2.5669	2.4495	18.8838	18.0197
7.6	0.8208	8/10	80	5.84	5.8	5.84	0.503	5.03	4.4305	3.9024	29.3752	25.9741
6.5	0.8129	5/10	50	5.00	5.1	5.00	0.634	6.34	5.1539	4.1897	31.7000	25.7694
5.5	0.7403	3/10	30	4.48	4.4	4.48	0.558	5.58	4.1312	3.0586	24.9984	18.5879
4.7	0.6721	1/10	10	3.72	3.8	3.72	0.370	3.70	2.4868	1.6713	13.7640	9.2508
				（查表 10-3 读出	（暂定线 10-4）	（查表 10-4）	（查表 10-4）	23.34	18.7693	15.2715	118.7214	97.4218

注：实验几率单位（ye）由表 10-3 查得；预期几率单位（Y）由图 10-3 中暂定线读出（以对数剂量 x 为横坐标，实验几率单位 ye 为纵坐标作图，得出暂定线）；权重系数（w）由表 10-4 查得

$$a = \bar{y} - b\bar{x} = 5.0866 - 10.96 \times 0.8042$$
$$= -3.729$$

校正线方程：$y = a + bx = -3.729 + 10.96 \cdot x$

$LD_{50} = \lg^{-1} 0.7963 = 6.26mg/10g$（可信限 5.74～6.81mg/10g）

$LD_5 = \lg^{-1} 0.6467 = 4.43mg/10g$

$LD_{95} = \lg^{-1} 0.9459 = 8.83mg/10g$

表 10-3　百分率与几率单位换算

反应率	0	1	2	3	4	5	6	7	8	9
0	—	2.674	2.949	3.119	3.249	3.355	3.445	3.524	3.595	3.659
10	3.718	3.773	3.325	3.874	3.920	3.964	4.006	4.046	4.085	4.122
20	4.158	4.194	4.228	4.261	4.294	4.326	4.375	4.387	4.417	4.447
30	4.476	4.504	4.532	4.560	4.587	4.615	4.642	4.668	4.695	4.721
40	4.747	4.773	4.798	4.824	4.849	4.874	4.900	4.925	4.950	4.975
50	5.000	5.025	5.050	5.075	5.100	5.126	5.151	5.176	5.202	5.227
60	5.253	5.279	5.305	5.332	5.358	5.385	5.413	5.440	5.468	5.496
70	5.524	5.553	5.583	5.613	5.643	5.674	5.706	5.739	5.772	5.806
80	5.842	5.878	5.915	5.954	5.995	6.036	6.080	6.126	6.175	6.227
90	6.282	6.341	6.405	6.476	6.555	6.645	6.751	6.881	7.054	7.326

表 10-4　权重系数和校算几率单位

Xx-pected problt Y	Maxlmum Conectcd Problt Y+Q/Z	Ranac 1/Z	Mlnlmum Cencctcd Problt Y-P/Z	Wolght-lng coemdent Z/pq	Maxtmurn conected Problt Y+Q/Z	Range 1/Z	Mlnlmum Cotrcctod Problt Y-P/Z	Xx-problt Pectod Y
5.0	6.253	2.507	3.747	0.6366	6.253	2.507	3.747	5.0

续表

Xx – pectcd problt Y	Maxlmum Conectcd Problt Y + Q/Z	Ranac 1/Z	Mlnlmum Cenccted Problt Y − P/Z	Wolght – lng coemdent Z/pq	Maxtmurn conected Problt Y + Q/Z	Range 1/Z	Mlnlmum Cotrcctod Problt Y − P/Z	Xx – problt Pectod Y
5.1	6.259	2.519	3.740	0.6343	6.260	2.519	3.741	4.9
5.2	6.276	2.557	3.719	0.6274	6.281	2.557	3.724	4.8
5.3	6.302	2.622	3.680	0.6161	6.320	2.622	3.698	4.7
5.4	6.336	2.715	3.620	0.6005	6.360	2.715	3.664	4.6
5.5	6.376	2.840	3.536	0.5810	6.464	2.840	3.624	4.5
5.6	6.423	3.001	3.422	0.5579	6.578	3.001	3.577	4.4
5.7	6.475	3.203	3.272	0.5316	6.728	3.203	3.525	4.3
5.8	6.531	3.452	3.079	0.5026	6.921	3.452	3.469	4.2
5.9	6.592	3.758	2.834	0.4714	7.166	3.758	3.408	4.1
6.0	6.656	4.133	2.523	0.4386	7.477	4.133	3.344	4.0
6.1	6.723	4.590	2.132	0.4047	7.867	4.590	3.277	3.9
6.2	6.793	5.150	1.643	0.3703	8.357	5.150	3.207	3.8
6.3	6.865	5.835	1.030	0.3350	8.970	5.835	3.135	3.7
6.4	6.939	6.679	1.621	0.3020	9.739	6.679	3.061	3.6
6.5	7.016	7.721	—	0.2691	—	7.721	2.934	3.5
6.6	7.094	9.015	—	0.2375	—	9.015	2.906	3.4
6.7	7.174	10.633	—	0.2077	—	10.633	2.826	3.3
6.8	7.255	12.666	—	0.1799	—	12.666	2.745	3.2
6.9	7.338	15.340	—	0.1544	—	15.340	2.662	3.1
7.0	7.421	18.522	—	0.1311	—	18.522	2.579	3.0
7.1	7.506	22.736	—	0.1103	—	22.736	2.494	2.9
7.2	7.592	28.189	—	0.0918	—	28.189	2.408	2.8
7.3	7.679	35.302	—	0.0756	—	35.302	2.321	2.7
7.4	7.766	44.654	—	0.0617	—	44.654	2.234	2.6
7.5	7.854	57.05	—	0.0498	—	57.05	2.146	2.5
7.6	7.943	73.62	—	0.0398	—	73.62	2.057	2.4
7.7	8.033	95.96	—	0.0314	—	95.96	1.967	2.3
7.8	8.123	126.34	—	0.0246	—	126.34	1.877	2.2
7.9	8.213	168.00	—	0.0190	—	168.00	1.787	2.1
8.0	8.305	225.6	—	0.0146	—	225.6	1.695	2.0
8.1	8.396	306.1	—	0.0110	—	306.1	1.604	1.9
8.2	8.488	419.4	—	0.0083	—	419.4	1.512	1.8
8.3	8.581	580.5	—	0.0061	—	580.5	1.419	1.7
8.4	8.673	811.5	—	0.0045		811.5	1.327	1.6

【方法评价】

LD_{50} 的测定方法简便，是药物的重要特征性参数之一。可用同一种动物、同一给药方式测得的 LD_{50} 和 ED_{50}（半数有效量，即半数动物出现疗效的剂量）来计算药物的治疗指数（TI），从而初步估计该药的安全性。

$$TI = LD_{50}/ED_{50}$$

TI 值越大，则越安全，一般认为 TI 在 3 以上的药物才可能具有实用意义。目前用于临床的药物，其治疗指数多在 10 以上。

但无论是 LD_{50} 还是 TI 都不能绝对地、完整地揭示某一特殊的毒性作用机制。致死效应是一个质反应过程，累积反应的几率与剂量呈双曲线函数（S 形曲线）关系，而累积反应的几率与剂量的对数呈线性关系。因此，对数剂量 – 反应曲线的斜率揭示了剂量变化与致死效应之间的关系，这种关系在安全性评价中有时比 LD_{50} 更为重要，尤其在比较同系列化学物时显得更为重要。两个化学物质 LD_{50} 可能相同或相近，但斜率却可以不同，因此在相同的剂量范围内，表现出不同的毒理学特征，如图 10 – 4 中 A、B 两药；而具平行的量 – 效曲线的两药尽管 LD_{50} 不同，却可能表明具有相近的毒性作用机制，如图 10 – 4 中 A、C 两药。斜率小（量效曲线较平坦）反映安全范围较大。根据斜率，还可将反应外推至低剂量范围，求出 LD_1、LD_{10} 等。

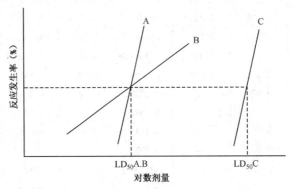

图 10 – 4　不同药物毒效应量 – 效关系比较

TI 值通常仅适用于比较治疗效应和致死效应的量效曲线相互平行的药物，对于两种效应的量效曲线斜率不同的药物，还应适当参考其他参数来补充其不足，比如安全指数（SI）、可靠安全系数（CSF）。

$$SI = LD_5/ED_{95}$$

SI 值说明药物的临床安全性，其应用虽不及 TI 值普遍，但近年来已受到重视。

$$CSF = LD_1/ED_{99}$$

CSF 与 TI 并不平行，如图 10 – 5 所示，在评价 A、B 两药时，从 TI 来看 A 药优于 B 药。但从 CSF 来看，A 药 CSF 小于 1，说明在 99% 有效时已有相当毒性发生，而 B 药 CSF 大于 1，说明 99% 有效时，还没有一例死亡。

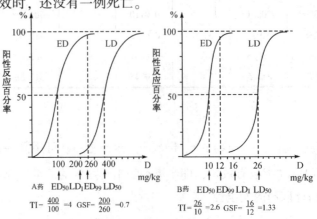

图 10 – 5　致死量、有效量与药物安全性的评价

【思考题】

1. 什么叫 LD_{50}？测定 LD_{50} 的意义和根据是什么？

2. 试讨论 Bliss 法和改进寇氏法计算 LD_{50} 的根据和优缺点。

（二）重复给药毒性试验

重复给药毒性试验主要观察动物因连续用药而产生的毒性反应，根据动物的毒性资料来判断一个新药是否有进一步开发研究的价值，并为选择临床初始剂量提供依据。

重复给药毒性试验的目的及意义决定了其试验设计的基本原则应是全面、严谨、合理。整个试验过程中必须严格控制条件，尽可能排除药物以外的其他影响，观察指标应能有针对性地反映供试药物毒性性质，最终结果应能解释供试药物长期应用时可能出现的毒性反应及作用特征和安全剂量的范围等。

一般而言，重复给药毒性试验至少应在两种动物身上进行，兼顾性别，剂量分高、中、低，同时设立不给药的空白对照组，必要的时候设溶剂对照。下面具体地叙述长期毒性实验设计时应考虑的几个重要方面。

1. 动物 至少两种动物，包括啮齿类和非啮齿类。啮齿类动物首选大鼠，起始周龄为 6 周，饲养观察 1 周后开始试验，每剂量组、每个性别一般不少于 15 只。非啮齿类动物首选犬，起始月龄为 6 至 12 个月，每剂量组、每个性别不少于 5 只。

各种实验动物应注明来源、品系。饲养条件必须严格控制，并始终恒定，如室温、湿度、光照、通风条件、饮水质量及营养平衡饲料等。

2. 剂量 选择无明显毒性反应的剂量水平是重复给药毒性试验设计中最为困难的任务。一般需要 3 个剂量，第一个是足以引起肯定的毒性症状的高剂量，这种毒性症状包括该组动物试验结束时死亡率不高于 10%；第二个是基本安全剂量，应高于整体动物最佳有效剂量而又不出现毒性反应；第三个是为表明毒性作用的量 – 效关系，在上述两个剂量之间插入一个中间剂量，应使动物产生轻微或中等程度的毒性反应。总之，高剂量的原则是在不造成过多动物死亡的情况下得到毒性作用的明确资料，低剂量则高于预计人临床用剂量。以上是剂量设计的原则。在实际工作中，常在急性毒性试验基础上，参考药代动力学资料，或进行一些短期蓄积毒性试验，将急性毒性参数外推于长期试验。最好的办法是先用少量动物进行剂量摸索试验。

3. 给药途径 应尽量与预期临床使用的途径一致。临床用药途径为静脉或肌内注射的，可用腹腔或皮下注射代替，口服给药的则可用灌胃或拌在食物中给药代替。

4. 试验周期 新药的重复给药毒性试验期限对不同国家和各类不同药物都有不同的要求。我国规定重复给药毒性试验大鼠最长为 6 个月，犬最长为 9 个月。

5. 观察指标 在整个试验阶段，至少应每天或每两天作一次详细的观察。一般日常观察的主要内容有动物的行为活动、外观、粪便等，记录每日食耗量，每周或每两周称记体重一次。在最后一次给药后 24h，剖杀部分（1/2 ~ 2/3）动物，进行血液学（红细胞或网织红细胞计数、血红蛋白、白细胞计数及其分类、血小板计数、凝血时间等）及血液生化学（天门冬氨酸氨基转移酶、丙氨酸氨基转移酶、碱性磷酸酶、尿素氮、总蛋白、白蛋白、血糖、总胆红素、肌酐、总胆固醇等）检测，并进行系统尸检，剖取各主要器官进行脏器系数测定和病理组织学检查。留下的部分动物继续观察 2 ~ 4 周，再活杀检查，了解毒性反应的可逆程度和可能出现的延迟性毒性反应。试验期长于 3 个月时，可在试验中期活杀少量动物（高剂量组和对照组）以检查各项指标。重复给药毒性试验应伴随进行药物毒代动力学试验。

（三）特殊毒性试验

特殊毒性试验包括遗传毒性试验、生殖毒性试验和致癌试验，这些毒性反应常常在经过较长的潜伏期以后或在特殊条件下才会表现出来，发生率虽较低，但造成的后果都较严重，并难以弥补。因此，特殊毒性试验日益受到重视。

1. 遗传毒性试验 又称致突变试验，目的是通过一系列试验来预测受试物是否有遗传毒性，在降低临床试验受试者和药品上市后使用人群的用药风险上发挥重要作用。由于致突变试验方法较多，且简便、快速、经济，其结果与致癌试验有一定的相关性，因此成了致癌试验的短期筛试手段。根据受试物的化学结构、理化性质及对遗传物质作用终点（基因突变、DNA 损伤、染色体畸变）的不同，要求新药必须做微生物回复突变试验，哺乳动物培养细胞染色体畸变试验和动物微核试验。前两者为离体试验，后者为整体动物试验，各有其优缺点，可用来互相补充和印证。上述试验如遇阳性或可疑阳性时，可选择其他试验，如哺乳动物培养细胞基因突变试验或果蝇伴性隐性致死试验、啮齿动物显性致死试验或精原细胞染色体畸变试验、程序外 DNA 合成试验或 SOS 显色试验作进一步研究分析。

2. 生殖毒性试验 生殖毒性试验分为 I 段生育力与早期胚胎发育毒性试验、II 段胚胎–胎仔发育毒性试验和 III 段围产期毒性试验。

（1）I 段生殖试验 在动物交配前给药，评价生殖细胞接触药物后对胚胎、胎儿、围产期以及断奶期的影响。实验动物通常选用小鼠或大鼠，雄性动物在交配前 60 至 80 天连续给药，雌性动物在交配前 14 天至受孕后器官形成期连续给药，观察动物的一般状况、体重变化、受孕率、死胎数、活胎数、活胎重量、外观、内脏及骨骼的变化，必要时进行组织学检查。

（2）II 段生殖毒性试验 在器官发生期给药，主要观察母体在接受药物之后，是否有胚胎毒性和致畸性。实验动物首选 Wistar 或 SD 大鼠，也可用小鼠或家兔。选用 2~3 个剂量，高剂量应有母体毒性反应，或为最大给药量，低剂量应为无母体和胚胎毒性反应剂量，另设溶剂对照，必要时设阳性对照。给药时间在胚胎器官形成期连续给药，如大鼠孕后 6~15 天，家兔孕后 6~18 天，全部动物于妊娠末期剖检，观察妊娠的确立，有无死胎和吸收胎及子宫内活胎发育情况，约 1/2 胎仔固定于 Bouin 氏液，作内脏检查，另 1/2 固定于酒精作骨骼畸形检查。并将数据汇总成表，各项数据经统计处理后判定药物的胚胎毒性和致畸潜力。

（3）III 段生殖毒性试验 在围产期和产后给药，检查药物对胎儿生长后期、产程、分娩、哺乳、新生儿存活及生长发育的影响。实验动物通常选用大鼠或家兔。大鼠于妊娠第 15 天开始给药，至分娩后 28 天；家兔于妊娠第 22 天开始给药，至分娩后 31 天。观察动物一般状况，记录胎仔数，一般发育状况和外观畸形等。取一定数量幼仔配对饲养，继续观察其存活、生长发育，包括行为、生殖功能及其他异常症状，必要时可对 F1 代动物进行运动和学习能力的测定。根据上述结果结合病理组织学检查，判断围产期给药的毒性影响及程度，并做出综合评价。

3. 致癌试验 它是特殊毒性试验中最为耗资费时的动物试验，因此对某种试验药物，往往只在致突变试验结果为阳性，或在长期毒性试验中发现有细胞毒及能使组织异常活跃者，或该药的结构和已知致癌物有关及相似的情况下才要求进行致癌试验。致癌试验分为短期致癌试验和动物长期致癌试验。

（1）短期致癌试验 又包括哺乳动物培养细胞恶性转化试验和动物短期致癌试验。前者为离体试验，培养细胞需经代谢活化，根据细胞恶性转化率判定结果；后者为整体动物试验，通常采用小鼠肺肿瘤诱发短期试验，实验动物推荐使用 6～8 周龄的 A 系小鼠，设高、中、低三个剂量，最高剂量组应是每周给药 3 次，连续 8 周的最大耐受剂量，另设阴性对照组。观察时间通常为 30～35 周或可更短些。符合下列情况可判为阳性：实验组肺肿瘤的均数比对照组显著增加；有剂量效应关系；阴性对照组肺肿瘤的平均数与文献报道的同龄未染毒小鼠肺肿瘤发生率大体相符。

（2）长期致癌试验 是一项极为持久的动物试验，因此，在实验前需进行详细周密的实验设计。下面就其动物要求、剂量设计及分组、给药方式、观察期限、观察指标等问题作一些说明。

1）动物：要求品系敏感性高，寿命期限不太长，能在相对较短时间内完成终身实验，抗病力强，自发肿瘤率低，动物体型小易满足实验所需数量等。首选小鼠、大鼠和仓鼠等啮齿类动物。动物年龄，一般认为采用刚断乳或幼年动物，这样对某些致癌物更敏感。

2）剂量设计及分组：剂量设计是整个试验的关键，剂量过低，可能出现假阴性的结果，难以下结论；偏高有可能造成动物死亡而使实验无法继续进行，或者使偏高的剂量组数据不能使用。

设计多剂量组虽好，但增加人力财力，因此通常设计 2～3 个剂量组。一般最高剂量可用 LD_{10} 作 3～8 周预试，要求 10%～20% 的动物出现轻度慢性中毒而不致死亡，这些毒性常表现为体重增加受到轻度抑制或血清酶的改变（这种情况表明剂量较适宜）。低剂量可参照临床拟用剂量折算，原则是不影响动物的正常生长、发育和寿命，一般不应低于最高剂量的 10%。在高、低剂量间可插入一适当的中间剂量，另外还要设一个阳性对照组，以及溶媒和空白对照组。每组动物数量，雌雄至少各 50 只，因考虑最终进行生物统计处理时有足够的数目。

3）给药方式：原则与长期毒性试验相同，即选择与临床用药相同的途径。具体有喂饲和灌胃法、皮肤涂抹、皮下或肌内注射等。

4）观察期限：一般要求给药期应占有动物寿命的较大部分时间，如小鼠 18 个月，大鼠 24 个月，这样保证使致癌作用较弱、潜伏期较长的致癌物有机会表现致癌活性。总之，当给药组与阴性对照组间肿瘤发生率已有明显差别时，可结束致癌试验。

5）观察指标和病理学检查：至少每天观察一次动物的行为活动、摄食量等，开始时每周称一次体重，13 周后至少每 4 周称一次，试验结束时全部动物进行剖检及血常规检验。对肉眼观察到有肿瘤性病变或可疑者时，对以下器官进行病理学检查：皮肤、乳腺、淋巴结、唾液腺、胸骨、脊椎及大腿骨、胸腺、气管、肺及支气管、心、甲状腺、舌、食管、胃、十二指肠、大肠、小肠、肝、胰、脾、肾、肾上腺、睾丸、卵巢、性腺、眼球、垂体、脊髓等。

6）结果评定：符合下列情况之一者判断为阳性：试验组肿瘤阳性，对照组阴性；试验组和对照组虽均有肿瘤发生，但试验组肿瘤发生率高于对照组；试验组肿瘤发生的部位多于对照组；试验组和对照组肿瘤的发生率虽无明显差异，但试验组的肿瘤出现早（潜伏期短）。

二、制剂的安全限度试验

为了控制制剂质量，确保安全用药，除了进行必要的理化检验外，常常还需要从药理学的角度对制剂进行质量检查，这些检验统称为制剂的安全限度试验。限度试验主要用于检验注射剂，通常包括下列项目：热原检查、刺激性检查、过敏性检查、降压物质检查、溶血性检查等。在实际工作中，对于常规产品，通常根据药典或生产规程上的要求，来决定检查项目。对于新产品或中草药制剂，则根据药品的性质和制剂的生产工艺特点而决定检查项目。下面介绍的试验方法仅供参考，如果用于申报新药，请参考国家药政部门的相关规定和政策法规。

实验 10.2   热原试验

【目的】

学习用家兔法检查注射液内热原的步骤与判断标准。

【原理】

某些微生物（尤其是革兰阴性杆菌）的遗体或其代谢产物注入体内（特别是经静脉注入体内）以后，能引起发热等反应。这些能引起发热等反应的物质统称为热原或致热质，其化学成分有蛋白质、脂多糖、核蛋白及它们的水解产物等。

【材料】

家兔 3 只，体重 1.7～3.0kg，雌兔应无孕。

兔固定箱、磅秤、肛门温度计、小型铝盒、注射器、注射针头、镊子、酒精棉球、干棉球。

25% 或 50% 葡萄糖注射液、含热原的同种注射液（作为阳性对照）、液状石蜡。

【方法与步骤】

1. **器具的准备**　试验中用的注射器及其他一切与试验品直接接触的器物均须事先经去热原处理。方法是：注射器、针头及镊子等物可置铝盒内，在 250℃ 烘箱中加热 30min，或 180℃ 加热 2h，冷却后待用。

2. **家兔的选择**　凡未经用于热原检查的家兔应在试验前 7 天内预测体温，进行挑选。停食 2～3h 后用肛门温度计测量，每隔 30min 1 次，共测 4 次。如 4 次体温都在 38.3～39.6℃ 范围内，且最高与最低体温的差值不超过 0.4℃，即可以认为该兔适合于热原检查之用。已经用于热原检查的家兔，如上次检查时供试品判断为符合规定，休息 2 日以上即可供第二次检查之用，如上次供试品判断为不符合规定，至少在 2 周内不得供第二次检查用。

3. **实验前准备**　热原检查前 1～2 日，供试家兔应尽可能处于同一温度的环境中，试验前给家兔停食 2～3h。用肛门温度计测量家兔体温，每 30min 1 次，共测 2～3 次，末两次体温的差值不得超过 0.20℃，即以此两次体温的平均值作为该兔的正常体温。供试家兔的正常体温应在 38.3～39.6℃ 的范围内，各兔间的温差不得超过 1℃。

4. **检查方法**　取适用的家兔 3 只，于测定其正常体温后 15min 内自耳缘静脉缓慢注入预热至 37℃ 左右的供试溶液。然后每隔 1h 按前法测温 1 次，共测 3 次。从 3 次测温中所得的最高值减去正常体温，即为该兔的体温升高度数。

【结果处理】

1. 若3只家兔中，体温升高均在0.6℃以下，并且3只家兔体温升高总度数在1.4℃以下，应认为该供试品符合规定。

2. 若3只家兔中仅有1只体温升高0.6℃或0.6℃以上；或3只家兔体温升高均低于0.6℃，但升高总数达1.4℃或1.4℃以上，应另取5只家兔复试。如在复试时，5只家兔中，体温升高0.6℃或0.6℃以上的家兔数不超过1只，并且初、复试合并8只家兔的体温升高总数不超过3.5℃，也应认为供试品符合规定。

3. 若在初试的3只家兔中，体温升高0.6℃或0.6℃以上的家兔数超过1只，或在复试的5只家兔中，体温升高0.6℃或0.6℃以上的家兔数超过1只；或在初、复试合并8只家兔的体温升高总数超过3.5℃，应认为供试品不符合规定。

4. 按表10-5要求做好记录。

表10-5　家兔法检查注射液内热原实验结果

检查日期		室温		检查者	
检查名称		理化性状含量		批号	
兔号	1	2	3	4	5
体重					
第1次测量					
第2次测量					
平均体温					
注射检品时间					
第1次测温					
第2次测温					
第3次测温					
注射前后温差					
检查结论					

【注意事项】

1. 供试家兔应健康无伤，体重1.7~3.0kg，雌兔应无孕，测温前7天应同一饲料饲养。在此期间，体重应不减轻，精神、食欲、排泄等不得有异常。

2. 测温时动作要轻，尽量避免对家兔刺激。温度计插入家兔的肛门前应先用液状石蜡涂抹温度计的水银球。插入的深度各兔应当一致，一般约5cm，保留1.5min，取出读数。

3. 测温时最好每只家兔用同一肛门温度计，以减少误差。

4. 注射供试品时动作也应快，以免引起家兔挣扎而使体温波动。注射速度宜缓慢，剂量较大者控制在10~15min内注射完毕。注射剂量：等渗大型输液为10ml/kg；中草药注射液为1~2ml/kg。

5. 影响热原检查的因素很多，必须严格操作。试验最好在15~25℃的环境中进行，整个试验过程中室温变化不宜超过5℃。

6. 常需进行热原检查的药品及用量可参考表10-6。

表 10 – 6　需进行热原检查的药品及用量

药　　物	注　射　量
注射用水	加无热原氯化钠制成 0.9% 溶液，静注 10ml/kg
氯化钠或复方氯化钠注射液	直接静注 10ml/kg
葡萄糖氯化钠注射液	直接静注 10ml/kg
25% 或 50% 葡萄糖注射液	直接静注 10ml/kg
枸橼酸钠注射液	以注射用水稀释成 0.5% 浓度，按 10ml/kg 缓慢注射
肝素注射液	以氯化钠注射液溶解成 100U/ml 溶液，静注 5ml/kg
注射用盐酸土霉素	以氯化钠注射液溶解成 5000U/ml 溶液，静注 1ml/kg

【方法评价】

注射剂，特别是大型输液如葡萄糖液及生理盐水等，热原检查已成为生产过程中的常规工作。一般而言，5～10ml 以上的静脉注射剂应做热原检查。中草药注射剂由于配制时间较长，污染机会也多，一般也应进行热原检查。目前我国药典规定的热原检查即为将一定剂量的供试品静脉注入家兔体内，在规定时间内，观察家兔体温升高的情况，以决定供试品中所含热原的限度是否符合规定的一种方法。热原检查的另一种方法叫鲎试剂法，此法可以在试管内进行，节省材料与时间，灵敏度较高，有条件时可采用。

【思考题】

1. 什么是热原？其化学本质是什么？在器皿上的热原可用何种方法将其破坏？

2. 用家兔法检查热原时对供试动物有何要求？哪些因素会影响动物体温的变化？试验中需注意什么？

实验 10.3　刺激性试验

【目的】

了解刺激性试验的意义，掌握试验方法和判断标准。

【原理】

一般供皮下或肌内注射的新产品或滴眼、滴鼻、栓剂等制剂需进行刺激性试验。试验的方法为将药物用于局部组织，观察它是否引起组织红肿、出血、变性、坏死等刺激症状。所获得的结果可供了解该制剂的毒性以及选择合理给药方法时的参考。

【材料】

家兔 2 只，体重 2.0～3.0kg，雌雄不限。

注射器及针头、滴管、解剖刀、手术剪、兔固定箱、酒精棉球。

1% 酒石酸锑钾注射液、灭菌生理盐水。

【方法与步骤】

1. **家兔股四头肌法**　本法适用于检查供肌内注射用制剂的刺激性。股四头肌在后肢大腿的前面，正中为股直肌，股直肌之下为股中间肌，股直肌外侧为股外侧肌，股直肌内侧为股内侧肌，四块肌肉合并称股四头肌。

试验时取健康家兔 2 只，分别于一侧后肢股四头肌处注射 1% 酒石酸锑钾注射液 1.0～2.0ml，于另一侧后肢的对应部位注射同容积的灭菌生理盐水作为对照。48h 后将家兔放血处死，解剖取出股四头肌，纵向切开，观察注射部位肌肉组织的反应。

一般将肌肉组织的反应分为六级：

0级（–）：注射供试品部位的肌肉组织与对照部位肌肉组织无明显差异。

1级（+）：注射供试品部位的肌肉组织有充血，直径在0.5cm以下。

2级（++）：注射供试品部位的肌肉组织红肿、充血，直径在1cm左右。

3级（+++）：注射供试品部位的肌肉组织红肿、发紫、光泽消失，可见坏死点。

4级（++++）：注射供试品部位的肌肉组织红肿、发紫、光泽消失、坏死范围直径达0.5cm左右。

5级（+++++）：注射供试品部位肌肉组织的各项反应更重，有大片坏死。

凡2只家兔的平均反应级数在2以下者，可供肌内注射之用；平均反应级数超过3者，不能供肌肉内注射之用；平均反应级数在2~3之间者，可进行复试或结合其他项目考虑其临床试用问题。凡刺激性试验不能达到肌内注射要求的制剂，一般也不宜供皮下注射或黏膜面给药和创面给药之用。

2. 家兔眼结膜法　本法主要用于试验滴眼剂和其他黏膜用药的刺激性。试验时取健康家兔1只放入固定箱中，待安定后观察正常时结膜的色泽及血管分布。然后将下眼睑拉成环形，并用手指压住鼻泪管（以防药液流入鼻泪管而吸收）。分别将供试品药液和生理盐水0.1ml（或2滴）滴入左、右眼结膜囊内。如供试品为软膏，则挤入约0.1g，另一侧挤入等量的软膏基质，作为对照。

给药后30min内，每隔5min检查一次眼泪分泌情况。给药后3h内，每隔1h轻轻翻开眼皮，观察结膜的反应，以无明显的充血、流泪、畏光、水肿等刺激症状者为合格。

3. 家兔耳壳法　家兔的耳壳比较薄，将药物注射于耳壳皮下，其刺激反应容易在透光检查中发现，不需将动物杀死，因而适用于注射液刺激性的初步试验。

试验时取健康家兔1只，放入固定箱中，透光检查耳壳的正常情况。选取耳壳近基部少血管处，皮下注射供试品0.1~0.2ml。在另一侧耳壳的对应部位皮下注射等量灭菌生理盐水，作为对照。30min内每10min观察兔耳1次，注意有无出现红肿及影响范围。30min后每1h观察1次，直至给药后3h。24h后查看供试品部位有无组织坏死现象。以无明显刺激反应者为合格。

【结果处理】

按下述要求做好记录：

1. 供试品的名称、主药含量、理化性状、生产单位及批号。

2. 家兔的性别、体重与健康状况。

3. 试验的方法、给药途径及剂量、给药时间、结果观察及试验结论。

【注意事项】

1. 兔股四头肌法　注射时必须注意严格消毒以防感染。注射器及针头高压灭菌，用药部位应用碘酒、酒精消毒。必要时可取一小块组织做病理切片，观察有无炎症现象。

2. 家兔眼结膜法　对有刺激性的药物应观察到作用完全消失，结膜完全恢复正常为止。

3. 家兔耳壳法　注射时应避开小血管。有刺激反应时应观察到作用完全消失，注射部位完全恢复正常为止。

【思考题】

家兔的股四头肌法、眼结膜法和耳壳法各适用于哪几种制剂的刺激性试验？其主要步骤和判断指标是什么？

实验 10.4　降压物质试验

【目的】

学习注射液的降压物质检查法。

【原理】

某些脏器制剂和生化制剂（如抗生素类等），因生产过程中混入组胺、腐胺、尸胺以及其他降压物质，故对这类制剂（特别是供注射给药用的）须进行降压物质检查。

【材料】

猫（犬）1只，体重2~3kg（犬10kg左右），雌雄不限，如雌者须无孕。

手术台、手术刀、手术剪、止血钳、气管插管、动脉插管、静脉插管、动脉夹、压力换能器、生理压力监测仪、注射器、铁支架、螺旋夹、双凹夹、棉线、纱布、婴儿秤、橡胶管。

组胺（0.5μg/ml）、链霉素（1.5万/ml）、3%戊巴比妥钠溶液（麻醉用）。

【方法与步骤】

1. **手术**　给猫腹腔注射3%戊巴比妥钠溶液（1ml/kg），麻醉后固定于保温手术台上。切开气管，插入气管以备必要时人工呼吸用。分离静脉，插入静脉插管并连接输液装置，供注药用；分离颈总动脉，插入充满抗凝剂的动脉插管，并与压力换能器和生理压力监测仪相连，以描记血压。

2. **描记正常血压**　调节生理压力监测仪的零点和量程后，打开动脉夹，记录一段正常血压。

3. **灵敏度检查**　待血压稳定后，按体重分次静脉注入不同量的组胺对照品稀释液，0.05μg/kg、0.1μg/kg和0.15μg/kg，每个剂量重复3次。如0.1μg/kg剂量所致血压下降均超过2.7kPa，同时各剂量组间所致反应的平均值有差别，且这一差别又大于任一剂量所致各次反应间的最大差别时，则认为该动物的反应灵敏度合格，可开始进行试验。

4. **给药**　静脉注射组胺0.1μg/kg（dS），按药典规定，供试品（dT）注入容量应与对照品相同，照下列次序注射8个剂量：dS_1、dT_1、dT_2、dS_2、dS_3、dT_3、dT_4、dS_4，每剂量间隔5min。以 dS_1 与 dT_2、dT_1 与 dS_2、dS_3 与 dT_4、dT_3 与 dS_4 所致的反应分别作比较。

【结果处理】

如 dT 所致反应均小于 dS 所致反应，即可认为供试品的降压物质限度符合规定，如 dT 所致的反应均大于 dS 所致的反应，即可认为供试品的降压物质不符合规定。如 dT 所致的反应不是均小于 dS 所致的反应时，应另取动物重复试验。如重复试验的结果仍然如此，则认为供试品的降压物质限度不符合规定。

实验报告记录以下主要内容：

（1）供试品的名称、含量、理化性状、生产单位及批号。

（2）实验动物的种类及性别、体重与健康状况。

（3）组胺对照品溶液和供试品溶液的稀释度、各次注射组胺对照品溶液和供试品溶液所致血压下降值（kPa）、检查结论。结果用完整的图像表示出来。

【注意事项】

1. 注射速度应相同，每次注射后立即注入一定量的生理盐水。相邻两剂量注射的间隔时间应固定（3～5min），但每次注射应在前一次反应恢复稳定以后进行。

2. 用磷酸组胺配制组胺对照品溶液及稀释液时，其用量要按组胺计算。加水配成1.0mg/ml的溶液，分装后于4～8℃下贮存，如无沉淀析出，可在3个月内使用。临用前，用生理盐水配制成0.5μg/ml的稀释液。

3. 供试品要求配制成适当浓度，其注射体积应与对照品稀释液的注射体积相等。

【方法评价】

本法是将一定量的供试品与一定量的组胺对照品轮流注入麻醉猫（或犬）的静脉中，以比较两者引起的血压下降程度，而判断供试品中降压物质的限度是否符合规定，是目前普遍使用的一种方法。

【思考题】

1. 制剂中可能混有哪些降压物质？哪几类药物需考虑作降压物质检查？

2. 4个dS和4个dT必须按照一定顺序、交替注射和比较降压效果，这是为什么？

实验10.5　溶血性试验

【目的】

通过本实验认识溶血现象，并掌握溶血性试验的基本操作。

【原理】

溶血指红细胞破裂、溶解的一种现象。皂苷是一类表面活性剂，有很强的乳化力，具有溶血作用，如多种中草药（如党参、桔梗、夹竹桃、远志、三七等）含有皂苷。另外大量输入低渗溶液以及含有某些甾体化合物的注射液也可以引起溶血。在溶血性检查中尚可附带观察供试品有无红细胞凝集作用。

【材料】

家兔1只，体重2.5～3.0kg，雌雄不限（供采血之用）。

烧杯、竹签（去纤维蛋白）、试管、试管架、滴管、吸管、离心机、恒温水浴。

5%远志煎剂或4%桔梗片煎剂、生理盐水、蒸馏水。

【方法与步骤】

1. 取新鲜兔血10～20ml，用竹签搅拌以除去纤维蛋白，再用生理盐水冲洗3～5次。每次加生理盐水5～10ml，混匀后离心，弃去上清液，再加入生理盐水，离心，直至上清液不呈红色为止。然后按所得红细胞的容积，用生理盐水配成2%的红细胞悬液。

2. 取试管7支（15×150mm），编号，按下表依次加入各种溶液，第6管不加供试品，作为空白对照，第7管不加供试品且用蒸馏水代替生理盐水，作为完全溶血对照。轻轻摇匀后置37℃的水浴中保温，观察0.5h、1h、2h、3h内各管的溶血情况。

试管	1	2	3	4	5	6	7
远志溶液（ml）	0.1	0.2	0.3	0.4	0.5	—	—
生理盐水（ml）	2.4	2.3	2.2	2.1	2.0	2.5	蒸馏水 2.5
2%红细胞悬液（ml）	2.5	2.5	2.5	2.5	2.5	2.5	2.5

【结果处理】

1. **全溶血** 溶液澄明，红色，管底无红细胞残留。

2. **部分溶血** 溶液澄明，红色或棕色，底部尚有少量红细胞残留。镜检红细胞稀少或变形。

3. **不溶血** 红细胞全部下沉，上层液体无色澄明。镜检红细胞不凝集。

4. **凝集** 虽不溶血，但出现红细胞凝集，经振摇后不能分散，或出现药物性沉淀。

一般认为凡1h后第3号试管以及第3号以前的各管出现溶血、部分溶血或凝集反应的制剂均不宜供静脉注射用。

实验报告记录以下主要内容：供试品的名称、含量、理化性状、生产单位及批号、保温后各号试管的结果以及试验结论。

【注意事项】

1. 供采血的动物除家兔外，羊、犬、大鼠等均可使用。

2. 本实验用的2%红细胞悬液，也可用2%全血的生理盐水混悬液。两种混悬液的实验结果基本一致。但前者溶液澄明，易于观察，而后者操作较简便。

3. 如在0.5h内溶液澄明，变成黄或棕黄色，并有棕黄色絮状沉淀，表示药液中有凝集血细胞蛋白的因素。这时可取凝集液一滴置于载玻片上，在显微镜下可见红细胞凝集，在载玻片边缘滴加生理盐水，凝集的红细胞能被冲散则为假凝集，不被冲散则为真凝集。有真凝集现象者不可供临床注射用；有假凝集者可结合局部刺激试验结果，考虑谨慎使用。

4. 如有假凝集现象，而必须进行溶血试验，可在药液中先加入1%鸡蛋清或明胶液，以除去凝集因素，再进行实验。

【方法评价】

本试验是考察受试物有无溶血和凝集反应常用的一种方法。为了保证用药安全，以中草药制成的注射剂，特别是供静脉注射的供试品，都应考虑做溶血性检查。

【思考题】

1. 什么叫溶血现象？与药物有关的哪些因素可以引起溶血现象？

2. 如何进行溶血性试验？其结果如何判断？

英 文 部 分

Chapter 1 Basic knowledge and techniques in pharmacological experiments

Ⅰ. Aim and objective of pharmacological experiments

The pharmacological experiment practically plays an important role in developing the theory of pharmacology, discovery of new drugs, and promoting the development process of clinical medicine. It is one of the most important part of pharmacology teaching, and its objectives are as follows:

1) To verify some important pharmacological theories and concepts in order to understand them completely.

2) To master the basic techniques and methods used in pharmacological experiments, and develop the scientific attitudes toward the experiments.

3) To develop the ability to observe, compare, analyze the objects, and solve practical problems.

4) To learn the research methods of pre – clinical studies of new drugs to have proper knowledge of their pharmacology and toxicity.

To get the objective mentioned above students are required as follows:

1) Conduct each experiment seriously, observe the phenomena carefully, record the data in detail and analyze the data scientifically to assure the accuracy and reliablity of the results.

2) Keep the objective, method, process and principle in mind in order to avoid mess and errors in the experiment.

3) Develop the ability to conduct the experiments while learning the basic use of instruments and apparatus along with proper handling and administration of drugs to animals under the instructions of a teacher.

4) Wash and arrange the used apparatus properly; meanwhile cleaning the lab and handling the alive and dead animals accordingly.

5) Develop the skills to write experimental reports while analyzing the problem and expressing thoughts clearly. Experimental report should consist of title, method, result and discussion on reporting notebook.

Ⅱ. How to handle and administer drugs to animals

Experiment 1. 1   How to handle and administer drugs to mice

Objective

To learn how to handle and administer drugs to mice.

扫码"学一学"

Materials

Animal required：3 - 4 mice, 18 - 22g, male or female.

Apparatus required：mouse cage, balance, syringe, needle, box for fixing mouse.

Chemicals required：saline.

Methods

1. Handling   The mouse can be handled by two methods.

Method Ⅰ：first of all, catch the mouse's tail with right hand and put the mouse on a rough object at the same time slightly pulling it backward. Later, pinch two ears and head skin with thumb, forefinger and middle finger of left hand. Finally, clamp the dorsal and tail skin with ring finger, little finger and center of the palm to make its head forward and neck straight but pay attention to its breath (Fig. 1 - 1).

Method Ⅱ (only with left hand)：Catch the tail with forefinger and thumb, clamp the tail with palm, little finger and ring finger and then catch two ears and back skin with thumb and forefinger (Fig. 1 - 2).

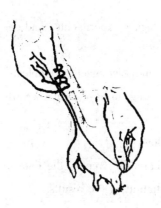 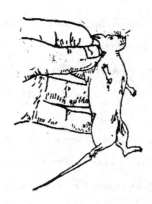 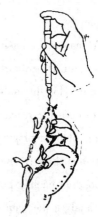

| Fig. 1 - 1   The method Ⅰ to catch mouse | Fig. 1 - 2   The method Ⅱ to catch mouse | Fig. 1 - 3   The method of oral administration to mouse |

The first method is easy to learn, while the second method of handling mice is good for quick drug administration.

2. Oral administration   First of all, hold the mouse in left hand with its head forward and neck fully straight. Later, insert a needle for oral administration into the stomach along the route of angle of mouth, upper palate, gullet, stomach sequentially (Fig. 1 - 3). Whether the needle enters smoothly indicates the correct route or incorrect one through which the needle may enter the air track. The administrative volume is no more than 1. 0 ml.

3. Subcutaneous administration   First of all, hold the mouse with left hand and pinch up the dorsal skin. Secondly, insert a needle (5# or 6#) into the dorsal skin and pull back the needle reelinly in case the drug solution leaks (Fig. 1 - 4). Another way can be adopted through two persons' cooperation. Firstly, one person holds the head skin with left hand and pulls the tail with right hand. Secondly, the other person pinches the dorsal skin with left hand and inserts a needle under the skin with right hand and then pulls back the needle reelingly to prevent any leakage of the drug solution.

4. Intramuscular administration   First of all, hold the head skin with thumb and forefinger of

left hand. Later, clamp the tail and hindlimb of one side with little finger, ring finger and palm and then insert a needle ($4^{\#}$ or $5^{\#}$) into the lateral muscle of the hindlimb with right hand. If two persons cooperate, one person holds the head skin with left hand and pulls the tail with right hand and the other person inserts a needle into lateral muscle of the back leg with right hand. The administrative volume is not more than 0.2ml each leg.

5. Intraperitoneal administration   First of all, hold the mouse (see oral administration)   with its abdomen upward and head down, later, insert subcutaneously a needle ($5^{\#}$ or $6^{\#}$) into the inferior belly either from left or right side (avoiding the bladder) at an angle of 10° towards the head and then insert it further into abdomen at an angle of 45° (Fig. 1 − 5). The advantage of this method is that it can prevent the drug leaking outside. Notes: ① Adjust the angle of syringe needle twice to avoid injecting the drug subcutaneously. ② Avoid inserting the needle from the middle belly in case the bladder is pierced. ③ Avoid inserting the needle too deep or too close to the upper abdomen in case the internal organs are damaged. The usual administrative volume is 0.5ml and not more than 1.0ml.

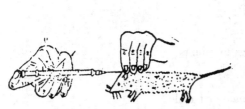

Fig. 1 − 4   The method of subcutaneous injection to mouse

Fig. 1 − 5   The method of intraperitoneal cavity injection to mouse

6. Intravenous administration from the caudal vein   First of all, fix the mouse inside the retrainer with its tail outside and wipe the tail using 75% alcohol solution to dilate the vein. Later, select an obviously dilated vein and hold the tail tip with thumb and middle finger and then press the tail with forefinger to keep the vein dilated all the time. Lastly, insert a needle ($4^{\#}$) into the vein at an angle of $3 - 5^{°}$ (almost parallel to tail) and give the drug (Fig. 1 − 6). Note: ① That resisting force occurs and the tail becomes white locally when injecting the drug indicates that the needle is inserted subcutaneously instead of intravenously. ② Insert the needle from the far end of the tail to ensure that the vein can be injected repeatedly for several times if the failure occurs. The usual administrative volume is 0.2 − 1.0ml.

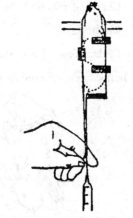

Fig. 1 − 6   The method of caudal vein injection to mouse

Experiment 1.2   How to handle and administer drugs to rats

Objective

To learn how to handle and administer drugs to rats.

Materials

Animal required: 2 rats, 180 − 250g, male or female.

Apparatus required: rat cage, balance, syringe, needle, needle for oral administration, box for fixing rat, a pair of operation glove.

Chemicals required: normal saline.

Methods

1. Handling   Wear a protection glove on the left hand. Other details can be referred to related contents in Experiment 1. 1. As for bigger rats, left hand is used to hold the rats by putting thumb and middle finger under the front oxters and forefinger on the neck to make rats stretch their forelimbs.

2. Oral administration   Similar to the method used for mice. The administrative volume is no more than 2. 0ml.

3. Intraperitoneal injection   Similar to the method used for mice.

4. Intravenous administration   The anesthetized rat can be administrated from either the sublingual vein or the caudal vein. Intravenous administration from the caudal vein can be conducted successfully only when the caudal vein is dilated by sufficiently heating or wiping it with dimethylbenzene.

Experiment 1. 3   How to handle and administer drugs to rabbits

Objective

To learn how to handle and administer drugs to rabbits.

Materials

Animal required: 1 – 2 rabbits, 2 – 3kg, male or female.

Apparatus required: box for fixing rabbit,   mouth – gag for rabbit, platform balance, bladder catheter, syringe.

Chemical required: normal saline.

Methods

1. Handling   Raise the rabbit slightly by holding the nuchal skin with one hand, and support the buttock with the other hand (Fig. 1 – 7) .

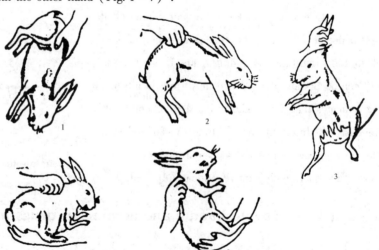

Fig 1 – 7   The methods to catch rabbit

Notes: 1, 2, 3 all are not properly catching method: 1. The kidneys will be injured, 2. The bleeding under the skin of rabbit will be made, 3. The ears will be injured, 4, 5 Those are the correct catching method: to catch the skin of neck back that has thick skin, and hold the rabbit body at the same time

2. Fixation　Lay the rabbit on its back by holding the jugular skin with one hand and knee joint - with the other hand. Then fix the rabbit on the operation platform by binding the extremities with ropes by another person. Fix the head with special device for fixing the head of the rabbit.

3. Oral administration　First, fix the rabbit into the special box and insert horizontally the wood - made mouth - gag into the mouth of the rabbit and roll it upward until the tongue is stretched out. Second, insert slightly the bladder catheter into the stomach instead of air track as long as 15 - 20cm

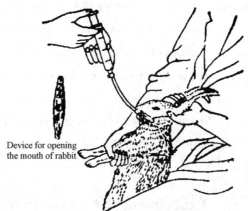

Device for opening the mouth of rabbit

Fig. 1 - 8　The method of oral administration to rabbit

following the route of small hole in the device, back upper palate, gullet (Fig. 1 - 8). The way to check whether or not the bladder catheter goes into the air track is to observe whether or not the air bubble goes out if put the other end of the bladder catheter into the water. Third, inject drug or saline followed by 4 - 5ml of water or air which aims to push all drug inside into the stomach. Last, pull fast the bladder catheter out by holding tightly the end of the bladder catheter in case the water inside drops into the air track.

4. Intravenous administration　First, fix the rabbit into a special box and make the vein in the back and external ear seen clearly by plucking the fur. Second, hold the tip of the ear with the

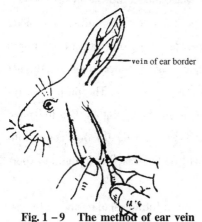

vein of ear border

Fig. 1 - 9　The method of ear vein injection to rabbit

thumb and middle finger and support under the vein with the forefinger of the left hand. Third, insert needle ($6^\#$) into the vein from the tip (having another chance in case failing to do it) at an angle of 5° and fix the needle inside by pressing it outside with thumb, forefinger, and middle finger of the left hand in case the needle goes out of the vein when the rabbit moves its head. Lastly, inject about 10ml of the drug slowly and pull out the needle followed by pressing the vein with cotton in case the blood blows out (Fig. 1 - 9). The way to check whether or not the needle goes into the vein is to observe whether or not the drug goes into smoothly or the bubble appears.

5. Subcutaneous, intramuscular and intraperitoneal administration　Similar to administration of mice in experiment 1 - 1 except that a bigger needle is needed and more volume including 2ml, 2ml and 5ml of the drug respectively is needed

Appendix　How to handle and administer drugs to guinea pigs?

1. Methods of handling　Make the abdomen of the guinea pig upward by holding the forelimbs, neck and chest with the right hand and the hindlimbs with the left hand, not too tight or it will suffer from asphyxia.

2. Oral, subcutaneous, intramuscular and intrperitoneal administration　Similar to the administration of mice in experiment 1 – 1 except that more volume of the drug is needed.

3. Intravenous administration　Either the vein in lateral of the sole of the foot or the external jugular vein can be selected. The former method is as follows. First, hold one hind leg of the guinea pig by one person. Second, cut the fur in the leg and make the vein seen clearly by wiping it with alcohol cotton by another person. Last, insert the small needle for children head injection into the vein. The latter method is adopted such as the following. Make the external jugular vein exposed by cutting a little piece of skin and insert the small needle into it. Be careful when inserting the needle into the vulnerable vein.

Experiment 1. 4　How to handle and administer drugs to dogs

Objective

To learn how to handle and administer drugs to dogs.

Materials

Animal required: 1 dog, 5 – 10kg, male or female.

Apparatus required: special iron tongs,　mouth – gag for dog, platform balance, bladder catheter, syringe, needle, rope.

Chemicals required: normal saline.

Methods

1. For the tameless dog, in order to prevent being bitten, push it down by holding the head and

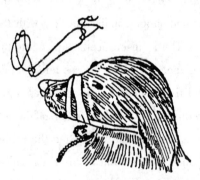

Fig. 1 – 10　The method of binding the dog mouth

neck with special iron tongs and tie up the mouth quickly and delicately with rope as following routes: first node from lower jaw to upper jaws; second node from upper jaw to lower jaw and third node added another slipknot from lower jaw to neck (Fig. 1 – 10). The purpose of tying up the mouth is to avoid being bitten. For the tame dog (trained for about 1 week), tie up the mouth with rope only, or the dog will be too irascible to do the experiment.

2. Oral, subcutaneous, intramuscular and intraperitoneal administration　Similar to administration of rabbit in experiment 1 – 3 except that bigger equipment and more volume of the drug is required.

3. Intravenous administration　Either the small saphenous vein of the hindlimb (this vein goes from the anterior of the lateral malleolus to the external upper side) (Fig. 1 – 11) or the subcutaneous cephalic vein of the forelimb (this vein is at the right anteposition of the upper of the claw at the back side) (Fig. 1 – 12) can be selected. Cut the fur locally and wipe the skin with alcohol cotton. Make the vein seen clearly by holding tightly the superior extremity of the leg for injection by one person; insert the small needle into the vein and drug should be injected by some body else.

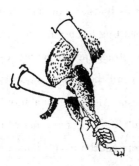
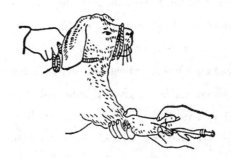

Fig. 1 – 11　The method of small saphenous vein injection to outside of dog's hindlimb

Fig. 1 – 12　The method of cephalic vein subcutaneous injection to backside of dog's forelimb

Ⅲ. Anesthesia of animals widely used in experiment

Anesthesia of animal is often needed in both acute and chronic experiments. As anesthetic not only has the inhibitory effects on central nervous system but also can change other physiological function, its proper selection plays an important role in both making the experiment smoothly carried out and getting the scientific results. Anesthetics and anesthesia protocols vary depending on the objective and type of animals in different experiments.

1. Ether　Ether is the most widely used inhalation anesthetic which is suitable for all types of experimental animals. Its advantages are: ① good therapeutic index. ② controllable depth of anesthesia. ③ Post operative rapid recovery. Its disadvantages are: ① It can stimulate upper respiratory tract to secrete more mucus which may cause postoperative pneumonia because of its strong local stimulatory effect. This can be avoided by subcutaneous injection of atropine (0. 1mg/kg) 20 – 30 minutes before anesthesia. ② It can disturb the functions of respiration, blood pressure and heart, even cause asphyxiation by nervous reflection. This can be overcome by subcutaneous injection of hydrochloric or sulfate morphine (5 – 10mg/kg) 20 – 30 minutes prior to anesthesia because it can decrease excitability of central nervous system, increase pain threshold, reduce the volume of ether, and avoid the excitation period.

When anesthetizing animals such as rats, mice and frogs with ether, put them into glass bell jar or beaker and then throw the ether cotton or carbasus into it. The animal will be anesthetized quickly after inhalation of ether vapours.

When anesthetizing pigeon or chicken with ether, first put ether cotton into a beaker of 25ml and then place its head into it to absorb the ether vapours by holding the animal with a piece of operation scarf.

When anesthetizing cat or rabbit with ether, place the animal into anesthesia glass box and then press ether vapours from ether bottle into the box through a plastic tube till the animal lies down. The signs to be good anesthetized are obviously reduced tensity of all extremities, dull brady – corneal reflex, and disappeared skin pain sensation.

When anesthetizing dog with ether, first of all, bind mouth of dog in order not to be bitten during the excitatory phase. Select the suitable anesthesia mask with carbasus containing ether in it according to the size of the dog. Fix the anterior and hindlimbs by one person, press the chest and neck with right knee, hold the head and neck with one hand, cuff the mask on the mouth of the dog with another hand by another person. More ether is needed when starting to anesthetize and reduced gradually. Pay more attention to the excitatory state which includes struggling, irregular respiration, even asphyxiation that indicates to stop anesthetizing temporarily. Until the animal recovers the normal respiration, ether is given continuously to deepen the anesthesia. Alternate inhalation of the ether and air until the signs to be good anesthesia including gradually disappeared tensity of muscle, dull brady – corneal reflex, and sound sleep appear. Unbind the rope on the mouth immediately and operation can be performed.

2. Barbiturates Barbiturates, with features of weak acidity, white crystals, difficult to dissolve in the water except its sodium salt, are the derivatives of barbituric acid and can be used for intravenous injection. Prepare its water solution only before use because its sodium salt is not stable and easy to dissociate and precipitate.

Barbiturates have good anesthetic effect on animal. Sodium phenobarbital and amobarbital sodium are suitable for long – time operation; while short – acting sodium pentobarbital and pentothal sodium are fit for the recovery of animal after operation.

See Table 1 –1 to 1 –6 for usage and dose of barbiturates.

Table 1 –1   Sodium Barbital

Animal	Route	Concentration and dose	Action
dog	intravenous	10%, 1.8 – 2.2ml/kg	anesthesia
cat	oral	10%, 2.5 – 4ml/kg	anesthesia
cat	abdominal	10%, 5ml/kg	anesthesia
rabbit	intravenous	10%, 1.2 – 1.5ml/kg	anesthesia
rabbit	oral	0.1 – 0.12g/kg	minimal anesthesia
rat	subcutaneous	0.2g/kg	anesthesia
pigeon	abdominal	0.182g/kg	anesthesia
frog	lymph sack	0.18 – 0.2g/kg	minimal anesthesia

Table 1 –2   Phenobarbital （Luminal）

Animal	Route	Concentration and dose	Action
dog, cat	intravenous	10%, 0.8 – 1.0ml/kg	anesthesia
cat	abdominal	10%, 1.5ml/kg	anesthesia
rabbit	abdominal	10%, 1.5 – 2.0ml/kg	anesthesia
pigeon	intramuscular	10%, 3.0ml/kg	anesthesia
frog	subcutaneous	13mg/kg	anesthesia

Table 1 –3   Pentobarbital Sodium

Animal	Route	Dose	Action
dog, cat, rabbit	Intravenous, abdominal	25 – 40mg/kg	anesthesia
rabbit	intravenous	10mg/kg	sleeping
rat	oral	60mg/kg	anesthesia
guinea pig	abdominal	40 – 50mg/kg	anesthesia

Table 1 – 4　Amobarbital（Amytal）

Animal	Route	Dose	Action
dog	abdominal	60mg/kg	sleeping
dog	intravenous	30mg/kg	minimal anesthesia
cat	subcutaneous	100mg/kg	anesthesia
rabbit	intravenous	40 – 50mg/kg	anesthesia
rat	oral	70mg/kg	minimal anesthesia
rat	abdominal	100mg/kg	anesthesia
rat	intravenous	20mg/kg	minimal anesthesia

Table 1 – 5　Thiopental sodium

Animal	Route	Concentration and dose	Action
dog, cat	intravenous	20 – 30mg/kg	anesthesia
dog, cat	abdominal	30 – 50mg/kg	anesthesia
rabbit	intravenous	1%, 1 – 1.8ml/kg	anesthesia

Table 1 – 6　Evipan sodium

Animal	Route	Dose	Action
dog	intravenous	30mg/kg	anesthesia
dog	intravenous	25mg/kg	sleeping
dog	subcutaneous	120mg/kg	anesthesia
cat	intravenous	25mg/kg	anesthesia
rabbit	intravenous	15mg/kg	sleeping
rabbit	intravenous	25mg/kg	anesthesia
rabbit	abdominal	70mg/kg	anesthesia

3. Carbamates（Urethane）　Ethyl carbamate（urethane）, derivative of carbamide, is a kind of mild hypnotic with features of colorless crystal, water – soluble, with strong and rapid effect on animal. It can decrease the blood pressure of both rat and cat and slightly increase CO_2 threshold in respiratory center and reduce oxygen demand. It can cause toxicities if the dose is too high.

4. Chloraloze　Chloraloze, featured by only anesthetizing kinesthetic sense spinal center without any effect on reflection, is particularly suitable for the experiment such as heart and lung assembly. It can also enhance the exciting action of adrenaline on uterus, decrease parasympathetic action and increase or decrease blood pressure.

Cat and rabbit can be anesthetized by intravenous or abdominal injection of mixtures of 1% chloraloze and 3% urethane with dose of 7ml/kg.

IV. How to collect blood from experimental animals

1. Rat or mouse

1）Caudal vein: First of all, fix the animal into a special box with its tail outside and make the caudal vein full of blood by such means as rubbing with hands, heating with warm water（45 – 50℃）or wiping with dimethylbenzene. Later, dry the tail and shear the tip of the tail（5 – 10mm for rat, 1 – 2mm for mouse）to collect the blood by pressing heavily the tail with hands from root to tip of the tail. Finally, press the wound with cotton to stop bleeding and smear 6% collodion on the wound at once in order to protect it by forming a layer of collodion diaphragm on it.

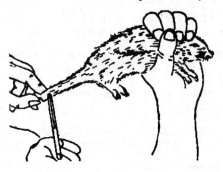

Fig 1 – 13　The second method of taking blood from mouse's tail

In addition, to get 0. 3 – 0. 5ml of blood for route blood test by cutting the 3 caudal veins alternatively from tip to root of the tail. This way is relatively suitable for rat (Fig. 1 – 13).

Sometimes animal anesthetized with thiopental (50mg/kg) is needed in case of failing to get enough blood when the animal is awake. Pay more attention to: ① Add anticoagulant into the tube prior to collecting the blood to avoid blood coagulation. ② If blood cell suspension is needed, blood should be mixed with saline immediately.

2) Orbital artery and vein: First of all, hold the rat with left hand and make its eye exposed outside by pinching tightly the skin on the head with thumb and index finger. Later, pick out right eyeball with a corner pincet without claw with right hand. Finally, place the rat head upside down and the blood drops into the glassware with anticoagulant in it. Blood of 4% – 5% of the body weight can be acquired because of its beating heart but this way is only suitable for one – off blood collection.

3) Venous plexus in the post – orbit: This way is suitable for small animal. The post – orbit venous plexus lies between eyeball and post – orbit. A specially made 7 – 10cm long hard glass straw consisting of 1cm long, 0. 1 – 1. 5mm inner diameter capillary and 0. 6cm diameter tube is needed. First of all, make the eyeball fully exposed outside by holding tightly the head skin between the two ears with index finger and thumb and pressing downward two sides of the neck, which aims to cause difficult blood re – flow of head vein. Later, insert a dry capillary dealt with 1% heparin solution into the orbit venous plexus through the routes of inner side of the eye, between the blepharon and eyeball, 4 – 5mm towards fundus of eye and roll the capillary slightly so that the blood flows out automatically. Finally, stop bleeding by pulling out the capillary and relaxing the neck. This process can be repeated only after several minutes depending on the demand of the experiment (Fig. 1 – 14、1 – 15).

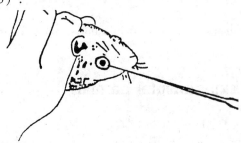

Fig. 1 – 14　The method of taking blood from the venous plexus of the fundus of eye of mouse

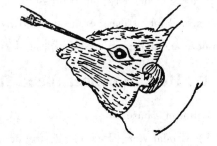

Fig. 1 – 15　The method of taking blood from the venous plexus of the fundus of rat eye

4) Decollation: Hold the back of the mouse with little finger, ring finger and palm and fix the head with thumb and index finger of the left hand with cotton glove. Shear off the head from the neck with scissors in the right hand and turn the mouse downward so the blood drops into the vessel with anticoagulant in it (Fig. 1 – 16).

5) Heart: First of all, place the animal lying on the back and fix it onto the fixation board. Later, shear the fur in the precordial region with scissor and then sterilize the skin with iodine tincture and alcohol. Finally, feel the beat of the heart between the third and fourth ribs of left side with index finger of the left hand and insert a needle ($4^{\#} - 5^{\#}$) into heart at the strongest position of the heartbeat with right hand. The blood will enter into the syringe automatically due to the pressure of the heartbeat (Fig. 1 – 17).

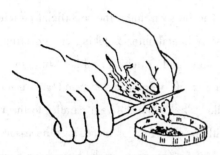

Fig. 1 – 16　**The method of shearing head of mouse**

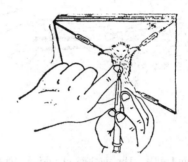

Fig. 1 – 17　**The method of taking blood from the heart of mouse**

6) Carotid artery and vein: First of all, place the animal lying on its back and fix it onto the fixation board, shear the fur in the lateral neck of one side and then conduct the operation to separate and expose the artery and vein in the neck. Later, insert a needle into the artery or vein parallel to it and collect the blood needed.

Another way is to cut apart the artery or vein and collect the blood with a syringe without needle or get it with tube. Ordinarily, 0.6ml from mouse (20g) or 8ml from rat (300g) of the blood can be collected.

2. Rabbit and guinea pig

1) Heart of rabbit: First of all, place the rabbit lying on its back and fix it onto the operation table. Later, shear the fur in the precordial region with scissors and then sterilize the skin with iodine tincture and alcohol. Finally, feel the heart beat between the third and fourth ribs of left side with index finger of the left hand and insert a needle with right hand into the ventricle at the strongest position of the heart beat. The blood will enter the syringe automatically due to the pressure of the heartbeat. This process can be repeated after 6 – 7 days. 1/6 – 1/5 the total blood in rabbit can be obtained once.

2) Central artery on the ear of the rabbit: Fix the rabbit into the box and a thick and bright red central artery full of blood can be seen soon after rubbing with hands or heating with lamp. Stabilize the ear with left hand and insert a needle into central artery towards heart from the end of it with right hand so that the blood enters the syringe immediately. Pay more attention to: ① Stop bleeding after pulling out the syringe. ② Withdraw blood at once before spasmodic contraction of

artery occurs which can be avoided by fully expanding the artery. ③ 6$^{\#}$ needle is necessary. ④ The position for insertion starts from the end of the artery.

Another way is to cut the branch of the central artery slightly with a sharp knife so that the blood flows out and is collected with a tube with anticoagulant in it.

3）Vein on the ear border of rabbit: Insert the big needle into the vein to collect blood after the vessel is expanded by clamping the ear root with small vascular clamp and applying dimethylbenzene and alcohol（Fig. 1 – 18）. A small quantity of blood for route blood test can also to be collected by cutting the vein with needle（5½$^{\#}$）.

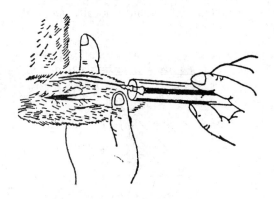

Fig. 1 – 18   The method of taking blood from the ear border of rab bit

4）Subcutaneous vein in the shin of the hindlimb of rabbit: Fix the rabbit lying on it back onto the fixation board and subcutaneous vein can be seen under the superficial cuticle of the shin lateral after plucking fur covering on the shin and pricking rubber tub on the thigh. Fix the vein with left hand and insert a needle（5½$^{\#}$）into the vein parallel to the vein to withdraw 2 – 5ml of blood. It is necessary to stop bleeding by pressing the wound for a sufficient time after collecting the blood in case of formation of subcutaneous hematoma that can affect another withdrawal.

5）Femoral and cervical vein of rabbit: Do an operation to separate and expose the femoral vein or cervical vein fully. Insert a needle（5½ or 6$^{\#}$）towards the heart into the femoral vein parallel to the vein to collect blood. Be careful to stop bleeding by pressing the wound with dry carbasus after collecting the blood and select the position as far away from the heart if the process will be repeated.

Insert a needle（6$^{\#}$）towards the head（2 – 3cm away from branch of cervical vein）into the extra – cervical vein parallel to it as deep as to reach the branch of the cervical vein because the blood vessel here is big and 10ml of blood can be easily acquired. Stop bleeding by pressing the wound with dry carbasus after collecting the blood.

6）Femoral artery and common carotid artery of rabbit: Perform an operation to separate and expose fully the femoral artery or common carotid artery and place a piece of thread under the artery for raising it. Raise the thread and pad under the vessel with the index finger of left hand and insert towards the heart into a needle（6$^{\#}$）paralleling to the vessel. After fixing the needle and vessel together with thumb and index finger of left hand, the blood can be acquired by drawing the syringe core. If a large quantity of blood is needed, shear a small open on the common carotid artery and insert into a flexible plastic tube which is connected to a large syringe with a thin rubber tube（both syringe and rubber tube is added into anticoagulant prior to）and the blood enters the syringe by drawing the syringe core.

7）Eye fundus of rabbit: Insert a needle or a capillary into the veins of eye fundus and about 1 – 2ml blood comes out automatically.

The way to collect blood from a guinea pig is basically similar to that of rabbit.

3. Dog

1) Heart: First of all, fix the dog lying on its back by fixing the forelimb onto the operation table after anesthetizing. Later, shear the fur between the third and fifth rib on the left and then sterilize the skin with iodine tincture and alcohol. Finally, feel the heartbeat between the third and fifth ribs of left side with index finger of the left hand and insert vertically a needle ($8^{\#}$) with right hand into the heart at the position of strongest heartbeat. The blood will enter the syringe automatically due to the pressure of the heartbeat. Pay more attention to: ①The position and direction of insertion can be adjusted according to the sense of touching the heart if failing to collect blood once. ②Do not move the needle left and right in the heart to avoid the damage to the heart. ③The total volume of blood in dog is 80ml/kg.

2) Lateral small saphenous vein of hindlimb and inside subcutaneous vein of head of forelimb: The latter is more widely used than the former. First of all, hold the dog and tie up the mouth with rope. Later, shear the fur on the skin of lateral small saphenous vein of hindlimb or inside subcutaneous vein of head of forelimb and sterilize the skin with iodine tincture and alcohol. Finally, the vein can be seen clearly by holding tightly the upper leg to block the blood reflu by one person and insert into a needle paralleling to the vein to collect the blood by another person (Fig. 1 – 19, 1 – 20, 1 – 21). Pay more attention to: ①Stop bleeding by pressing with cotton after that. ②If a large quantity of blood is needed, collect the blood to use syringe without the needle. ③Remember to relieve the hand that holds the upper leg.

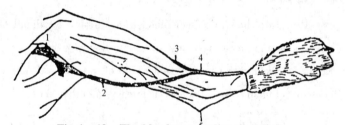

Fig. 1 – 19　The blood stream direction of the smallsaphenous vein to outside the dog's hindlimb

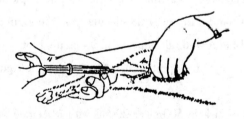

Fig. 1 – 20　The method of taking blood from the small saphenous vein to outside the dog's hindlimb

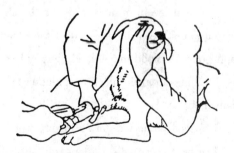

Fig. 1 – 21　The method of taking blood from the cephalic vein to backside of dog's forelimb

3) Vein of neck: Fix the dog with sidelying position, shear the fur on the neck about 10cm × 3cm and sterilize skin with iodine tincture and alcohol. Pull straight the neck, press vein near to the

heart with thumb of left hand to make it clear and insert towards the heart into a needle ($6\frac{1}{2}^{\#}$) paralleling to the vein with right hand (Fig. 1 – 22). Pay more attention to: 1) Press the vein because of its easy movement, and 2) Stop bleeding after that.

4) Femoral artery: Fix the dog lying on its back with or without anesthesia and make the artery in the inguinal trigone exposed by pulling straight the hindlimb outward. After shearing the fur and sterilizing the skin on it with iodine tincture and alcohol, find from the beat of the femoral artery and fix it with middle and index finger of left hand and insert into a needle ($5\frac{1}{2}^{\#}$) from beating position with right hand and collect the blood needed (Fig. 1 – 23). Pay attention to stop bleeding.

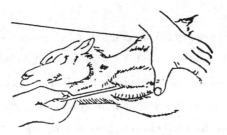

Fig. 1 – 22   The method of taking blood from the cervical vein of dog

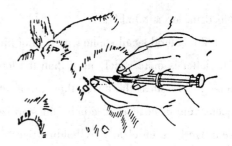

Fig. 1 – 23   The method of taking blood from the femoral artery of dog

5) Vein in the edge of ear: This way is suitable for small quantity of blood for RT. Refer to "how to collect blood from rabbit" for detail (4.2.3).

6) Carotid artery: Refer to "how to collect blood from rabbit" for detail (4.2.6).

The way to collect blood from cat is basically similar to that of dog.

4. Sheep   The vein of neck and the subcutaneous vein of fore or hind limb can be used to collect blood but the former is common – used because it is easy to collect more blood (generally 50 – 100ml at one time).

Pull down the sheep by tying up the limps and fix the head by holding the lower jaw upward. Shear the fur on the neck for 5cm and sterilize the skin with iodine tincture and alcohol. Press the vein of neck with the thumb of right hand and insert into a needle with an angle of 30° towards the heart and collect the blood with right hand. Pull away the needle from the syringe and pour the blood immediately into either a sterilized bottle with glass pears in it agitating for several minutes to avoid blood coagulation by separating from fibrous protein or a flask with anticoagulant in it.

Special bottle for storing blood, which is a trigone flask of 500ml or 200ml with a tampon on it, can be used to collect a large quantity of blood with no pollution. There is a hole as big as a glass duct in the tampon and the bottle should be sterilized with high pressure before to collect the blood. This bottle is suitable for separating the fibrous protein. The common used plastic bag in the hospital also can be used for collecting blood except to adding anticoagulant (100ml blood needs 4ml of 10% sodium citromalic acid saline) in it prior to and the blood can be stored for one week.

The equipment for collecting blood is made of glass tub, rubber tub, glass connecting tub and needle. It should be sterilized before use (Fig. 1 – 24).

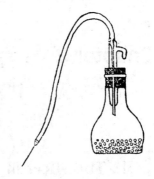

Fig. 1 – 24　The equipment of collecting blood for sheep

Method: ①Fix the sheep into the fixation device. ②Shear the fur on the neck and sterilize the skin with iodine tincture and alcohol. ③Make the vein clear by tying a rubber strap around the neck near the heart. ④Install the bottle for collecting the blood. ⑤Insert into a needle and the blood enters the bottle placed lower than the sheep, shake the bottle continuously. Shake the bottle a little if the anticoagulant is already added. Shake the bottle for 5 minutes to remove the fibrous protein after pulling out of the needle.

Chapter 2　Experiments related to introduction of pharmacology

I. The effect of drugs on the body

The effect of drug on the body is mainly divided into two types, excitation and inhibition. The original physiologic function of the body can be enhanced by some drugs, which is called excitation; and it can also be weakened by some drugs, which is called inhibition. For example, respiratory system can be excited by pentetrazole, and the smooth muscle of gastrointestinal (GI) tract can be relaxed by atropine.

Also, the effect of one drug is different on individual organ or tissue of the body. Functions of some organs or tissues are affected more as compared to other organs or tissues, which is the selective action of drug. For example, digitalis has high selective action on the heart and phenobarbital on the central nervous system. Drugs with high selectivity usually have good curative effects and little side effects.

When a drug acts on the body, the effect it causes can be divided into local action and systemic action according to the part it affects. The former refers to the effect that appears on the site where drug is applied, such as the local anesthetic action of procain; while the latter refers to the effect that occurs after drug is absorbed throughout the body, for instance, the heart rate decreases after propranolol is given.

The reason why drug can exert effects is that it combines with a certain site of body effectors. That site is called receptor. Many classes of receptors have been discovered besides adrenaline receptor and acetylcholine (Ach) receptor. It is generally believed that most drugs exert their effects by binding with receptors. But there are also some drugs whose effects are produced through other mechanisms. For example, ether and chloroform produce general anesthetic effect probably because they can dissolve into liquid easily, and mass into the nervous tissue full of liquid, which changes the permeability of nerve cell membranes and thus cause disturbance of conduction of nerve impulse.

Experiment 2. 1　The local and systemic action of drugs

Objective

Learn the local and systemic action of the drug in this experiment.

Principle

The direct action on the administrative site before the drug is absorbed into blood is called local action, for instance, magnesium sulfate taken orally is difficult to be absorbed and has cathartic effect; injecting local anesthetic in nerve endings or nerve trunk can block the conduction of nerve impulse. The effects exerted when the drug is distributed to every part of the body after entering blood circulation is called systemic effect. For example, after being absorbed in gastrointestinal - tract, drugs cross the portal vein to the liver from blood vessel of intestinal system, and then enter the blood circulation. A few drugs can be applied sublingually and rectally, and they can be absorbed into blood through oral cavity, mucus of rectum and colon respectively. After hypodermic and intramuscular injection, drugs spread along connective tissue at first, and then go through capillary or lymphoid endothelial cell to blood. After intravenous injection, drugs go straight into the blood circulation without being absorbed.

Oral administration and injection of drugs lead to the absorption in digestive tract and injection site respectively. Local application mainly causes local effect such as inunction, poudrage, nebulization, gargling, wet pack, cleaning and drip. Although, inhalation, implantation, iontophoresis, sublingual, anal and vaginal application belong to local administration, but they must get absorbed to produce effect.

Materials

Animals required: 2 mice, 18 – 22g,   male or female.

Apparatus required: mouse cage, beaker, glass plate, hemostat.

Reagent required: chlorethyl spray (or chlorethyl solution) .

Methods

Take two mice and mark them. Observe the mobility, color and luster of tails. Clip the part of tail and hind limb of both mice by hemostat, observe their response to pain, then operate as follows: The first mouse, spray chlorethyl to its tail or drop about 1ml chlorethyl, observe the change of the color and luster of the tail's skin, clip its tail and hind limb by hemostat immediately, observe its response to pain and mobility, and compare these situations to that before administration. The second mouse, put it into a beaker, place a cotton ball soaked with 1ml chlorethyl, then cover the beaker with glass plate, bring out the mouse from the beaker as soon as it falls down from anesthesia, check if its tail has the similar change of the color and luster to the first mouse, then clip its tail and hind limb by hemostat, observe its response to pain.

Results

Make table to compare the results.

Table 2 – 1   The experimental results of local action and systemic action of choloroethyl

Number	Administration method	Reactions				Local or system action
		Color change of tail's skin	Reaction of clipping tails	Reaction clipping limbs	Moving ability	

Notes

1. The grip of clipping tails and hind limbs of mice by hemostat to examine their reaction to pain must be moderate and consistent, and don't exert too much strength to injure the tissue.

2. Concentrate on the response of mice. Both local and systemic actions of chlorethyl are easy to disappear after administration, so they must be quickly observed.

Evaluation

1. The purpose of this experiment is to primarily learn the local and systemic action of drug. The observation index is positive or negative reaction, and the experiment is simple, with reliable results.

2. In order to further explain the type of action of drug, measurement of the blood concentration after administration will be more accurate.

Question

1. What are the local action and systemic action of drug and what are their characteristics? With examples further explain them.

2. Through the effect chlorethyl has on the two mice, analyze which ones are local actions and which ones are systemic actions, and infer from these the pharmacological effect of chlorethyl.

Experiment 2. 2　Indirect effect of drugs

Objective

Understand the indirect effects of drugs.

Principle

The effect that drug directly produces on the tissue or organ it contacts is called direct effect. The effect on other organs caused by direct effect is called reflex action. For example, antiacid ⟶decreased gastric acid (direct effect) ⟶stomachache alleviated (indirect effect); cardiac glucosides ⟶ heart power enforced (direct effect) ⟶ circulation developed (indirect effect) ⟶diuresis (indirect effect), etc.

Materials

Animal required: 1 rabbit, 1. 8 – 2. 2kg, male or female.

Apparatus required: biological signal acquisition system, operation table, pulley block, myodynamia transducer, iron Keepe set, frog heart clasp, and cotton thread.

Reagent required: 10% ammonia water, 2% dicaine hydrochloride solution.

Methods

Take a rabbit, tie the animal in supine position on a table, and fix its head with rabbit head clasp. Clip where respiratory is the most obvious on abdominal wall by frog heart clasp, which is linked to myodynamia transducer through pulley block by thread and then connected to biological signal acquisition system, so as to record the rabbit's respiration. Record the normal respiratory for some time, then place a cotton ball absorbing ammonia water near the rabbit's nostril, make it inhale ammonia, and observe the influence on the rate and range of respiratory. Take away the cotton ball, wait till the rabbit's respiratory is normal again, then apply 2% dicaine hydrochloride with a cotton ball absorbing it to the mucosa of the nostril, and make the rabbit inhale ammonia by the same way . 5 minutes later, observe the influence on the respiration. Compare the reaction of the rabbit when inhaling ammonia before applying dicaine hydrochloride with that of ammonia, after administration.

Results

Record the respiratory curve, and explain it.

Notes

1. Fix the rabbit on the table tightly so it can't struggle, otherwise it will affect the record of the respiratory curve.

2. The situation of inhaling ammonia, such as the volume of ammonia solution being absorbed, inhaling time and the distance between the cotton ball and the nostril, should be as same as possible.

Dicaine should be applied evenly on both nostrils' mucosa with a depth of 1cm.

Evaluation

This experiment is carried out by a simple way, but it can illustrate the indirect effect of drug and the factors that affect it easily.

II. The effect of the body on drug

The effect of body on the drug is generally called pharmacokinetics, which aims to evaluate the process of drug absorption, distribution, metabolism and excretion in the body and provides an important reference to clinical drug administration design. Generally, there are two types of research methods, *in vitro* experiments such as the research on hepatic metabolic enzymes and drug metabolism and plasma – protein binding rate, and *in vivo* experiments, such as measuring blood concentration, making $C - t$ curve of fit according to the concentration at every time point, and then obtaining a series of pharmacokinetic parameters.

Experiment 2. 3　Estimation of pharmacokinetic parameters of BSP

Objective

With sodium bromsulphalein (BSP), study the usual method of estimating pharmacokinetic parameters.

扫码 "学一学"

Principle

Some drugs are eliminated from the body following first order kinetics. When they are intravenously injected and pharmacokinetic mode belongs to one – compartment, the relationship between the concentration of drug in plasma and the time is given by

$$C = C_0 e^{-kt} \quad (1)$$

Where K is constant of elimination rate, C_0 is initial concentration (ie. $t = 0$, $C = C_0$).

After logarithm transform, (1) yields

That is to say, plotting the logarithms of concentration vs time yields a straight line. Its slope b $= k/2.303$, its intercept a $= \log C_0$. Thus we obtain $k = 2.303 \times b$ and $C_0 = \log^a$.

$$\lg C = \lg C_0 - \frac{K}{2.303} \times t$$

Pharmacokinetic parameters may be estimated according to following equations:

$$k = -\,2.303 \times b \qquad\qquad (\text{time}^{-1})$$

$$t_{1/2} = 0.693/\text{k} \qquad\qquad (\text{time})$$

$$V = X_0/C_0 \qquad\qquad (\text{volume/kg})$$

$$\text{Cl} = kV = 0.693/\,t_{1/2} \cdot V \qquad\qquad (\text{volume/time/kg})$$

Where $t_{1/2}$, V and Cl are half – life, apparent volume of distribution and clearance, respectively.

BSP is a dye used to determine the function of the liver. It is pink in a basic solution and colorless in an acidic solution. It may be determined by colorimetric method.

Materials

Animal required: 1 rabbit.

Apparatus required: 722 colorimeter, test tubes, centrifuger, pipetts, syringes, operation table, venous cannulation.

Reagent required: solution Of BSP 2%, saturated solution of potassium citrate, heparinized Saline (10U/ml), 2.5mol/L NaOH, 0.01mol/L HCl, 1% Procaine hydrochloride.

Methods

1. Take a rabbit and weigh it, fix the animal on a table in supine position.

2. Shave the hair in the groin on one side where throbbing can be seen, subdermal local anesthesia with 1% Procaine hydrochloride.

3. Cut the skin 3 – 4cm vertically, separate the femoral vein and pass double threads under the vein, tie the distal end up with one thread, make a incision on the vein, insert a venous cannula (already connected to a syringe filled with heparinized saline) into the femoral vein and fix it with another thread, and make sure blood can be taken smoothly.

4. Blood samples (1.5ml) are taken from femoral vein at 2, 4, 6, 10, 15, 20min following iv 20mg/kg of BSP. The blood samples run freely into the tubes containing $K_2C_2O_4$. Shake them gently to make $K_2C_2O_4$ dissolve evenly in the blood.

5. Every time before taking blood sample, discard about 0.2ml blood at first, and after sampling blood, inject the same capacity of Saline to rabbit to make up the blood for loss.

6. Separate the plasma by centrifuging at 3000rpm for 5min.

7. Transfer 0.5ml plasma from each sample to various dry tubes.

8. Add 5.5ml of 0.01mol/L HCl to each tube and shake it thoroughly.

9. The optical densities A_{H^+} are measured with colormeter (540nm). Distilled water serves as a blank.

10. Measure the optical densities A_{H^+}, add one drop of 2.5mol/L NaOH to each tube and shake it. Then measure optical densities A_{OH^-}.

11. With the difference between two optical densities $\Delta A = A_{OH^-} A_{H^+}$, the concentration of BSP in plasma is determined from the standard curve.

$$\lg C = \lg C_0 - \frac{K}{2.303} \times t$$

12. Make a linear regression of lgC vs t, ie.

13. Using equations mentioned above, estimate pharmacokinetic parameters.

Preparation for standard curve: compound 200μg/ml BSP solution with distilled water, take 7 test tubes, number them with 1, 2, 3, ...7, perform as following Table 2 – 2.

Make a linear regression of ΔA vs C and obtained.

Standard curve of BSP ie $\Delta A = A + B \cdot C$.

Make a graph of ΔA vs C (of BSP) and get the standard curve.

Table 2 – 2   Plotting of the standard curve of BSP

No	1	2	3	4	5	6	7
ml of 200μg/ml BSP	0.025	0.05	0.075	0.10	0.15	0.20	0.30
ml of 0.01mol/L HCl	5.975	5.95	5.925	5.90	5.85	5.80	5.70
optical densities A_{H^+}							
drop of 2.5mol/L NaOH	1	1	1	1	1	1	1
optical densities A_{OH^-}							
$\Delta A = A_{OH^-} - A_{H^+}$							
concentration (μg/ml)	5	10	15	20	30	40	60

Notes

1. Perform it softly, and wash the hemolystix by drawing Saline so as to be sure to avoid hemolysising when sampling.

2. Every time, while taking sample, take 0.2ml blood and discard it at first, the process of taking sample should be as quick as possible to be sure that the time of blood sample is accurate.

3. Samples should be balanced before centrifuging, and the speed of centrifuging should be moderate.

Evaluation

Taking blood via femoral vein is quick, convenient and not easy to hemolysis compared to other ways such as that via veins of ear border. The method introduced here is only a rough one to estimate pharmacokinetic parameters.

Experiment 2.4   Measurement of plasma – protein binding rate

Objective

Understand the method of measuring plasma – protein binding rate.

Principle

The plasma – protein binding rate is an important pharmacokinetic parameter, for binding of drug and protein at a high level (about 80%) has a significant clinical value. There are many experimental methods of evaluating drug – protein binding. At present, balanced dialysis, ultrafiltration and gel filtration are often used. Here we make a detailed introduction of balanced dialysis. Put protein solution in a semipermeable membrane, then put into buffer solution involving drug, let the drug molecule diffuse freely through the semipermeable membrane, measure the drug concentration inside and outside of the membrane as the diffusion reaches balance. Subtract the concentration outside the membrane from that inside the membrane, and the result divided by the concentration inside is the rate of protein binding.

Materials

Apparatus required: tubular semipermeable membrane (about 5cm round – long, 10cm long).

Reagent required: 0.2ml pH 7.4 phosphoric acid buffer solution (involving 0.15mol/L NaCl), 3% sulfosalicylic acid solution.

Methods

1. Fold one end of the tubular semipermeable membrane, tie it tightly with a thread to make a sack, add 2.5ml plasma sample into it with pipette fold and tie the mouth of the sack, with a little air in the sack.

2. Place the semipermeable membrane sack in a wide – mouth bottle with volume of 30ml which has 10ml dialysate in it, adjust with the thread of both ends of the sack the surface of the liquid inside and outside of the sack to make them remain at the same level.

3. Place the wide – mouth bottle in the refrigerator (4℃) to balance it more than 60h, draw out a little dialysate outside of the sack after reaching the dialysis equilibration, add equal capacity of sulfosalicylic acid solution to examine if any plasma – protein has leaked from the sack.

4. Measure the concentration of drug of the solution both inside and outside of the sack.

Results

The method of calculating βp and K_{dp}

$$[D] = \beta p \times \frac{P[D]}{[D] + [PD] - [D]W} - K_{dp}$$

$[D]$ and $P[D]$ is mol concentration of free and bound drug respectively, P is the concentration of protein (g/L), W is water involving rate of plasma, βp is the maximum of apparent ability of drug – protein binding (μmol/L), K_{dp} is dissociation constant of drug – protein compound (μmol/L). Make a graph of $[D]$ vs $P[D] / ([D] + [PD] - [D]W)$, β_p and K_{dp} can be calculated through linear regression. And use the following equation to calculate the protein – binding rate of every concentration.

Protein binding rate = $1 - [W + P\beta p / ([D] + K_{dp})]$

Evaluation

This method is easy and suitable for determining many samples at the same time, but it needs a relatively long time to attain equilibrium.

III. Factors that influence drug action

The factors that influence drug action involve two aspects: drug and body.

1. The aspect of drug

1) The chemical structure and physicochemical properties of drug not only directly decide the nature and intensity of drug action, but also decide the absorption, distribution, metabolism and excretion of drug in the body. Drugs that have similar chemical structure usually have similar pharmacological activity.

2) The dose of drug can produce both intensity change and quality change, so for drugs that have narrow therapeutic window, the dose must be seriously controlled and medication should be individualized if necessary so as to be sure of safe administration.

3) Different routes of administration can directly influence the quantity and speed of drug absorption, and also the distribution and excretion of drug, and thus influence the effect of drug.

2. The aspect of body   The difference of age, sex, weight and race can lead to different reactions to drug, especially the babies and the old who have obvious different reactions to the same dose of drug comparing to the average person. In addition, other factors such as inheritance, pathologic condition and even the tolerance to some drugs can affect the development of drug effect.

Experiment 2. 5   Factors affecting drug action

A. Effects of preparations on drug action

Objective

Compare the effects of two preparations of strychnine on toads.

Principle

Strychnine is a central stimulant, and the animal will produce convulsion and even die as dose increases. The pharmacological effect has direct relationship to rate of absorption of drug.

Materials

Animal required: 2 toads.

Reagent required: strychnine, 0. 2% solution W/V, strychnine, 0. 2% colloidal solution W/V (in 2. 5% carboxymethyl cellulose sodium solution) .

Methods

1. Tie the paws with a ligature to mark the animal.

2. Each of them is treated by Pectoral lymph sac injection. One receives strychnine solution 10mg/kg, The other receives strychnine colloidal 10mg/kg.

3. Place the toads under a lamp. Observe their reflexes from time to time by touching them, until they experience tonic spasm.

4. Record the latent period and extent of spasm in both animals.

Results

Make two tables to compare the results, and make statistical analysis of the latent period of all teams of class (Table 2 −3, 2 −4) .

Table 2 −3   The effect of two preparations to toads

Preparation	Sex	Weight (g)	Latent period (min)	Extent of spasm
water				
colloidal				

Table 2 −4   The influence of spasm latent period of two preparations

Preparation	Team number								$\bar{x} \pm SD$
	1	2	3	4	5	6	7	8	
water									
colloidal									

B. The influence of administrative route on drug action

Objective

Observe the influence of administrative route on the pharmacological action of remeflin.

Principle

Remeflin is a central stimulant; it can cause excitation, convulsion or death on animals.

Materials

Animal required: 3 mice.

Reagent required: Remeflin 0.04 % (W/V).

Methods

1. Mark three mice, preferably uniform weight and sex.

2. Each animal receives 8mg/kg of remeflin by oral, subcutaneous or intraperitond rove respectively.

3. Record the latent period of action (from the administration to convulsion), lethal period (from the administration to death) and living condition (alive or died).

Results

Make two tables to compare the results, compare the appearing period and action degree of drug reaction in the three routes of administration. Statistical analysis is recommended (Table 2 – 5, 2 – 6).

Table 2 – 5   The influence of administrative route on drug action

Number	Dose (mg/kg)	Route of administration	Latent period (min)	Extent of spasm
A				
B				
C				

Table 2 – 6   The influence of latent period on administration

Route	Team number								x ± SD
	1	2	3	4	5	6	7	8	
Oral									
Subcutaneous									
Intraperitoneal									

C. The influence of liver function on drug action

Objective

Observe the effects of sick liver functions on drug action.

Principle

Carbon tetrachloride (CCl_4) is a hepatotoxic compound often used to produce toxic hepatitis in animals for screening compounds that can prevent liver damage.

Materials

Animal required: 2 mice, 18 – 22g, same sexuality.

Reagent required: Carbon tetrachloride (CCl_4) 100% (W/V), Pentobarbital sodium, 0.3% (W/V), normal saline.

Methods

1. Mice, preferably uniform weight and sex are arranged in 2 groups.

2. 24h before experiment, inject one mouse subcutaneously with 0.1ml of CCl_4 solution and other mouse with 0.1ml of normal saline.

3. Two mice receive pentobarbital of 30mg/kg by ip.

4. Watch the symptoms closely and assess the righting reflex gently.

5. Carefully time the latent period (from administration to disappearance of righting reflex) and last period (sleeping time) of drug action.

6. Carry out the post – mortem examination and compare the alterations in the color and surface of the liver.

Results

Make two tables to compare the results (Table 2 – 7, 2 – 8).

Table 2 – 7   The influence of liver function on drug action

Number	Dose (mg/kg)	Liver function	Latent period (min)	Sleeping time (min)	Post – mortem examination of liver
A					
B					

Table 2 – 8   The influence of latent period on liver function

Liver function	Team number								x ± SD
	1	2	3	4	5	6	7	8	
Normal saline									
CCl_4									

Chapter 3   Experiments of drugs affecting the central nervous system

Drugs affecting the central nervous system include general anesthetics, sedative – hypnotics, Narcotic analgesics, anti – epileptics, anticonvulsants, anti – psychotics, central stimulants, etc.

Traditionally, general anesthetics can be divided into inhaled anesthetics (ether, halothanes, nitrous oxide, etc), intravenous anesthetics (sodium thiopentone, ketamine, γ – hydroxybutyrat, etc) and Chinese traditional herbal anesthetics (datura flower). Inhaled anesthetics and intravenous anesthetics can widely inhibit the electrocerebral action in CNS, and reach phase Ⅲ of anesthesia, therefore consciousness and pain reflex disappear and muscles relaxe, so they are called inhibitory anesthetics. A few anesthetics such as ketamine can selectively block the pain sense, but show exciting effect on reticular formation and limbic system, so they are defined as excitatory anesthetics. During anesthesia patients experience complete loss of pain sensation, but incomplete loss of consciousness.

Sedatives and hypnotics have inhibitory effect on CNS. The degree of their effect on CNS divides them into low effect sedatives and high effect hypnotics depending on the dose administered. Those drugs include barbiturates (such as phenobarbital), benzodiazepines (such as chlordiazepoxide, diazepam, etc) and other sedatives and hypnotics. In addition, antihistamines (such as diphenhydramine, promethazine, etc), antisychotics (such as chloropromazine), analgesics and some Chinese herbal medicines also have sedative and hypnotic effects.

Analgesics can relieve pain selectively, and can be divided into strong analgesics and weak analgesics. Strong analgesics, which can inhibit the CNS pain – sensor area, include addictive analgesics or narcotic analgesics (such as opiates including pethidine, fentanvl, methadone, etc). Weak analgesics are the analgesics acting on the peripheral pain – receptor and called as NSAIDs (such as aspirin).

Epilepsy, a kind of cerebral function disturbance syndrome caused by abnormal discharge of some hyperexcitability cranial nerves, can be divided into grand mal, petit mal, psychomotor seizures and localized seizures. Clinically, we carry out controlled treatment with the drugs that inhibit abnormal discharge of impulse or prevent its diffusion. Convulsion, a kind of hyperexcitability symptom of CNS caused by various reasons, is featured by involuntary, incoordinate, stiff and clonic tic of total body skeletal muscle. It generally occurs in high fever of children, eclampsia, tetanus and acute poisoning, and can be controlled by central motor inhibitor or some peripheral muscle relaxant.

Mental disorder is a disease of psychomotility (such as thinking, sentiment, behavior, etc) disorder having various reasons, which include schizophrenia, mania, depression and anxiety neurosis. Antipsychotics are the drugs having therapeutic effect on schizophrenia, mania, depression and anxiety state, etc. and can be divided into: ① antischizophrenia drugs (or antipsychotics);

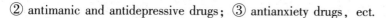

② antimanic and antidepressive drugs; ③ antianxiety drugs, ect.

Central stimulants are a class of drugs that can raise the functional activity of CNS. Usually they can be divided according to different site of action into cerebral stimulants (such as caffeine, nikethamine, lobeline, dimefline, bemegride, pentetrazole, etc) and spinal cord stimulants (such as strychnine). This class of drugs, with therapeutic dose, mainly affect on medulla oblongata respiratory center, so they are also called bulbar stimulants. At the same time, they can excite medulla oblongata vasomotor center to raise blood pressure and improve breathing and circulatory function. In clinical practice, they are mainly used in the treatment of respiratory failure caused by various reasons. But if the dose is too high or over frequently used, it can cause convulsion because of the over-excitation of cerebrum and medulla oblongata. Because energy in cerebrum is exhausted, toxic doses of central stimulants can lead to coma and death.

I. Experiment of general anesthetics

Experiment 3. 1   Activity determination of volatile fluid anesthetics

Objective

Observe the characteristics of ether anesthesia, and learn the activity determination method of general anesthetics.

Principle

Usually use the loss of righting reflex of small animals and the head pendency of big animals (loss of head righting reflex) as the index of anesthetic activity determination.

Add volatile fluid anesthetics of known molecular weight and relative density into a capacity – known container, and we can count out vapor concentration of anesthetic in the container with this formula:

$$\text{vapor concentration}\% = \frac{\text{fluid volume (ml)} \times \text{relative density} \times 22.4 \text{ (L)} \times 100}{\text{molecular weight of drug} \times \text{capacity of container (L)}}$$

The concentration calculated by that formula is volume in the standard status, the practical volume need to be corrected with this formula, according to the situation of experiment:

$$PV/T = P'V'/T'$$

P、V、T are pressure, volume and temperature of the gas in the standard status.

P'、V'、T' are pressure, volume and temperature of the gas in the experimental status.

Materials

Animal required: mouse, 18 – 22g, no restriction on sex.

Apparatus required: box for animal anesthetization.

Reagent required: ether.

Methods

1. The box for animal anesthetization is a sealed box made of glass with the capacity of 4 – 10L (Fig. 3 – 1). A plate with sodalime is placed in this box to absorb carbon dioxide and moisture in the box. Upper side of the box is openable. An electric fan can be fixed in the box to accelerate evaporation of drugs.

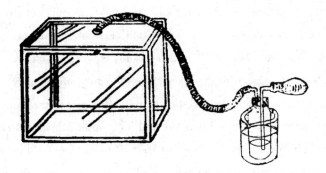

Fig. 3 – 1　Box for animal anesthetization

2. Calculate the dose of drug according to the requirement of drug vapor concentration in the box, shake the box to volatilize drug fluid, and then throw the mice into the box. If 50% anesthetic concentration (AD_{50}) is required to be reckoned, increase drug vapor percentage concentration by 4 – 6 dosages according to geometric progression. Each group has 5 – 10 mice. In this way we can get the dose – effect curve, and calculate AD_{50}.

3. Induction period of anesthesia should be 0.5 – 5 minutes. Adjust the vapor concentration of anesthetic, if beyond that range.

4. Loss of righting reflex and pain sensation is deemed as the anesthetic indexes. If animals cluster together or lean against each other, it is difficult to determine the result. At this time, the suspected mice should be observed in supine position. When measuring the pain sensation, we can stab the hind foot with pin or clip the root of mouse of tail near nausea with alligator clamp.

5. Continue to observe for 10 – 30 minutes after anesthetization, to survey whether the process of anesthetization is steady.

Results

Calculate the value of AD_{50}.

Notes

1. Ether is combustible and easy to explode, and it is heavier than air. Exercise caution during the experiment.

2. Examine whether the box for anesthetization is air tight before the experiment.

3. Control the anesthetic index strictly, that is where righting reflex disappears.

Evaluation

There are two major methods of general anesthetic experiments, small animal method and big animal method. The former is simple, economical, and suitable for initial drug screening. The latter is usually used in review study. Mice are usually used in small animal method. We can primarily estimate the safety of drugs by the difference between anesthetic concentration/dose and lethal concentration/dose, and it can be used to compare the potency and efficacy of the same kind of anesthetics. But the result of big animal method is more close to the response of clinical patients, so it has better reference value, and easy to measure induction period of anesthetics, process of anesthetization, restoration period, and influence to breath, blood pressure, ECG, all kinds of reflection, de-

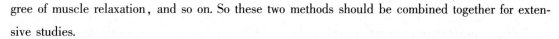

gree of muscle relaxation, and so on. So these two methods should be combined together for extensive studies.

Questions

1. What are the advantages and disadvantages of ether anesthetization?

2. What is its role in the clinical application?

II. Experiment of sedatives and hypnotics

Experiment 3. 2　Comparison of the actions of barbiturates

Objective

Compare the intensity of effect, latent period, duration of effect of some barbiturates.

Principle

Liposolubility of barbiturates is the main factor of their rapid absorption to brain tissues. High liposoluble drugs penetrate blood – brain barrier easily, so the latent period is short and more drugs can enter the brain. High liposoluble drugs are metabolized mainly by liver microsomal mixed-function oxidase system (MFOS), so their duration of action is short. But low liposoluble drugs excrete from kidney mainly on prototype, so the duration of effect are longer.

Materials

Animal required: 3 mice, 18 – 22g, male or female.

Apparatus required: balance, syringes.

Reagent required: Luminal 0. 6% solution W/V, pentobarbital sodium 0. 2% solution W/V, thiopentone sodium 0. 2% solution W/V, picric acid.

Methods

Mark and weigh three mice, each of which is treated by intraperitoneal injection. Mouse A receives 0. 6% Luminal 150mg/kg (0. 25ml/10g); Mouse B receives 0. 2% pentobarbital 50mg/kg (0. 25ml/10g); Mouse C receives 0. 2% thiopentone 50mg/kg (0. 25ml/10g). Observe the behavior of the mice after administration, assess the righting reflex gently, and record the latent period and duration of anesthesia.

Results

Record the result of experiment in Table 3 – 1.

Table 3 – 1　Result of comparing the actions of some barbiturates

Number	Weight (g)	Drug& Dosage (mg/kg)	Change of Behavior	Righting reflex (min)		Character of action
				Latent period	Duration	

Notes

1. Keep quiet during the course of experiment.

2. Put a mouse on its supine position. When it keeps lying on the back means loss of righting

reflex.

3. Keep surrounding temperature constant after the disappearance of mouse righting reflex.

Evaluation

Sedatives, hypnotics and tranquilizers can change the behavior of animals to different degree such as quietness, aggression, eyes closure, drowsiness, loss of righting reflex, etc. According to the characteristics, intensity, latent period and duration of drug actions, we can compare the efficacy of this kind of drugs. This method is simple, but all the central depressants possess the aforementioned effects. So this method has poor specificity, and can be used only in initial qualitative study. If we want to study further characters of drug effects, we should choose the methods with higher specificity, such as experiment of taming, the action of confronting central stimulants, and experiment of conditioned reflex, etc.

Question

Discuss the difference of barbiturates in intensity, latent period and duration, and the reason of difference.

Experiment 3.3 Synergism of sedatives and hypnotics and their antagonistic actions to central stimulants

Objective

Through the experiment, study the drug – drug interaction——synergism and antagonism, and learn the screening method of sedatives and hypnotics.

Principle

The effects of sedatives and hypnotics are, in turn, sedation, hypnosis and barbiturates also have anesthetic effects, with the increase of the dosage. Combined use of sedatives and hypnotics can produce additive action and inhibit convulsion caused by central stimulants.

Materials

Animal required: 5 mice, 18 – 22g, male or female.

Apparatus required: balance, syringes and bell jar.

Reagent required: diazepam 0.04% solution W/V, sodium pentobarbital 0.2% solution W/V, remeflin 0.04% solution W/V.

Methods

Mark and weigh five mice of the same sex and weight. Then dispose as follows:

Mouse A is treated with intraperitoneal injection with 0.04% Diazepam 8mg/kg (0.2ml/10g).

Mouse B is treated with subcutaneous injection of sodium pentobarbital 40mg/kg (0.2ml/10g).

Mouse C is treated with intraperitoneal injection of 0.04% Diazepam 8mg/kg (0.2ml/10g), 10 minutes later, inject with sodium pentobarbital 40mg/kg (0.2ml/10g) subcutaneously.

Mouse D is treated with subcutaneous injection of 0.04% remeflin 8mg/kg (0.2ml/10g).

Mouse E is treated with intraperitoneal injection of 0.04% Diazepam 8mg/kg (0.2ml/10g), 10 minutes later, inject with 0.04% remeflin 8mg/kg (0.2ml/10g) subcutaneously.

Put the five mice in the bell jar individually. Compare the drug effects and the final results. Observe the effects of per – treating with Diazepam to pharmacological effects of sodium pento-barbital and remeflin.

Results

Record the result of experiment in Table 3 – 2.

Table 3 – 2　Experiment result of drugs synergism and antagonism

Number	Sex	Weight (g)	First treatment		Second treatment		Type of drug interaction
			Drug & Dosage (mg/kg)	Drug effect	Drug & Dose (mg/kg)	Drug effect	

Notes

1. Wash the needle clearly before injection, in order to avoid effect of drugs interaction on the result.

2. Sedatives and hypnotics belong to central depressants, so it is difficult to distinguish their effects in animal experiments. The main index of sedation is reduction of spontaneous activity; the main index of hypnosis is incoordination of animals, and falling asleep gradually in quiet surrounding. Loss of righting reflex can represent hypnosis and reflect anesthesia of barbiturates.

3. Keep quiet during the course of experiment, and the suitable room temperature is 15 – 20℃.

Evaluation

Praxiology experiments are usually used in initial drug screenings of sedatives and hypnotics, which can enhance mice falling asleep when pentobarbital of subthreshold dose is given simultaneously. Evaluate the drugs effect by the index of the number of mice losing righting reflex. In addition, we can also screen with the reduction of over – activity resulting from central stimulants. And evaluate the drugs effect by the resistance to toxicity of central stimulants or the rising range of LD_{50}.

But the specificity of all those methods is low, which makes it difficult to distinguish action characters of drugs. So they are always used in initial screening and qualitative analyse.

Question

What manners can drugs interact with each other during combination of drugs? What results do they cause respectively?

Experiment 3. 4　Effects of drugs on spontaneous activity of animals

Objective

Observe the effect of Diazepam on spontaneous activity of mice, and learn the screening methods of sedatives and hypnotics.

Principle

Spontaneous activity is a physiological character of animals, its frequency can usually indicate the status of central excitation or inhibition. Sedatives and hypnotics and other central depressants

扫码 "学一学"

can all reduce the frequency of spontaneous activity obviously. The degree of reduction of spontaneous activity is directly proportional to the intensity of central depressants.

Materials

Animal required: 3 – 4 mice, 18 – 22g, with the same sex.

Apparatus required: mouse spontaneous activity recording equipment, balance, syringes and mouse cage.

Reagent required: diazepam 0. 04% solution W/V, normal saline, picric acid.

Methods

Connect mouse spontaneous activity recording equipment with power and set the recording period at 5 minutes. Mark and weigh two mice with close activity.

Put mouse A into the box of spontaneous activity recording equipment and allow it to adapt the surrounding for 5 minutes. Then count the time, record the number of of activity showed on the digital display, as the control value before administration. Take out the mouse, treat it by intraperitoneal injection of 0. 05% Diazepam 4mg/kg (0. 1ml/10g), put it back to the box, and record its activity within 5 minutes at 15, 30, 60, 90 and 120 minutes by the previous method.

Test mouse B by the previous method and measure the times of spontaneous activity within 5 minutes, then administer ip. Saline 0. 2ml/10g, observe and record its activity every 5 minutes for 25 minutes.

Results

Record the result of experiment in Table 3 – 3.

Table 3 – 3   Effect of diazepam on spontaneous activity of animals

Number	Drug & Dose (mg/kg)	Number of spontaneous activity in 5 minutes					
		Before drug	after drug				
			15min	30min	60min	90min	120min
normal saline							
diazepam							

Notes

1. Keep quiet during the course of the experiment, and carry it out in a sound – insulated room if possible.

2. Activity of animals is related to diet, day and night, living environment, etc. So this experiment should be conducted in the similar conditions.

3. The animals should fast for 12 hours before the experiment, in order to increase search for foods.

Evaluation

The effects of sedatives and hypnotics and nueroleptic are usually measured by the degree of reduction in frequency of spontaneous activity. The commonly used method is to put the mouse into a specially made cage, record its activity by shaking or covering the path of light, and compare the difference between pre – adminstation and post – administration. But the spontaneous activities of animals are easily affected by environmental factors, and are changeable. So it is necessary to have a control group.

Question

What should be observed in this experiment? The method apply to which type of drugs?

Ⅲ. Experiment of antiepileptics and anticonvulsants

Experiment 3. 5　Effects of drugs on electric shock

扫码"学一学"

Objective

Observe the protective effects of phenytoin sodium and phenobarbital on electric shock

Principle

Stimulating head of mouse with a strong electric current can cause general tetanic convulsion. If a drug can prevent the occurrence of general tetanic convulsion, we could initially suspect that it has antagonistic effect on grand mal.

Materials

Animal required: 3 – 4 mice, 18 – 22g, no restriction on sex.

Apparatus required: balance, syringes, bell jar, pharmacological and physiological multipurpose apparatus.

Reagent required: phenytoin sodium, 0. 5% solution W/V, phenobarbital sodium, 0. 5% solution W/V, normal saline.

Methods

Adjust the stimulator. Stimulating parameters are as follows: working condition electric shock, output voltage maximum, model of stimulating single, frequency 8 Hz.

1. Connect the outlet with clips and plug the connection for power.

2. Select convulsion mice. Attach the clips moistened with Saline to the mouse ears. A current is applied to the head of the mouse, then cause tonic convulsion that is the state of flexing forelimb and straightening hind limb. If the animals don't fall into convulsions with 1 Hz, modulate to 4 Hz, and start again. Replace another one to test if have no reaction, yet.

3. Select three mice in which convulsions occur typically. Mark and weigh them. Treat them by intraperitoneal injection of 0. 5% phenytoin sodium 75mg/kg (0. 15ml/10g), 0. 5% phenobarbital sodium 75mg/kg (0. 15ml/10g) and normal Saline 0. 10ml/10g separately.

4. 40 minutes after injection, stimulate the mice again with previous – threshold. Record the responses.

Results

Collect all experiment results in your laboratory, fill in table 3 – 4, and do the statistical analysis.

Notes

1. Because of individual difference of animals, stimulating parameters should be set with experiment. Don't set it over – strong, in order to prevent animals from death.

2. Prevent short circuit of clips carefully, otherwise the stimulator would be damaged.

3. The convulsion of animals can be divided in five phases, latent period, stiff flexion phase, straightening hindlimb phase, clonic phase and restoration period.

Table 3 – 4   Protective effects on electric shock of some barbiturates

Drug		degree of reaction							
		1	2	3	4	5	6	7	8
Normal saline	pre – treating								
	post – treating								
Phenytoin sodium	pre – treating								
	post – treating								
Phenobarbital sodium	pre – treating								
	post – treating								

Evaluation

Convulsion is the state of involuntary and incoordinate movement of skeletal muscle resulting from hyperexcitability of CNS. We screen antiepileptics by the method of experimental convulsion produced by electric or sound stimulation. Maximum electroshock episode and psychomotor seizure are the two widely used electric shock method. The former is considered to be a good model of grand mal; the latter is correspondent with psychomotor seizure. So this method is mainly used in screening drugs of grand mal.

Question

Compare the effects of phenobarbital sodium and phenytoin sodium, according to the change of animals' activity after administration and the responses of electric stimulation.

Experiment 3. 6   Effects of drugs on convulsion produced by central stimulants

Objective

Observe the effects of sodium valproate on convulsion produced by dimefline.

Principle

Remeflin, a central stimulant which can directly excite respiratory center, can produce convulsion with overdose. The protective effects of drugs on convulsion produced by dimefline can be used to screen antiepileptics and anticonvulsants.

Materials

Animal required: 2 mice, 18 – 22g, no restriction on sex.

Apparatus required: balance, syringes, bell jar.

Reagent required: 0. 04% Dimefline, 2% sodium valproate, normal saline.

Methods

1. Mark and weigh two mice.

2. Treat them separately by intraperitoneal injection of 2% sodium valproate 600mg/kg

(0.3ml/10g) and normal Saline 0.3ml/10g.

3. 30 minutes after administration, inject them with dimefline 8mg/kg (0.2ml/10g) subcutaneously. Observe the speed and degree of reaction of each mouse (spasm, falling down, sttif or death).

Notes

If condition permits, pentetrazole (120mg/kg, sc.) is recommended to be substituted for dimefline because the convulsion caused by pentetrazole is more typical.

Evaluation

The method of producing convulsion by chemical substances has the advantage of operating easily and needs no special equipment. Now, the experiment of pentetrazole convulsion is a common method of screening effective drugs of absence seizures.

Question

Discuss the effects and clinical uses of those drugs according to the above results.

IV. Experiment of antipsychotics

Experiment 3.7   Tranquilizing effect of chlorpromazine

Objective

Observe the effect of chlorpromazine on aggressive mice.

Principle

Mouse will be enraged after stimulated with electric current of some intensity, and present the activities such as escape, squeak, fighting, confronting each other, biting each other, etc. Antipsychotics can inhibit those behaviors.

Materials

Animal required: 4 male mice, 20 – 22g, raised individually.

Apparatus required: electric stimulator, plastic cages, syringes, needles, balance.

Reagent required: chlorpromazine hydrochloride, 0.04% solution W/V.

Methods

Adjust the stimulator. Determine the stimulating parameters as follows: work condition aggressive, output voltage minimum, pattern of stimulating continuous B, time 1 second and frequence 8Hz.

1. Connect the stimulator with the enraging cage using a wire with an outlet and two alligator clips.

2. Select aggressive mice. Place two male mice raised individually into the enraging cage. Switch the stimulator on and modulate the output of the voltage progressively until the mice start squeaking and running to appropriate extent. If the enraged reaction appears, indicated by the phenomena that the mice stand face to face and bite each other, record the latent period of enraged reaction and the threshold voltage. If not, discard them. Select two pair of enraged mice (Fig. 3 – 2).

3. Inject one pair of mice intraperitoneally with 4mg/kg of chlorpromazine (0.1ml/10g of

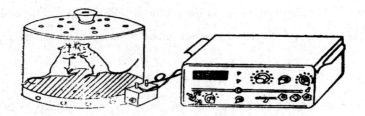

Fig. 3 – 2　The test instrument to enrage mice

0. 04% solution), the other 0. 1ml/10g of normal saline.

4. 20 minutes after the injection, stimulate the mice again with the same stimulating parameters as before. Observe the mice responses (aggressive behaviour, threshold voltage and latent period).

Results

Record the result of experiment in Table 3 – 5.

Table 3 – 5　Effects of chlorpromazine (CPZ) on aggressive mice

Group		Threshold voltage (V)	Latent period (min)
Saline	Pre – treating		
	Post – treating		
CPZ	Pre – treating		
	Post – treating		

Notes

1. Typical fighting of the mice in experiment is not fewer than 3 times in 3 minutes. After administration, stimulate the mice with pre – parameters. If the typical fighting is fewer than 3 times, the mouse is inhibited.

2. The box of stimulation should be kept dry, wipe off excrement and urine of mice in time, to prevent short circuit that influences the output of normal voltage.

3. Shut the source of electricity immediately after appearance of typical fighting reaction. Check up whether there is output voltage when taking mice out of the box, to prevent any accident.

Evaluation

Antipsychotics affect on dopaminergic system in brain, so they can produce many reactions related to dopaminergic system, such as rigor, antivomiting, antianhydromorphine, etc. Those effects are side effects or minor effects of antipsychotics, but they are proved to have some parallel relationship with therapeutical effect by many experiments. The effect of antipsychotics on experiment – based enraged activity has important clinical significance. This method is simple, and suitable for initial screening on a great quantity. If possible, the method of radioligand – receptor binding analysis can be adopted with behavior test together to screen antipsychotics. The intensity of antipsychotics is predicted mainly based on the results of the two experiments.

Question

Discuss the character of sedative effect and the use of chlorpromazine from the above results.

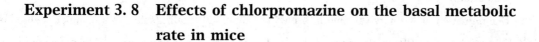

Experiment 3. 8　Effects of chlorpromazine on the basal metabolic rate in mice

Objective

Through this experiment, observe the effects of chlorpromazine on the basal metabolic rate in mice.

Principle

The surviving time of mouse in a sealed container can reflect its oxygen consumption ability. Reducing the basal metabolic rate (such as central depressants) can lengthen the surviving time of mouse in a sealed container.

Materials

Animal required: 20 similar weight female mice.

Apparatus required: wide mouthed bottle with glass stopper, Vaseline, granulated sodalime.

Reagent required: 0. 1% chlorpromazine hydrochloride, 0. 9% solution w/v, normal saline.

Methods

1. Take 20 female mice with similar body weight and divide them into two groups averagely.

2. All mice are treated by intraperitoneal injection.

Group I receive 0. 1% chlorpromazine hydrochloride 15mg/kg (0. 15ml/10g).

Group II receive normal Saline 15ml/kg.

3. 20 minutes after administration, each mouse is placed into a wide mouthed bottle containing 25g sodalime to absorb the expired carbon dioxide.

4. The bottle is sealed by a stopper covered with vaseline. Turn the stoppers left and right to keep from air and start observing immediately.

5. Watch the mice carefully until they die and record the dead time. Collect all the results in the laboratory and then carry out the statistical calculation by t – test.

Results

Record the results in the table below.

Table 3 – 6　Effects of chlorpromazine on the tolerance of hypoxia

Group	Survival time (min)										$\bar{x} \pm SD$
	1	2	3	4	5	6	7	8	9	10	
Control											
Chlorpromazine											

Notes

1. Sodalime should be fresh. The device should be enclosed and of equal capacity.

2. The weight of mice in each group should be near as far as possible, because the metabolic rate of energy has direct ratio to body surface area.

3. Observe the death time of mice for 5 minutes after breath stops, to make sure the death of mice.

4. Keep the surrounding temperature constant and coincident.

Evaluation

Determination of the survival time in sealed containers of small animals is a common method of initial screening some effects of central depressants, such as increasing cerebral blood flow and enhancing the oxygen uptake ability of central neuron. This method is simple, but has poor specificity.

Question

From the effect of chlorpromazine on the basal metabolic rate, and its effect of reducing body temperature, discuss the clinical use of chlorpromazine in this field.

V. Experiments of analgesics

Experiment 3.9   Analgesic action of drugs (the hot plate method)

Objective

Study the hot plate method of screening analgesic drugs and compare the analgesic potency of drugs.

Principle

扫码"学一学"

Various trauma and injuries such as thermal stimulus initiate sensory stimulation of impulses transmitted to spinal cord through sensory nerve fibers, which reach sensory area of cerebral cortex to produce pain. Central analgesics (such as morphine) and peripheral analgesics (such as acetyl salicylic acid) relieve pain by reducing the pain sensation. The effects of central analgesic are easily testified through animal experiments, but the effects of some peripheral analgesic such as acetyl salicylic acid are not easy to be determined.

Materials

Animal required: 3 – 4 mice, 18 – 22g, female.

Apparatus required: electric hot plate, mouse cage, balance, syringes, needles, beakers.

Reagent required: 0.1% (*W/V*) morphine hydrochloride, 2% (*W/V*) sodium salicylate, 0.9% (*W/V*) normal saline.

Methods

1. Choose animals. Place a mouse on the hot plate which is heated to constant temperature of 55℃ ±0.5℃. Remove it from the hot plate until the mouse licks its hindpaws or raises its hindpaws and turns the head. The duration is the latent period (LP) of the pain response. Each mouse will be tested twice at an interval of 5 minutes. Select three mice each of whose mean latent period is shorter than 30 seconds.

2. All mice are administered by intraperitoneal injection.

Mouse A receives morphine hydrochloride 15mg/kg (0.15ml/10g of 0.1% solution).

Mouse B receives sodium salicylate 300mg/kg (0.15ml/10g of 2% solution).

Mouse C receives normal Saline 0.15ml/10g.

3. Determine the LP of pain response of the mice at 15, 30, 45, and 60 minutes after administration according to the method mentioned above.

4. Calculate the increased percentage of pain threshold according to the following equation.

Increased percentage of pain threshold =

$$\frac{Post - treatment\ latent\ period - Pre - treatment\ latent\ period}{Pre - treatment\ latent\ period} \times 100\%$$

Results

Record the experimental results according to Fig. 3 – 3 and Table 3 – 7.

Table 3 – 7   Compare the analgesic effects of morphine and sodium salicylate

Group	Weight (g)	Drugs & Doses (mg/kg)	The latent period to the pain (s)						
			Pre – treating			Post – treating			
			1	2	mean	15min	30min	45min	60min
A									
B									
C									

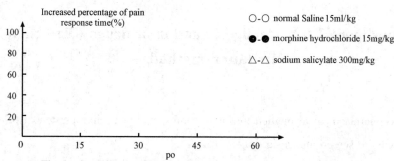

Fig. 3 – 3   **Effect – time relationship of morphine and salicylate**

Notes

1. Take the mouse away from the hot plate immediately, when it presents typical pain reaction, or has no reaction after 60 seconds, in order to prevent scald.

2. Male mice are not suitable for this experiment, because the scrotum will droop when heated and the skin of scrotum is sensitive to pain.

3. The room temperature will influence this experiment to some degree. The suitable temperature is 15 –20℃. The reaction of mouse is dull at too low temperature. And if it is too high, mouse is hypersensitive leading to jumping. This will affect the accuracy of the result.

4. Normal mice will show the activities of restlessness, raising forelimb, lapping forefoot, kicking hindlimb, jumping, etc, within 10 – 15 seconds after put on the hot plate. But licking hindlimb is the only indicator of pain.

Evaluation

The common methods of screening analgesics are physical (heat, electric, mechanical) stimulation and chemical stimulation. Among those methods, heat stimulation, electric stimulation and potassium subcutaneous penetration are relatively widely used. The commonly – used animals are rat, mouse, guinea pig, rabbit, dog, etc. and the common indices of pain reaction are roar, licking foot, flinging tail, struggling, and tic of skin or muscle.

The advantages of the hot plate method are: ①the device is simple. ②the index is clear. ③tissues are less injured. ④animals can be repeatedly used. ⑤the latent period of pain reaction is relatively long. Therefore, we can compare the slight difference of drugs, and thus compare the intensity, latent time and duration of analgesics. Due to these factors, it is a commonly – used method. But drugs that have sedative, muscle relaxation or psychotomimetic actions usually present false – positive results, and especially the results of partial agonists of opiate receptors are always unreliable. So the temperature of hot plate should be lower than 49.5℃ when partial agonists are assessed.

The various methods of producing pain have different use. Electric and mechanical stimulation are suitable for screening of narcotic analgesics, but not fit for screening antipyretic – analgesic drugs. Heat stimulation is also used to screen narcotoic analgesics. Chemical stimulation is fit for screening and testing antipyretic – analgesic drugs.

Question

Discuss the clinical use of those two types of analgesics according to the above – mentioned results.

Experiment 3.10   Analgesic action of drugs(The chemical irritation method)

扫码 "学一学"

Objective

Study the pharmacological method that makes mice writhe by intraperitoneal injection of some irritant chemicals to screen analgesic drugs.

Principle

Intraperitoneal injection of some irritant chemicals, such as acetic acid, can stimulate peritoneum and cause large – area, deep and persistent pain. The mouse will present writhing reaction, which is featured by invaginating abdomen, extending trunk and hindlimb, lifting buttocks.

Materials

Animal required: 3 mice, 20 – 25g, female or male.

Equipment required: balance, syringes, and plastic cage.

Reagent required: morphine hydrochloride 0.1% solution W/V, sodium salicylate 4% solution W/V, acetic acid 0.8% solution W/V, normal saline.

Methods

1. Weigh three mice and mark them.

2. Mouse A is treated with 0.1% morphine hydrochloride 15mg/kg (0.15ml/10g) subcutaneously. Mouse B is treated with 4% sodium salicylate 400mg/kg (0.15 ml/10g) intragastrically. Mouse C is treated with normal Saline 15ml/kg subcutaneously.

3. 30 minutes later, each mouse is rendered 0.2ml 0.8% acetic acid intraperitoneally.

4. In 15 minutes, record the number of writhing mice or the writhing numbers of each mouse.

5. Collect the results of the whole laboratory and compare the analgesic action of the two drugs.

Results

Record the results in the Table 3 – 8.

Table 3 – 8   Effects of analgesic drugs on the pain induced by ip 0. 6% acetic acid in mice

Group	Doses (mg/kg)	No. of mice (n)	No. of writhing mice (n)	Writhing incidence (%)	No. of writhing ($\bar{x} \pm SD$)	Writhing inhibition rate (%)
Normal saline						
Morphine Hydrochloride						
Sodium Salicylate						

Notes

1. Antimony potassium tartrare solution can be substituted for acetic acid, but it must be newly dispensed because its effect will be weakened after a long time. Acetic acid must also be newly dispensed to prevent evaporation.

2. Keeping the room temperature at 20℃. The times of writhing will decrease at too low temperature. The presenting rate of writhing reaction will also decrease when the body weight of the mouse is too low.

3. The result can be disposed by the number of writhing or non – writhing mice, or the times of writhing.

Evaluation

This method is suitable for screening central analgesics and peripheral analgesics, especially for antipyretic – analgesic drugs. But it has poor specificity in that many non – analgesics can present positive results, such as H_1 – receptor blocker, pseudocholinergic drugs, anticholinergics, clonidine and haloperidol, etc. So the analgesic effect must be decided combining with other methods. Some reports consider that the drug possesses no analgesic effect when the writhing inhibition rate (writhing incidence of control group – writhing incidence of treatment group), is lower than 70%.

Question

Discuss the difference between hot plate method and chemical irritation method from the results of this experiment and experiment 3. 9.

VI. Experiments of central stimulants

Experiment 3. 11   Comparison of convulsive type and site of action of strychnine and picrotoxin

Objective

Observe the different convulsive types produced by strychnine and picrotoxin, and learn the method of analyzing action site by damaging the CNS sectionally.

Principle

Strychnine and picrotoxin both act on the CNS. The former mainly affects spinal cord, and produce symmetric incoordinate tetanic convulsions. The behavior is continuous stiff spasm of double limbs, and the part above spinal cord has nothing to do with convulsion. The latter mainly affects midbrain, and produce asymmetric coordinate clonic convulsion. The behavior is interactive expansion and relaxation spasm of double limbs, and the convulsion disappears when midbrain is damaged（Fig. 3 – 4）.

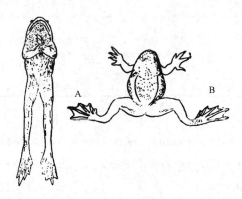

Fig. 3 – 4　The comparison of convulsion type of strychnine and picrotoxin

A. Convulsion produced by strychnine　　B. Convulsion produced by picrotoxin

Materials

Animal required：2 toads，body weight above 70g, no restriction on sex.

Apparatus required：glass separation needle, syringe, beaker, pincette probe, scissors, balance, and cotton line.

Reagent required：0. 03% strychnine nitrate solution, 0. 3% picrotoxin solution.

Methods

1. Take two toads . fix them on the frog plate in supine position. Cut out the skin of right thigh, separate sciatic nerve between semimembranosus and biceps femoris, cross a bold line under it, and tie up all muscle and vessel of this leg except the nerve to block blood stream.

2. Take down toads from frog plate. Toad A is injected 0. 03% strychnine nitrate from chest lymph – capsule 3mg/kg（0. 1ml/10g）. Toad B is injected 0. 3% picrotoxin. 15 minutes later, stimulate with various ways, and observe the difference about convulsions of two toads and the types. The stimulation can be：①touch the skin suddenly. ②blow the skin with mouth. ③clap hands to produce sound. ④pull the hindlimb.

3. Steps of analysis of action site：

1）Amputate the sciatic nerve of one leg, and compare its reaction with the other normal leg when convulsion occurs?

2）Cut off cerebrum from posterior border of eyes, and observe whether convulsion stops or not?

3）Cut off medulla oblongata from posterior border of ear drum, and observe whether convulsion stops or not?

4）Destroy spinal cord, and observe whether convulsion stops or not?

Results

Record the result of the experiment on Table 3 – 9.

Table 3 – 9   The comparison of convulsion type about strychnine and picrotoxin

Number	Weight (g)	Drug & Dose (mg/kg)	The reaction and type of stimulations				Cut off the sciatic actionsites nerve of one leg		Cut off cerebrum	medulla	Cut off oblongata	Destroy spinal cord	Main site of action
			touch	blow	clap	P	cut off	reserve					
A													
B													

P: pull hands hindlimb

Notes

1. Close to the spinal cord side when separating sciatic nerve. Cut off the branch, too, when cutting off the sciatic nerve.

2. If picrotoxin is not available, remeflin can be used to obtain similar results. The dose is 24mg/kg (0.2% solution 0.12ml/10g).

Evaluation

The screening methods of central stimulants mainly consist of observation of the activities of animals (such as spontaneous activity, conditioned reflex activity, spirography and reflex time determination, etc), antagonism of central depressants (such as enhancing the LD_{50} of central depressants or inhibiting the intoxication of respiratory depressants), and analysis of action site, for instance, a classical method of localization is to treat the toad with high dose, and observe the site of action from the type of convulsion and the influence of destroying CNS sectionally on drug action. Analysis of action site is suitable for the study of the principle of central stimulants and drugs causing convulsion. These methods are applicable differently and should be chosen according to the specific requirement and different stages of experiment.

Question

Analyze the central action site of strychnine and picrotoxin from the result.

Experiment 3.12   The antagonistic effect of nikethamide on the depression of respiration by morphine

Objective

Study the commonly used recording method for respiration and observe the antagonistic effect of nikethamide on the depression of respiration by morphine.

Principle

Morphine with high dose can inhibit the respiratory center of the medulla oblongata, and respiratory center stimulants can inhibit the depression of respiration caused by morphine.

Materials

Animal required: 1 rabbit, 1.8 – 2.2 kg, no restriction on sex.

Apparatus required: operation platform for rabbit, suture needle, suture, tension transducer, biological signal acquisition system, syringes, needles.

Reagent required: morphine hydrocloride, 1.5% solution *W/V*. nikethamide, 2% solution *W/V*.

Methods

1. Weigh and place the rabbit lying on its back and fix it onto the operation platform. Using suture needle and thread to connect xiphold of the rabbit with tension transducer. Then connect the transducer with biological signal acquisition system to record respiration curve.

2. Allow the breath to become steady. Trace a segment of normal breathing activity by the recorder.

3. Treat the rabbit with fast intravenous injection of 1.5% morphine 45mg/kg (3ml/kg). When the depression of respiration is observed, give 2% nikethamide 50mg/kg (2.5ml/kg) by slow intravenous injection. Record the respiration on the drum and notice the rate of respiration.

Results

Record the result of experiment according to Table 3 – 10.

Table 3 – 10 The result of antagonistic effect of nikethamide on the depression of respiration caused by morphine

Item	Pre – treating	After iv. Morphine	After iv. nikethamide
respiration amplitude (mm)			
respiration rate (times/min)			

Notes

1. Inject morphine quickly so as to rapidly reach the concentration that can inhibit respiratory center.

2. The speed of injecting nikethamide should be slow to prevent convulsion.

Evaluation

The method of observing the effect of stimulating respiratory center and antagonistic effect of central stimulants is mainly used to screen and study the awakening drugs which can relieve depressive state and selectively stimulate respiratory center. Central stimulants can be divided into different types, and the experimental method cam be chosen according to the purpose of the study.

Question

Why nikethamide is suitable for saving acute poisoning of morphine? What should be noticed in the usage?

Experiment 3. 13 The promotive effect of nimodipine on acquired memory of mouse

Objective

Observe the process of producing acquired memory of mouse trained by Y – maze. Learn the commonly used method of screening drugs affecting learning and memory.

Principle

The equipment of Y – maze consists of starting area, electric shock area and safety area. The mouse which is given electric stimulation escapes and obtains the memory of finding the safety area because of unconditioned reflex. In this way the effects of drugs on the memory can be observed.

Materials

Animal required: 8 mice, 18 – 22g.

Apparatus required: mouse cage, syringes, and equipment of Y – maze.

Reagent required: 0. 1% nimodipine solution, normal saline.

Methods

1. Connect the equipment, fix the starting point, and train each mouse separately. Put the mouse at starting area, let it adapt the surrounding for 1 minute, then open the gate and push the button to give the mouse electric stimulation. Adjust the voltage to the degree that can cause the mice to run and escape. (The voltage is too high if the mouse squeaks, and too low if the mouse have no reaction.) If the mouse fled into safety area (without electric stimulation), let it stay here for 10 seconds to consolidate its memory.

2. Take the mouse out from safety area and put it back on starting area. One minute later, give e-lectric stimulation for the second time, the mouse flee into safety area again. Train the mouse repeat-edly in this way. If the mouse runs into safety area directly when shocked, the reaction is "true"; if it runs to other areas or go here and there before entering safety area, it is "false" . When the mouse gets 9 "true" in continual 10 shocks, it obtains memory. Record the total times of electric shock the mouse need to get 9/10 "true" reactions.

3. Treat 4 successfully trained mice with nimodipine (10mg/kg, ip). Treat the other 4 mice with normal Saline of equal rolume, and then shock them continually until they get 9/10 "true" reactions. Record the total times of electric shock and calculate the preservation rate of memo-ry. Compare the results of two groups to evaluate the effect of drugs.

$$\text{preservation rate of memory} = \frac{A - B}{A} \times 100\%$$

A——the total times of electric shock to get 9/10 "true" reactions before administration

B——the total times of electric shock to get 9/10 "true" reactions after administration

Results

Calculate the result of the experiment in Table 3 – 11.

Table 3 – 11   The effect of nimodipine on the faculty of memory of mouse

Group		Dose (mg/kg)	Number of animals	Total times of shock		Preservation rate of memory
				Pre – treating	Post – treating	
Saline	1					
	2					
	3					
	4					
Nimodipine	1					
	2					
	3					
	4					

Notes

1. Grown – up mice are generally used in this experiment. Electric resistance between two fore-limbs skin is measured and the mice whose electric resistance is $150 - 300$ kΩ is suitable.

2. Fast and interrupting shock is better, and continuous electrification can not be used.

3. Don't drive the mouse back to starting point following its way, and be sure to take it out from safety area and put back to starting area directly.

4. Keep quiet in the laboratory, the light should be dim, and the suitable room temperature is $18°C - 30°C$.

5. We can also use piracetam ($20 - 40$mg/kg, ig) instead of nimodipine.

Evaluation

Learning and memory is one of the important functions of the brain. But the mental process of humans and animals can't be observed directly and can only be guessed from the visible reaction to stimulation. The mental learning process can only be studied by measuring the operational results to execute a certain task. The common methods are step – down, step through, shuttle box and maze tests. Rodents are experts of interspaced recognition, and can master only if trained a few times. Y – maze, as a maze method, is a simple, single experiment of training interspaced recognition, and usually used in initial screening of nootropics. But the activity of animals can be influenced by various internal physiological factors. So this method is only a nonspecific index to evaluate the systemic effects of drug on general physiological function of animals. At the same time, the result of experiment can be affected by various external factors, so the experiment conditions must be strictly controlled to reduce experimental error. And it should be combined with the results of other learning and memory experiment to evaluate nootropic effect of drug.

Question

What is the correct method of training mice in Y – maze?

Chapter 4   Experiments of drugs affecting the peripheral efferent nervous system

The peripheral efferent nervous system consists of the vegetative nervous system and the motor nervous system. The vegetative nervous system mainly controls effectors including heart, smooth muscles and glands, and can be further divided into two subdivisions based on their different functions, the sympathetic and the parasympathetic nervous system. The effects of parasympathetic stimulate the gastrointestinal smooth muscle and bronchial smooth muscles. Parasympathetic stimulation also leads to increase of gland excretion and diminution fo pupil. The sympathetic nervous system usually acts to oppose the actions of the parasympathetic nervous system. Generally, the sympathetic nervous system tends to dominate heart and small vessels, whereas the parasympathetic nervous system obviously influences smooth muscles and glands. In the efferent motor nervous system a single motor neuron, originating in the CNS, travels directly to skeletal muscle without the mediation of ganglia.

There are large numbers of pharmacological experiments of the drugs affecting the peripheral efferent nervous system due to the extensive influence of the efferent nervous system. The methods and principles of the experiments are chiefly based on neurotransmitters, receptors and physiological effects they produce. The sympathetic postaganglionic nerve terminals release norepinephrine as neurotransmitter to bind with α and β receptors located on the target cell or postsynapitic membrane to react, while the parasympathetic nerve fibers discharge acetylcholine that acts on M receptors.

Two methods, drug effect method and radioligand binding assay of receptor (RBA), are often adopted in the study of what drugs do to the receptors. In the former method, *in vivo* or *in vitro* animal experiment models are generally employed to observe the drug effects on the receptors. For example, when a drug acts on adrenoceptors, excitation of a receptors can cause the rise of blood pressure, and stimulation of β receptors can result in the descent of blood pressure and increase of heart rate. To precisely distinguish the action of α receptor from that of β receptor, α receptor blockers (e. g phentolamine) and β receptor blockers (e. g. propranolol) can be used as tool drugs, and experiments such as nictiating membrane of cat and *in vivo* blood pressure and intestinal movement in cat or dog can be conducted. Sympathomimetic action of drugs canbe analyzed by *in vitro* experiments such as gastric fundus strips of rat, isolated ear of rabbit, tracheal chain and ileum of Guinea pig. Cholinoceptors, relevant to acetylcholine, can be pharmacologically divided into M and N receptors. The effect of activation of M receptors is to decrease heart rate and blood pressure, and to weaken heart contractility. It also results in constriction of gastrointestinal smooth muscles and miosis. N receptors can be further distinguished as N_1 and N_2. When N_1 receptors are activated, vegetative ganglions are excited and adrenal medulla sevretions are stimulated. If drugs withous contraction action of blood vessels can increase blood pressure of the atropine treated cat, they are N_1

receptors agonists.

RBA is a technique used to analyze the type of receptors that bind drugs and the affinity between drugs and receptors to provide experimental results of animal organs with further evidence through interaction of radioactive labeling ligands and receptors.

Drugs influence the efferent neurotransmitters mainly through the steps of synthesis, release, uptake and transformation of transmitters. There are also many experiment methods on the study of what drugs do to the neurotransmitter. In this category of experiments we utilize tool drugs (transmitter or transmitter mimic) to see whether the drugs block the reaction caused by nerve exitation without disturbance of the actions of tool drugs, and then analyze the steps through which drugs affect the transmitters.

On balance, there are various pharmacological experiment methods concerning the peripheral efferent nervous system. Here only some common experiments that students should grasp and understand are introduced.

扫码"学一学"

Experiment 4.1　Effects of drugs affecting the peripheral efferent nervous system on blood pressure, intestinal movement and gland secretion in anesthetized dog

Objective

Learn the methods and equipment used for recording BP, intestinal movement and glandular secretions accurately. Observe the effects of drugs affecting the peripheral efferent nervous system on above – mentioned physiological phenomena, and comprehend the interaction of this kind of drugs.

Principle

The vegetative nervous system, belonging to the peripheral efferent nervous system, is divided into two subdivisions, the parasympathetic nervous system whose chief transmitter is acetylcholine, and the sympathetic nervous system whose chief transmitter is norepinephrine. The two systems coordinate and oppose each other to maintain normal physiological functions. The drugs affect the parasympathetic and the sympathetic nervous system mainly through the transmitters and receptors. The drug actions can be qualitatively analyzed indirectly through the effects on blood pressure, smooth muscles movement and gland secretion in animals.

Materials

Animal required: 1 dog, 6 – 10kg, male or female.

Apparatus required: operation table, surgical instruments, physiological pressure detector, flatbed recorder, pressure transducer, syringes, and buret.

Reagent required: heparinized saline, normal saline, and pentobarbital sodium solution (3%, W/V).

Drugs used in this experiment may be found in detail afterward.

Methods

1. Anesthesia　Weigh the dog and administer 30mg/kg of 3% pentobarbital sodium (iv.) to anesthetize it. Then fix it on the operation table.

2. The procedure of operation is divided into 3 parts.

1) Neck: Cut off the fur on the front of the neck and open the skin along midline. Isolate and open the trachea, and insert the tracheal cannula and tie it firmly. Isolate right carotid artery and insert an arterial cannula filled with heparinized saline and connected to force – displacement transducer linking the physiological pressure detector. After the physiological pressure detector is well regulated, open the artery forceps and then record normal blood pressure.

2) Abdomen: Cut off the fur on the abdomen. Open the skin 5 – 8cm along midline below xiphoid, and then expose abdominal cavity by carving abdominal muscle along linea alba abdominis and find duodenum and jejunum. Make a tobacco bag structure on jejunum and make a small longitudinal incision in the suture. Insert the water sac that has been deflated beforehand towards the duodenum and fasten the tobacco bag. Fill the water sac full of water and connect its outlet with a titertube and another physiological pressure detector linking biological signal acquisition system.

3) Groin: In either side of groin, find the pulse position of femoral artery with fingers and cut off the fur on that position. Make a longitudinal incision of 3 – 4cm and isolate femoral vein. Insert a vein cannula linking the transfusion apparatus and check whether the cannula is unblocked.

3. Administration　After surgery, trace a portion of normal blood pressure and intestine movement curve and observe the salivary secretion. Then inject following drugs in turn. After administration every time, infuse 2ml normal saline through infusion tube immediately to make the drug enter the blood circulation entirely. Observe and record the alteration in blood pressure, intestine movement and gland secretion. Don't give next drug until above – mentioned physiological condition is back to normal or stable level.

A. Observe the effects of adrenergic drugs on blood pressure, intestine movement and salivary secretion.

1) adrenaline hydrochloride, 10^{-4}W/V, 10μg/kg or 0.1ml/kg

2) norepinephrine bitartrate, 10^{-4}W/V, 10μg/kg or 0.1ml/kg

3) isoprenaline hydrochloride, 5×10^{-4} W/V, 25μg/kg or 0.05ml/kg

B. Observe the effects of α – adrenoceptor blockers on the action of adrenergic drugs.

4) phentolamine, 2.5×10^{-2}W/V, 5mg/kg or 0.2ml/kg

5) repeat 1)

6) repeat 2)

7) repeat 3)

C. Observe the effects of β – adrenoceptor blockers on the action of adrenergic drugs.

8) propranolol hydrochloride, 10^{-3} (W/V), 0.1mg/kg or 0.1ml/kg

9) repeat 1)

10) repeat 2)

11) repeat 3)

D. Observe the effects of cholinergic drugs on the blood pressure, intestine movement and salivary secretion.

12) pilocarpine, 10^{-3} W/V, 0.1mg/kg or 0.1ml/kg

13) acetylcholine, 10^{-5} W/V, 1μg/kg or 0.1ml/kg

14) atropine, 5×10^{-3} W/V, 0.5mg/kg or 0.1ml/kg

15) repeat 13)

16) acetylcholine, 10^{-4} W/V, 10μg/kg or 0.1ml/kg

Results

Copy the curve of the blood pressure and intestine movement, and mark the value of blood pressure (mmHg), name and dosage of drugs administered. Analyze the interaction of drugs and explain the change of physiological phenomena after administration of drugs. The results of experiments may be recorded in the table showed below.

Table 4 – 1 Effects of drugs affecting the efferent nervous system on blood pressure, intestine movement and gland secretion of anesthetized dog

Animal		Weight		Gender		Anesthetic	
Drug	Dosage	Blood Pressure		Intense of intestine		Salivary Secretion	
		before	after	before	after	before	after
adrenaline	10μg/kg						
norepinephrine	10μg/kg						
isoprenaline	50μg/kg						
phentolamine	5mg/kg						
adrenaline	10μg/kg						
norepinephrine	10μg/kg						
isoprenaline	50μg/kg						
propranolol	0.1mg/kg						
adrenaline	10μg/kg						
norepinephrine	10μg/kg						
isoprenaline	50μg/kg						
pilocarpine	10μg/kg						
acetylcholine	1μg/kg						
atropine	0.5mg/kg						
acetylcholine	1μg/kg						
acetylcholine	10μg/kg						

Notes

1. Do not operate the neck close to thyroid otherwise it causes bleeding easily. Be sure to avoid damaging cervical vagus nerve and sympathetic nerve.

2. When the blood pressure is relatively low, clamp the arterial cannula to prevent excessive anticoagulant from flowing into the animal's body.

3. The drug dosage is calculated based on its salt form in this experiment. So the dosage may be adjusted according to the actual situation.

Evaluation

The blood pressure and gland secretion are very sensitive indices for testing the drugs affecting the peripheral efferent nervous system. Acute experiments of dog, cat, rabbit and rat are usually preferred. Relatively speaking, dog – used experiments have more advantages: ①The blood pressure of dog is constant, and more close to human body than that of rat, rabbit and such small animals. ②The dog is sensitive to the drugs, and its response is consistent with human on the whole.

③It has relatively thick blood vessels and nerves and elastic vascular wall, easy to operate on. ④It has a powerful heart pulsation force, which makes blood pressure curve better portrayed. ⑤The experiment is suitable for analysis of action mechanism of drugs effects on the circulation system. ⑥The dog can be repeatedly utilized for drug screening experiments. However, the costs of dog – used experiments are high, so they are unsuitable for the experiments requiring large quantities of animals.

Experiment 4. 2   Effects of drugs on the isolated aorta strip of rabbit

Objective

Observe the effects of adrenergic agonists and adrenergic antagonists on the isolated aorta strip of the rabbit.

Principle

The aorta strip of rabbit has α adrenergic receptors, so it is very sensitive to catecholamines. It is a good specimen for screening drugs acting on α adrenoceptors.

Materials

Animal required: 1 rabbit, 1. 8 – 2. 2kg, sexuality not limited.

Apparatus required: magrus glass organ – bath, superior thermostatic water bath, biological signal acquisition system, thermometer, iron stand, double clamp, scissors, eye forceps, beaker, Petri dish, needle, thread, syringe.

Reagent required: Krebs – Henseleit's (K – H) solution, norepinephrine, adrenaline, and phentolamine.

Methods

Kill the rabbit by knocking the head. Expose the heart quickly and then isolate the aorta. Cut off the thoracic aorta close to the heart as much as possible, and place it in a dish containing enough Krebs – Henseleit's solution saturated with oxygen. Remove the connective tissue around the blood vessel, and encase a glass rod (diameter 3 – 4mm) in the blood vessel, then use eye scissors to shear the blood vessel into spiral sheet with 4mm width and 3 – 4mm length. Attach threads on the both sides, one side is located on the ventilatory hook and the other is connected with the transducer linking the biological signal acquisition system. Control the conditions: preload 1g, volume of bath tank 20ml, temperature 37℃ ± 0. 5℃. Aerate constant oxygen during the experiment. 2h later when the specimen and the system are stable, observe the actions of the following drugs. Remember to wash the specimen 2 – 3 times with Krebs – Henseleit's solution each time after administration.

1. norepinephrine, 0. 01 percent solution, 10μg (0. 1ml) .

2. adrenaline, 0. 01 percent solution, 10μg (0. 1ml) .

3. phentolamine, 1 percent solution, 1mg (0. 1ml) 15 minutes later repeat step 1) and 2).

Results

Trace and copy the curve. Mark administered drug and dosage on the curve.

Notes

1. Don't hold the aorta strip by hand. Use eye forceps to take the specimen and avoid long exposure of it in the air in order to prevent it from losing sensitivity.

2. Krebs – Henseleit's solution should be fresh dispensed.

3. After the experiment, the aorta strip can be stored at 4℃ in a refrigerator and reused in the experiment within 1 – 2 days.

4. The specimen responds slowly to adrenergic agonists. It takes 1 – 15 minutes for the aorta strip to contract. And it is the same with relaxation of it.

5. The aorta strip of rat can also be applied to this experiment.

Evaluation

This method is one of the classical methods of screening α – adrenoceptor agonists and antagonists, because the aorta strip of rabbit mainly has α – adrenoceptors and the specimen can be easily shaped into ring, sheet and strip (the most suitable shape is helix), and one piece of aorta can be fabricated into 3 – 4 specimens for pair experiment. The specimen is very sensitive to agonists and antagonists of low concentration with good ruggedness and able to maintain activity for a long time. The relationship between agonist and antagonist can be judged from the alteration of the dosage – effect curve of the agonist. If the curve were shifted to the right with constant efficacy of the antagonist, the action should be called competitive antagonism and the intensity of the antagonist is indicated by pA_2.

Experiment 4.3   Effects of drugs on isolated intestine

Objective

Study the pharmacological experiment methods on isolated smooth muscles and organs. Observe the effects of cholinergic and anticholinergic drugs on isolated ileum of Guinea pig.

Principle

The contractile response of gastrointestinal smooth muscles is chiefly controlled by parasympathetic nerve. Intestinal smooth muscles contain M cholinergic receptors richly, so the contractile response of intestinal smooth muscles is obviously influenced by both M-cholinoceptor agonists and antagonists. Since the ileum specimen of Guinea pig is completely lax after the load is added, this method can be utilized to observe the actions of acetylcholine and cholinergic drugs.

Materials

Animal required: Guinea pig, 200 – 300g, sexuality not limited, on an empty stomach for more than 6h.

Equipment required: magrus glass organ – bath, thermostatic water bath, pressure transducer, biological signal acquisition system, iron stand, double clamp, scissors, eye forceps, graduated cylinder (10ml), syringe, beaker, dish, needle, thread.

Reagent required: Tyrode's solution, acetylcholine chloride solution (10^{-4} and 10^{-5}, W/V), atropine sulphate solution (0.1 percent, W/V), barium chloride solution (1 percent, W/V).

扫码"学一学"

Methods

Kill the animal by a blow on the head. Open the abdomen, remove a piece of ileum and place it in a dish containing Tyrode's solution. The length of the ileum piece should be 1.5 – 2cm. Attach a thread to each end by inserting a needle from inside to outside. Then fix the ileum piece in the organ bath with about 0.5g loading. Add 10ml Tyrode's solution into the organ bath and mark the level. The temperature of the organ bath should be constant at 38℃ ± 0.5℃. Connect the aerator to blow oxygen into the organ bath at the speed of 2 bubbles per second. Link the muscle strength transducer, turn on the biological signal acquisition system and record a length of base line until the base line becomes steady (the procedure usually needs more than 15 minutes). Then conduct the following steps.

Add 0.1ml acetylcholine chloride solution (10^{-5}, W/V) to the bath.

When the ileum piece contracts obviously, add 0.1ml atropine sulphate solution (0.1%, W/V) to the bath.

When the expected effects appear, add 0.1ml acetylcholine chloride solution (10^{-5}, W/V) to the bath and observe it for 3 minutes. If no obvious effects appear, then add 0.1ml acetylcholine chloride solution (10^{-4}, W/V) again.

Change Tyrode's solution 3 times. Allow the base line to be steady. Add 0.5ml barium chloride solution (1%, W/V) into the bath and observe the effects.

Again change Tyrode's solution 3 times. Allow the base line to be steady. Add 0.05ml atropine sulphate solution (0.1%, W/V), and then add 0.5ml barium chloride solution (1%, W/V) into the bath and observe the effects.

Results

Trace and copy the curve. Mark administered drug and dosage on the curve.

Notes

1. The ileum is located at the end distal end of intestine. Smooth muscular layer of the ileum is thin. It has relatively low autorhythmicity. The closer it approaches the ileocecal position, the lower its autorhythmicity is, and the steadier the base line is.

2. Control the temperature of the organ bath and the weight of the preload, or the specimen's contractile function and response to the drugs will be affected.

3. Don't seal the intestinal lumen when tying its both sides, or the potency of the drugs will be affected.

Evaluation

The isolated intestinal muscles of several kinds of animals can be used to conduct the experiments of drugs affecting the efferent nervous system. Guinea pig and rabbit are generally adopted. The ileum of Guinea pig is frequently used to screen and examine cholinergic drugs because the base line can be traced steadily due to its few spontaneous activities and it is sensitive to acetylcholine and cholinergic drugs. The jejunum of rabbit shows regular rocking movement, so it can be applied to observing the effects of drugs on the movement. The in-vitro experiments can be conducted conveniently and quickly and can be used to screen large quantities of drugs. However, the factors such as absorption and metabolism *in vivo* should be considered, and the drug action should be correctly analyzed.

Experiment 4. 4   Effects of drugs on *in vivo* spermaduct controlled by hypogastric nerve in Guinea pig

Objective

Study the pharmacological experiment method on *in vivo* spermaduct controlled by hypogastric nerve in Guinea pig. Observe the effects of several drugs including α-adrenoceptor agonists and antagonists, adrenergic nerve blockers on the animal model.

Principle

Hypogastric nerve, a branch of sympathetic nerve, can dominate visceral organs including spermaduct whose smooth muscles contain α-adrenoceptors. Either stimulation of hypogastric nerve or administration of α-adrenoceptor agonists can cause contraction of smooth muscles of spermaduct. α-adrenoceptor antagonists and adrenergic nerve blockers can oppose the contractile response by affecting the receptors and nerve conduction.

Materials

Animal required: 1 Guinea pig, 400 – 450g, male.

Apparatus required: physio – pharmacological electric stimulator, shield electrode, pressure transducer, flatbed recorder, thermos operation table, iron stand, transfusion needle, pulley, surgical scissors, hemostat, trachea cannula, thread, gauze, syringe.

Reagent required: norepinephrine bitartrate solution (10^{-5}, W/V), guanethidine sulphate solution (3×10^{-3}, W/V), phentolamine methanesulfonate phenol solution (10^{-3}, W/V), normal saline.

Methods

Weigh the animal. Inject 1. 2g/kg urethane intraperitoneally to anesthetize the animal, and fix its back on the thermos operation table. Cut open the skin on the front of neck; make a cut on the trachea; insert the trachea cannula and tie it. Expose external jugular vein, and insert the transfusion needle connected with a syringe. Then ligate it and prepare to inject the drugs.

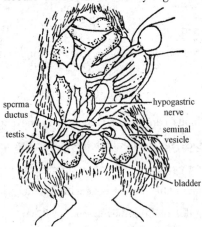

Fig. 4 – 1   The position of hypogastric nerve and spermaduct of Guinea pig

Cut open the skin of hypogastrium along midline. Push the intestine up to the right to find two strips of white fibrous (fine) hypogastric nerve roughly parallel to the ureter. Select either side of the hypogastric nerve and tie the end towards the center. Place the shield electrode under the ligation site to be ready for stimulation. Isolate the spermaduct on the same side. Cut off the spermaduct on the position near to the testicle and tie the stump. Raise the spermaduct and attach it to the pressure transducer. Then record its activity (Fig. 4 – 1).

The stimulating parameters of the physio – pharmacological electric stimulator are as follows: wave width 1ms, frequency 50 – 80Hz, voltage from 3V to the numeric value that can cause obvious contraction of the spermaduct, duration time of each stimulation is 5 seconds.

After the device is installed, do the experiment according to the following steps.

1) Inject intravenously 10μg/0.1ml norepinephrine bitartrate solution (10^{-5}, W/V) per kilogram of body weight.

2) Stimulate the hypogastric nerve for 5 seconds. Observe the response of the spermaduct until the effect disappears.

3) Inject intravenously 6mg/kg guanethidine sulphate solution (3×10^{-3}, W/V, 2ml/kg). Wait for 45 minutes after administration.

4) Stimulate the hypogastric nerve for 5 seconds. Notice the response of the spermaduct this time.

5) Inject intravenously 10μg/kg norepinephrine bitartrate solution (10^{-5}, W/V, 1ml/kg).

6) Inject intravenously 2mg/kg phentolamine methanesulfonate phenol solution (10^{-3}, W/V, 2ml/kg).

7) Inject intravenously 10μg/kg norepinephrine bitartrate solution (10^{-5}, W/V, 2ml/kg).

Results

Copy the contraction curve of the spermaduct. Mark the successive disposition and explain the experiment results.

Notes

1. The Guinea pig that just reaches sexual maturity is most suitable in this experiment because the spermaduct of the animal younger than 2 months is too thin to record its activity while that of the animal older than 5 months is insensitive to the drugs.

2. It is hard to find the hypogastric nerve because it is relatively fine. The general steps are as follows. ①Find the ureters of both sides. ②Push the ureters aside. ③See the white fibers as fine as a hair filament. That is the hypogastric nerve.

3. Be careful to protect the spermaduct from coldness and dryness during the course of the experiment.

4. The speed of injection should be slow because all the drugs administered can cause intense fluctuation of the blood pressure.

Evaluation

The hypogastric nerve, belonging to the sympathetic postganglionic fiber, can control the spermaduct whose smooth muscles contain α – adrenoceptors. Stimulation of the hypogastric nerve can cause contraction of smooth muscles of the spermaduct. This method is convenient to trace the action site of adrenergic nerve blockers. In addition, the spermaduct contracts quickly. So it is one of the most frequent methods of analysis of α – adrenoceptor agonists, antagonists and adrenergic nerve blockers.

Experiment 4.5   Acute intoxication by organophosphate compounds and its treatment

Objective

Observe the toxic symptoms of organophosphate compounds and the inhibition action of the compounds on cholinesterase in the blood. Analyze the mechanism of detoxication of atropine and pralidoxime (PAM) based on the antagonistic action of the two drugs on organophosphate compounds.

Principle

Under the normal physiological circumstances, the constant quantity of acetylcholine in the body is maintained by acetylcholinesterase in the synaptic space. Inhibitors of acetylcholinesterase have the capacity to cause noticeable accumulation of acetylcholine in the body, which results in a series of toxic symptoms. Cholinesterase reactivating drugs are able to reactivate inhibited acetylcholinesterase in a short time, so they can relieve or eliminate the toxic symptoms. M receptor blockers can directly antagonize various symptoms mediated by M receptors. As for the treatment of intoxication of organophosphate compounds, the synergistic action of the two kinds of drugs and their difference can be analyzed through the toxic symptoms and their remission.

Materials

Animal required: 2 rabbits, 2.0 – 2.5kg, male or female.

Apparatus required: rabbit boxes, syringes, ruler, alcoholic cotton, dry cotton, test kit of serum acetylcholinesterase activity.

Reagent required: dipterex (5%, *W/V*), atropine sulphate (0.1%, *W/V*), pralidoxime iodide (2.5%, *W/V*).

Methods

Weigh the two rabbits and fix them in the rabbit boxes. Observe and record the following indices: frequency and extent of breathing, diameter of pupil, saliva secretion, excretion of urine and feces, and tremor of skeletal muscles. Collect 1ml blood sample from marginal vein of the ear. Centrifuge the blood sample and collect the serum. Then assay the activity of acetylcholinesterase.

Scrub the ear with alcoholic cotton to dilate its marginal vein. Inject 120mg/kg (2.4ml/kg) dipterex (5%, W/V) intravenously. Observe the above – mentioned indices and record them when the toxic symptoms are obvious. Supply another 1/3 of the original dosage if 20 – 25 minutes later no toxic symptoms appear or the symptoms are not obvious. Collect 1ml blood sample from marginal vein of the ear and centrifuge the sample to obtain the serum. Then assay the activity of acetylcholinesterase.

Immediately inject intravenously one of the rabbits with 4.0mg/kg (4ml/kg) atropine sulphate (0.1%, *W/V*), and the other with 50mg/kg (2.0ml/kg) pralidoxime iodide (2.5%, *W/V*). Then observe whether their toxic symptoms are relieved. Record the indices when the toxic symptoms are obviously relieved. Administer another 1/3 of the original dosages if the toxic symp-

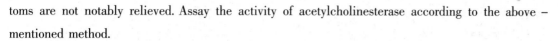

toms are not notably relieved. Assay the activity of acetylcholinesterase according to the above – mentioned method.

Results

Record the results according to Table 4 – 2. Compare and analyze the results.

Notes

1. Dipterex is a powerful toxicant, and it can be absorbed via skin. If your hands touch the drug, wash your hands with water immediately. Alkali soaps are not allowed to be used because dipterex can transform to dichlorvos whose toxicity is more powerful.

2. Clean up the saliva, urine and feces to prepare for the observation in the experiment.

3. Cut off the eyelashes of the rabbits beforehand to avoid their nictitating when the diameters of the pupils are measured.

4. Since the size of pupil is influenced by light, the rabbit box should not be moved optionally during the course of the whole experiment and the condition of the light should be kept with one accord.

5. This experiment is designed to analyze the mechanism of detoxication of atropine and pralidoxime iodide. In clinical practice, the two drugs should be applied together to obtain optimal effect of detoxication. Therefore, after the experiment the other drug can be administered. Then observe the result.

Table 4 – 2　Indices of acute intoxication of organophosphate compounds
and its treatment in rabbit

	Breathing	Diameter of pupil saliva secretion	Excretion of feces and urine	Tremor	Activity of cholinesterase
Normal					
After treated with dipterex					
After treated with atropine					
Normal					
After treated with dipterex					
After treated with PAM					

Evaluation

During the experiment, acute intoxication of organophosphate compounds and its treatment, the physiological and pharmacological knowledge of cholinergic nerve can be systemically reviewed. Not only can we observe M and N symptoms due to mass accumulation of acetylcholine in the body, but we can further understand M and N actions and analyze the kind of antidotes. In addition, the item of measurement of activity of cholinesterase in blood is added to the experiment. So, the experiment is one of the best *in vivo* experiments on the cholinergic nervous system.

Experiment 4. 6　Comparison of surface anesthetic action of procaine and tetracaine

Objective

Study the method of screening surface anesthetic drugs. Understand the difference of action of procaine and tetracaine.

Principle

Cornea is a kind of simple and uniform membrane which contains non – myelinated nerve fiber without any other sensory cells or blood vessels. Corneal reflex is the index frequently used to test the penetrability, anesthetic intensity and action duration of local anesthetics.

Materials

Animal required: 1 rabbit, 2. 0 – 2. 5kg, male or female.

Apparatus required: rabbit box, scissors, drip tube.

Reagent required: procaine hydrochloride solution (5mg/ml), tetracaine hydrochloride solution (6mg/ml).

Methods

Take 1 rabbit and examine its eyes. If there is no disease of the eyes, put it into the rabbit box. Cut off the eyelashes of the rabbit. Touch the corneas gently with its beard to test whether the corneal reflex is normal. Stimulate 6 sites with roughly equal strength according to the sequence of Site 1, 2, 3, 4, 2, 5. (Fig. 4 – 2) Record 6/6 when the results are all positive (that is, the rabbit does not wink) and 0/6 when the results are all negative (that is, the rabbit winks). The rest is on the analogy of this.

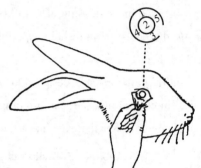

Fig. 4 – 2 The method of dropping drug in eyelid of rabbit and test order of Corneal reflex stimulation sites

Then pull its eyelids to form cup shape with your thumb and forefinger, and press its nasolacrimal duct with your middle finger. Drop 2 drops of procaine hydrochloride solution (5mg/ml) in the left eye and 2 drops of tetracaine hydrochloride solution (6mg/ml) in the right eye. Massage gently the eyelid to allow the cornea to contact the drug solution sufficiently. Keep the drug solutions in the eye sockets for 1 minute, and then let it go. Test the corneal reflex every 5 minutes for 30 minutes after administration. At the same time observe whether conjunctival congestion occurs. Record and compare the actions of the two drugs.

Results

Record the testing results of the corneal reflex according to Table 4 – 3.

Table 4 – 3 Comparison of surface anesthetic action of procaine and tetracaine

Eye of rabbit	Drug	Corneal reflex before administration	Corneal reflex after administration (min)					
			5	10	15	20	25	30
Left	procaine hydrochloride (5mg/ml)							
Right	tetracaine hydrochloride (6mg/ml)							

Notes

1. The nasolacrimal duct must be pressed when the drug is dropped. The aim is to prevent the drug solution from flowing into the nasal cavity and being absorbed via nasal mucosa because such things will lead to intoxication and affect the experimental results.

2. The hair of beard of the rabbit selected to stimulate the cornea should not be too hard or too soft. Using the same beard in the experiment to assure equal strength.

3. The eyelashes should be cut off before administration, or the wrong conclusion will be drawn because the corneal reflex still occur even if the cornea is already anesthetized.

Evaluation

The indices for studying local anesthetics are mainly as follows: potency (expressed by minimal effective concentration), efficiency of diffusing into nervous fiber and strength of penetrating mucosa surface (expressed by the initial time of action and efficiency of anesthetizing mucosa), anesthetic process (expressed by the initial time and duration of anesthesia). Therefore, the studying methods are various such as corneal anesthesia method, neuromuscular preparation method and *in vitro* nerve action potential observation method and so on. These methods evaluate local anesthetics from different standpoints. Corneal anesthesia method can only provide information of penetrability of drugs on superficial tissues. So, various methods should be adopted to obtain comprehensive information.

Chapter 5　Experiments of drugs affecting the splanchnic system

The splanchnic system is a general designation of different viscera systems in the thorax, abdominal cavity and pelvic cavity, it mainly includes the cardiovascular system, the respiratory system, the digestive system, the urinary system and the genital system, etc. Drugs acting on the hematic system are generally classified into the drug discussed in this chapter. Gonadal hormones act mainly on the genital system, so they are generally classified into "hormones". Because each viscera has its physiological and pathological characteristics, the kind of drugs acting on the splanchnic system are various, corresponding pharmacological experimental methods are different.

Cardiovascular agents include drugs for chronic cardiac insufficiency, anti – myocardial ischemia, antihypertensives, anti – arrhythmias and drugs for preventing atherosclerosis. Pharmacological experiments of cardiovascular system mainly test the effects of drugs on myocardium contractility, electrophysiologic characteristics, myocardial metabolism and vasoconstriction. Furthermore, we can prepare various animal pathologic models for experimental arrhythmia, hypertension, cardiac insufficiency, atherosclerosis and myocardial infarction to observe the experimental therapeutic effects of drugs.

Agents affecting the respiratory system include antitussive, anti – asthmatics and expectorants. The effects of antitussives could be evaluated by using animal tussive model. The methods of inducing tussis include chemical stimulation, mechanical stimulation, and electrical stimulation. Feline tussive reflex is very sensitive, so it is suitable for evaluating the antitussives. Anti – asthmatics are important and most of them can relax bronchial smooth muscle, so we can observe the relaxation effects of drugs on smooth muscle by using in – vitro trachea method and integral pneumo – overflow method. Experimental pathologic models generally consist of induced asthma by spraying bioactive or sensitized agents. Guinea pig is the most sensitive animal to anti – asthmatics. The main action of expectorants is to promote the movement of respiratory tract epithelia, to dilute or decompose sputum and actuate expectoration. The secretion output in respiratory tract can be utilized to evaluate expectorants.

Agents for the treatment of digestive diseases include anti – ulcer drugs, antiemetics, laxatives, antidiarrheals and choleretics, etc. The effects of antiulcer drugs are evaluated mainly using animal digestive tract ulcer model, observing the effect of drugs on gastro – acid secretion. Methods inducing experimental digestive tract ulcer include surgery, drugs, stress, artificial injury of digestive tract mucosa, etc. As for laxatives and antidiarrheal agents, we should observe their effects on the motor function of gastrointestinal smooth muscle and the conveying function of digestive tract besides fecal form, bowel evacuation amount and frequency.

The main agents affecting the urinary system are diuretics. In the evaluation of diuretics, not only the effect on urine volume but also the effect on electrolyte excretion in urine should be observed. The study of diuresis action situs is important for understanding the mechanisms of drug action. Renal clearance examination is an important method to understand renal functions.

Agents acting on the hematic system include drugs affecting hemopoiesis and clotting. Hematic cytology examination and clotting time determination are not only the fundamental experiments of agents acting on the hematic system but also one important part of toxicological experiments and have significance for new drug development. Antithrombotic drugs are an important kind of drugs for the prevention and treatment of cardiac diseases and cerebral diseases, and the corresponding methods include platelet function and hemorheology experiments. The study of platelet receptors, active substances and their functions is an active sphere.

Ⅰ. Experiments of drugs used for cardiac insufficiency

Cardiac insufficiency is a kind of syndrome in which the heart blood – pumping function comparatively insufficient and the blood flow can not meet the demand of tissue metabolism. Cardiac blood – pumping function is determined not only by myocardial contractility but also by pre – load, after – load and heart rate.

Myocardial contractility is the internal contractility of myocardial fibers which is determined by the interaction between myocardial contractile component (actin, myoglobulin) and Ca^{2+}. The average shortening velocity of myocardial peripheral fibers is a rational index for evaluating myocardial contractility, but its requirement of *in vivo* experiment is quite high, so its application is limited. Because intra – ventricular pressure can reflect ventricular wall tension, and the myocardial contraction which is opposite to isovolumic contraction is isometric contraction, myocardial contractility is generally reflected by elevation velocity indices (dp/dt_{max}, V_{pm}, V_{max}) of iso – volumetric contractile phase in practice. The index of iso – volumetric contractile phase is not suitable for the evaluation of myocardial contractile basal level since its individual difference is large. In *in vivo* experiments, myocardial contractility is affected by pre – load and after – load, whereas in *in vitro* experiments such as *in vitro* experiment of papillary muscles, pre – load and after – load could be controlled, and thus medical inotropic action could be accurately evaluated.

The increase of heart rate could induce the increase of cardiac output in some range as well as myocardial oxygen consumption. If the heart rate is over 160 – 180times/min, the cardiac output declines instead because the relaxing period is too short and the blood volume reentering the heart is insufficient. Drugs used for cardiac insufficiency should not increase heart rate to reduce myocardial oxygen consumption.

Pre – load is referred to the tension cardiac muscles bearing before contraction, and it can be indicated by ventricular diastole telophase stress in *in vivo* experiments.

After – load is referred to the tension cardiac muscles bearing during contraction and can be indicated by average arterial pressure or total peripheral vascular resistance. The vascular contraction and dilatation have great influence on after – load. The relaxation of arterial resistant vessel can lead to decrease in cardiac ejection resistance and increase in cardiac output.

Most of the drugs in treating cardiac insufficiency such as digitalis glycosides enhance the cardiac blood – pumping function by strengthening myocardial contractility. It should be pointed out that cadiac output is mainly determined by peripheral factors and their effects on pre – load and after – load, and it is affected a little by the actual level of myocardial contractility. When congestive heart failure loses compensation, peripheral blood vessels contract and pre – load and after – load increase, which make the burden of prostrated heart further exacerbated. That is because of neural and humoral actions. And the most important is to decrease the cardiac pre – load and after – load here.

In conclusion, when evaluating drugs used for cardiac insufficiency, we should consider the following three aspects: ①effect on myocardial contractility. ②effect on cardiac blood – pumping function. ③effect on hemodynamics (including heart rate, blood pressure, electrocardiogram and left ventricular function, etc.). Because cardiac diastole has important effect on cardiac blood – pumping, and cardiac diastolic function is more easily damaged than contractile function, now the effects of drugs on cardiac diastole are highly noticed. The effects of drugs on cardiac contraction and diastole could be evaluated by hemodynamics and experiments of papillary muscles of guinea pigs. Moreover, the evaluation of drugs used for cardiac insufficiency should be conducted not only in normal animals but also in heart – failure animals.

Experiment 5.1　Effect of cardiac glycosides on the isolated heart of frog

Objective

1. Study Yatsuki – Hartung's perfusion method of isolated heart of frog.

2. Observe the effect of cardiac glycosides on the isolated heart of frog (including contractile strength, frequency, rhythm and cardiac output).

Principle

The amphibian animals can live in the water, so their hearts can endure the environment lack of oxygen. Given suitable nutrient solution, the heart can survive for a long time and keep cardiac contraction. By adding drugs into the perfusion solution, the direct effect on the heart can be observed. The model of heart failure caused by low calcium – containing Ringer's solution can obviously manifest cardiotonic effect of drugs.

Materials

Animal required: 2 toads or frog, 70g, male or female.

Apparatus required: probe, a pin, frog board, clip, recording equipment, tweezers, scissors.

Reagent required: Ringer's solution, Ringer's solution containing low level of Ca^{2+} (1/4 $CaCl_2$ of Ringer's solution), 5% digitalis.

Methods

1. Take a toad or frog, and damage its brain and spinal cord with a pin. Put the animal on a frog board lying on its back. Open the thoracic cavity, and cut the pericardium to make the heart exposed adequately.

2. Put two pieces of thread under the left and right aorta respectively. Turn the heart upside

down and make the venous sinus and postcaval vein exposed. Separate the ligament between two sides of the liver. Free the postcaval vein and put a piece of thread under it. Make an incision under the site where the thread is placed.

Insert the venous cannulation from the incision and fasten it by thread to fix the cannulation. Wash the heart using Ringer's solution through the venous cannulation and remove the remaining blood.

3. Turn the heart back. Make an incision on the distal edge of the left aorta. Insert the artrial cannulation towards the heart. If the perfusion solution flows out fluently from the artrial cannulation, fasten the cannulation together with the right arota by a piece of thread placed beforehand. Use scissors to separate the heart from the peripheral tissues. Adjust the direction and angle to fix the artrial cannulation and the venous one together. Ligate all the blood vessels except the aorta and postcaval vein with the other piece of thread. Make the specimen of the frog's heart (Fig. 5 – 1) .

4. Wash the heart using Ringer's solution repeatedly until the effluent solution from the artery is colorless. Adjust the height of liquid level in the venous cannulation to 1.5 – 2 cm and keep the height constant during the course of the whole experiment. Clip the cardiac apex and link the recording equipment via the tension transducer.

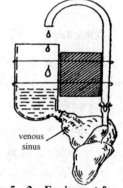

5. Trace a segment of normal curve. Observe the cardiac systolic range, heart rate and cardia output (drops/min). Then conduct the experiment according to the following steps:

1) Change solution with Ringer's solution containing low level of Ca^{2+}. Trace the curve after the systole weakens obviously. Observe the aforementioned indices.

venous sinus

Fig. 5 – 2　Equipment for isolated heart of frog

2) Add 1 – 2 drops of 5% digitalis into the venous cannulation, and observe and record the above indices sfter it acts obviously.

6. Compare the cardiac systolic strength, frequency, rhythm and the flow rate (drops/min) of the effluent solution from the artrial cannulation before and after administration.

Results

1. Copy the curve of heart contraction and mark administered drug and dosage.

2. Record the cardiac output before and after administration respectively.

Notes

1. During the course of surgery and experiment, be careful not to harm the venous sinus and prevent solution leaking out from the specimen.

2. The site of the arterial cannulation should be far away from the bulbus arteriosus.

3. During experiment, the height of the liquid level in the venous cannulation must be unchanged.

4. Add digitalis drop by drop as excessive dose may cause intoxication.

5. Keep the isolated heart moist.

Evaluation

1. The experiment is a classical method. The experimental materials are easily drawn, and the

instruments are simple to use. Experimental requirement is low and the success rate is high.

2. It can evaluate the effect of drugs on the isolated heart including systolic range, cardiac output and heart rate at the same time.

3. Because there are much differences of the cardiac response to drug between cold – blooded animals and warm – blooded ones, cold – blooded animals are rarely used in the experimental study. But it is an easy and clear experiment in teaching experiment.

Questions

1. In this experiment, what can we observe if the concentration of Calcium in Ringer's solution is increased gradually? Why?

2. What effect of digitalis has on isolated frog's heart?

3. Can we observe the effect of drug on pre – load and after – load circulation in this experiment? Why?

Experiment 5. 2   Effects of drugs on the contraction and relaxation of isolated papillary muscles

Objective

Study the preparation of isolated papillary muscles and observe the effects of drugs on myocardial contractility and relaxation with the specimen.

Principle

Papillary muscles, a special structure of the heart, possess various myocardial characteristics. Its muscle fibers align coincidently and are not interfered by the heart rate in vitro. Compared with the intact heart, it has special advantages in determination of myocardial tension change, tensive developing velocity (dT/dt) and diastolic function, so it is an important experiment for measurement of positive or negative myodynamic effect of drugs. With suitable temperature, oxygen supply and nutrient solution, driving papillary muscles with electric stimulation can maintain their fine activities of systole and diastole for several hours.

Materials

Animal required: 1 cat, 2 –3kg, male or female.

Apparatus required: super constant temperature water bath, bath tubes, iron cage, oxygen tank (be full of mixed gas of 95% O_2 and 5% CO_2), pharmacological physio multi – apply instrument, stimulating electrode, biological signal acquisition system, derivator, force – displacement transducer, operation instruments, syringe, beaker, plate.

Reagent required: modified Tyrode's solution (mmol/L): NaCl 137, KCl 5. 4, $MgCl_2$ 1. 05, NaH_2PO_2 0. 43, $CaCl_2$ 1. 8, $NaHCO_3$ 12, glucose 10. In general, all the components but $NaHCO_3$ and glucose are dispensed to mother solution 10 times condensed. The mother solution is 10 times diluted before use and then $NaHCO_3$ and glucose are added slowly. The pH of the solution prepared fresh is generally between 8. 1 and 8. 4. The pH value is decreased to 7. 35 – 7. 45 after mixed gas is aerated prior to use. K – H solution can also be used as the nutrient solution.

10^{-5} isoprenaline, 10^{-4} uabain, ether.

Methods

1. Anaesthetize the cat with ether and kill it by carotid bloodletting. Rapidly take out the heart and put it into the nutrient solution saturated with mixed gas, wash off remaining blood, and put it into a plate filled with the nutrient solution. Open the right ventricle, sufficiently expose papillary muscles, and choose a spindly one. Properly liberate its fundus, ligate it with a small quantity of cardiac muscles, ligate the tendinous cords of the papillary muscle using silk thread, and then cut down the tendinous cords and the fundus. Fix one end on the stimulating electrode hook, and quickly transfer it into the bath tube (containing 20ml nutrient solution). Link the other end with the force – displacement transducer. Resting load of the specimen is about 0.5 – 1g. Use electric stimulation (frequency 0.5Hz, wave width 3ms, 120% threshold voltage, square wave) to drive and stabilize it 30min, exchange solution 3 – 4 times during the stabilized period. After stabilization, adjust the load to maximize the contractile amplitude.

2. The contractile index is measured by recording single contractile curve and differential curve with paper speed of 100 – 200mm/s. Measure the following indices: ① peak tension (PT, mg) . ② time of peak contractile tension (TPT, ms). ③ maximum rising speed of tension (dp/dt_{max}, g/s). ④ time of maximum rising speed ($t – dp/dt_{max}$, ms). ⑤ time of PT to decrease 50% (1/2 PT, ms). ⑥ maximum descending speed of tension ($– dp/dt_{max}$, g/s).

3. Record the contractile curve before administration, add 10^{-5} isoprenaline 0.2ml, and then measure the contractile curve of post – administration after appearance of distinct action. Rinse the specimen three times with nutrient solution.

4. When contractile amplitude basically recovers, record the contractile curve, add 10^{-4} uabain 0.2ml, and then measure the contractile curve of post – administration after appearance of distinct action.

Results

Because the size of papillary muscles is various, the value of each specimen probably differs significantly, the diameter of the fundus of the papillary muscle can be measured and the cross section area can be calculated to revise the recorded PT, + (–) dp/dt_{max}. Also, the percentage of these parameters can be directly calculated to make the result of each specimen possess more comparability. Drug concentration should be calculated according to the final concentration in bath tubes.

Notes

1. During the preparation of the specimen of papillary muscles, be careful not to excessively pull and damage the specimen.

2. To keep the contractile amplitude of papillary muscles stable, pH of nutrient solution should be at about 7.4; stimulating frequency is generally 0.5 or 1Hz; temperature should be maintained at about 37℃.

3. Adjust the pre – load according to the size of the papillary muscle to maximize contractile amplitude.

4. Pay attention to the zero adjustment of the recorder's baseline.

5. Because the responses of atrium and ventricle to the effect of drugs are different, we had bet-

ter observe the effects of drugs on auricular and ventricular contractility simultaneously.

6. The volume of the added drug should not exceed 5% of nutrient solution and thus can be ignored when calculating drug concentration.

Evaluation

1. This method is used to study the effects of drug on the basic characteristics of cardiac muscle, which is important to elucidate nature of effects. If the method is combined with *in vivo* animal experiment such as hemodynamics, we could comprehensively understand the cardiovascular pharmacological action of drugs.

2. The specimen lack endogenous self – rhythmicity, so we can employ it to measure myocardial excitability, refractoriness, and self – rhythmicity, etc (the measurement of effective refractory period referred to auricle experiment).

3. Muscle fibers of papillary muscles align linearly, which makes the measurement of myocardial contractility more convenient than that of the intact heart.

4. The isolated specimen is not affected by heart rate, coronal vascular relaxation and contractility, etc, so it is suitable for observing the direct effects of drugs on cardiac muscles.

5. The introduction of $\pm dT/dt_{max}$, TPT, $t - dT/dt_{max}$, 1/2PT, and such mechanical index is advantageous to study of drugs' effects on myocardial contractility.

6. The sample is simply prepared and stabilized for a relatively long time but its technical requirement is higher than isolated atrial muscles.

Questions

1. Compared with *in vivo* experiments, what is the advantage when we measure the effects of drugs on myocardial contractility and relaxation using isolated papillary muscles? Could it replace *in vivo* experiment?

2. In this experiment, can we simultaneously observe the effects of drugs on myocardial excitability and refractory period?

Experiment 5. 3   Effects of drugs on left heart function and hemodynamics of rat

Objective

Study hemodynamic experimental method and left – ventricular intubation technique of rat. Understand various hemadynamic parameters and their actions on evaluation of drugs' effects on cardiac function.

Principle

In integral test, blood – pumping function of heart (including output, pulsatile power, blood – jet fraction, heart index, etc) are synthetic action of myocardial contractility, pre – , and after – load. In pharmacological experiments, it is generally necessary to evaluate the effects of drugs on integral myocardial contractility. Hemadynamics is a kind of frequently – used method to study the effects of drugs on cardiovascular functions, its index include blood – pump functions of heart, blood – flow, endocardial pressure, press – change velocity, volume of the cardiac chambers, blood pressure, vascular resistance and heart rate, etc. According to the changes in intraventricular pressure, pressure change velocity, and especially the index of isovolumic systole and period of relaxation, we can presume the change of myocardial systolic and diastolic functions.

Materials

Animal required: 1 rat, 200 – 250g, male.

Apparatus required: multi – channel physiological recorder (4 – 8 channels), double beam oscillograph, force – displacement transducer, direct current amplifier, PE – 50 polyethylene tube, operation instruments, beaker, syringe.

Reagent required: 0.4% pentobarbital sodium, 0.5% heparin – saline, 0.001% isoprenaline, 0.002% nifedipine.

Methods

1. Weigh the rat and anesthetize it with 40mg/kg 0.4% pentobarbital sodium. Fix the animal on back position, and cut jugular capillus. Fill the arterial cannula with heparin – saline.

2. Cut off the fur on the front of neck and open the skin along midline. Isolate left and right carotid, and insert the cannula into left ventriculus from right carotid. Measure the left ventricular pressure using force – displacement transducer, acquire the signal of $\pm dp/dt$ and $(dp/dt)\ p^{-1}$ by derivator and press processor. Connect left carotid cannula with another force – displacement transducer to record arterial blood pressure. Cannulate unilateral cervical vein for administration.

3. Adjust calibration value, record various indices of pre – administration after the animal stabilized for 15min.

4. Infuse drug from venous cannula and record various indices at 1min, 3min, 5min, 10min, and 20min after administration.

5. After each index basically recovers, render the next drug and record each index after administration at different time points. The sequence of administration:

1) 0.001% isoprenaline 0.01mg/kg, intravenous injection.

2) 0.002% nifedipine 0.02mg/kg, intravenous injection.

6. Calibration and measurement of each index:

1) LVP curve. The calibration sensitivity of LVP is 2.7mm/13.3kPa. It is generally suitable that LVEDP + $\triangle p$ is equal to 1.1 – 1.3kPa. We can acquire LVSP, LVDP and LVP signals from LVP curve, record them after 10 times amplification by direct current amplifier from which LVEDP can be read.

2) dp/dt curve. When the time constant of derivator is 1.0ms, high frequency filtered wave is 50 Hz, adjust signal amplitude of the standard triangular wave calibration pressure of derivator to equal that of LVP13.3kPa. Based on the curve, $+ dp/dt_{max}$, $- dp/dt_{max}$, $t - dp/dt_{max}$ can be measured.

3) $(dp/dt)\ p^{-1}$ curve. Dial the switch of press processor to $(dp/dt)\ p^{-1}$ side, its output scaling signal is a reverse hyperbola which culmination approaches actual measured left myocardial maximum decurtate velocity V_{pm}. $\triangle p$ is input to avoid the appearance of infinitely – great value, So actual curve value is $(dp/dt)\ /\ (p + \triangle p)$, we can multiply actual value with $(1 + \triangle p/p)$ to correct it. The correction is not needed if $\triangle p \ll p$.

4）LVP – （dp/dt）p^{-1} ring. Input the electric signals of LVP and （dp/dt）p^{-1} to x and y axes of SBR – 1 type twin line oscillograph to acquire the ring，take a photograph and record it. The nodical reading of ring's tangent of positive direction descending limb with y axes is the V_{max} of zero – load.

5）The measurement and calculation of T value. Read LVP on the corresponding LVP curve，adopt its natural logarithm（ln$p$），make linear regression according to x axes of ln$p$ and y axes of corresponding time t，the slope is T value.

Results

According to the above method，measure and calculate various parameters of pre – administration and post – administration，and then make analysis and evaluation.

Notes

1. The tubing system for pressure record should not have any bubble. The leakage and blood coagulation must be prevented to avoid anamorphosis of the wave form.

2. Left ventricular cannula shouldn't be too long（2 – 15cm is suitable），otherwise the pressure wave would be anamorphic because of the oversize internal pressure of cannula.

3. After left ventricular cannula is inserted to carotid，it should be slowly driven toward left ventricle under the monitoring of pressure wave by fluorescent screen to prevent damage of blood vessel or heart.

4. During the intubation，we should pull the blood vessel in front of cannula straight in order to make the cannula favorably propelled.

5. When the left ventricular cannula is difficult to enter left ventriculus at the entrance of aortic valves，we can drop out the cannula slightly，change angle and direction，or twitter the cannula and propel it toward to smoothly insert the cannula into left ventrcle.

Evaluation

1. All cardiovascular drugs should be evaluated through hemadynamics and integral cardiac functions，so the experiments of this aspect are requisite for the development of cardiovascular drugs. We can understand the effects of drugs on cardiac functions and peripheral blood vessels by the study of pharmaceutical hemadynamics.

2. The rat is small with a favourable tolerance，and the procedure of operation is simple，convenient，economical and substantial. We could measure various hemadynamic parameters from conscious rats by modifying the experimental method.

3. Cardiac output can't be determined by this method，so we can not acquire a series of important hemadynamic parameters such as pump function and change in peripheral resistance.

4. To acquire experimental data，we need to record，photograph，measure，and calculate，etc，and must spend a lot of time and manpower. These procedures could be spared if computer is available

5. Isovolumic systolic period is very suitable for evaluation of myocardial contractility before and after administration，but its range of normal value is too extensive to be suitable for evaluation of contractile basal level so blood – injecting phase should be used.

Questions

1. Which index should mainly be chosen to evaluate the effects of drugs on myocardial contractility in this experiment? Which index should be chosen to evaluate the effects on myocardial relaxation?

2. If a drug induces significant increase in dp/dt_{max}, $t - dp/dt_{max}$, and arterial blood pressure but no substantial change in V_{pm}, V_{max}, what are the main actions of the drug?

II. Experiments of antiarrhythmic drugs

Arrhythmia can be divided into tachyarrhythmia and bradyarrhythmia according to heart rate. Currently the commonly used antiarrhythmic drugs are used to treat tachyarrhythmia and the researching methods also aim directly at tachyarrhythmia. The researching methods of antiarrhythmic drugs are chiefly divided into two groups. One is to observe the effects of drugs on myocardial electrophysiological characteristics, such as excitability, autorhythmicity and conductivity. Glass microelectrode can be employed to record transmembrane action potential and contact electrode can be used to record monophasic action potential in order to study the effects of drugs on each phase of action potential and suspect the effects of drugs on ion channels. This kind of methods can be used to research the antiarrhythmic mechanism of drugs or screen the antiarrhythmic drugs bearing some electrophysiological characteristics. Another is to utilize arrhythmic model of animal to observe directly the antiarrhythmic action of drugs. The common methods of creating the arrhythmic model of animals are: ①drug – induced method. ②electric stimulation method. ③ligation of coronary artery.

Despite the various methods and models of inducing arrhythmia of animals, none has good correlation to the clinical or decisive significance. Therefore, in practice, antiarrhythmic action of new drugs is evaluated through various animal models. Corresponding models can be selected according to the possible mechanism of drug action. For instance, with regard to Class I drugs, arrhythmic models induced by cardiac glycoside or aconitine can be selected; as to Class II drugs, the models induced by adrenaline or chloroform can be adopted; and electricity – induced ventricular fibrillation model is suitable for anti – fibrillation drugs; for Class III drugs, in order to search and find the electrophysiological characteristics, myocardial action potential should be analyzed first and then arrhythmic model is used. As far as the animal is concerned, the cold – blooded animals are seldom applied because the arrhythmia of them is different from that of the warm – hearted animals. Rats are not sensitive to cardiac glycoside, so ouabain is inadvisable to induce arrhythmia of rats. The hearts of small animals such as rat, Guinea pig, rabbit and cat are possible to recover after ventricular fibrillation, so the ventricular fibrillation threshold can be determined repeatedly. The hearts of Guinea pig and rabbit are suitable for *in vitro* specimen. Cats are robust and have strong tolerance. The ventricular fibrillation of dog, pig and such large animals are difficult to recover and the defibrillator must be used. Dogs are very sensitive to arrhythmia – induced stimuli and thus easier to be caused ventricular fidrillation than humans. The coronary vascular system of pigs is quite similar to that of humans, so pigs are fit for the arrhythmia model caused by ligaturing the coronary artery.

Experiment 5. 4   The antagonistic effects of quinidine on aconitine – induced arrhythmia in rat

Objective

Learn the preparation method of aconitine – induced arrhythmic model of rat. Observe the protective effects of drugs on this type of arrhythmia.

Principle

Aconitine can cause an increase in excitability of cardiac muscle by direct action hence it causes arrhythmia. Aconitine can force sodium channels to open and increase Na^+ entry, resulting in depolarization of cell membrane, and therefore enhance the autorhythmicity of fast – response cells including artrial conductive tissues and AV bundles – Purkinje system to form unifocal or multifocal ectopic rhythm. Aconitine can produce ventricular or supraventricular extrasystole, ventricular tachycardia and ventricular fibrillation.

Materials

Animal required: 1 rat, 180 – 250g, male or female.

Apparatus required: electrocardiograph, electrocardioscope, operation table, surgical instruments, syringe, venous cannulation.

Reagent required: 20% urethane, 0.001% aconotine, 0.5% quinidine, normal saline.

Methods

1. Take the rat and weigh it. Inject the animal intraperitoneally with 20% urethane to anesthetize it. Fix it on the operation table on its back.

2. Incise the skin on the neck. Separate the external jugular vein on one side. Insert the venous cannulation into the vein. (This step can be replaced by inserting scalp acupuncture into the femoral vein.)

3. Link the lead wire of electrocardiogram with the electrocardioscope. Record the electrocardiogram of Lead Ⅱ. Then inject 0.001% aconitine (25μg/kg) from the venous cannulation quickly (about 5s). Observe and record the arrhythmia occurring now.

4. 5 minutes after the occurrence of arrhythmia, inject 0.5% quinidine (10mg/kg) intravenously. Observe the change of arrhythmia. Record the following time: reverting to sinus rhythm, reappearance of ventricular extrasystole, ventricular tachycardia, ventricular fibrillation and death (observational time limit: 60 minutes). In the control group equivalent saline is substituted for quinidine.

Results

The latent period of quinidine is the period from administration to the time when the ventricular tachycardia reverts to sinus rhythm. The duration of the drug action consists of two parts, the duration of sinus rhythm and the period from sinus rhythm – reverting time point to appearance of ventricular fibrillation. Clip and paste the electrocardiogram and compare it with the control group to evaluate antiarrhythmic effects of the drug.

Notes

1. The injection speed of aconitine should be controlled strictly to ensure that the injection is finished within 5 – 10 seconds.

2. Pay attention to heat preservation of the animal.

3. The aconitine solution cannot be refrigerated too long (generally not more than 2 weeks).

Evaluation

1. The arrhythmia induced by aconitine can last for more than one hour and is not easy to revert to sinus rhythm. The experimental method is easy and reliable. Due to the long duration of arrhythmia, not only preventive administration but therapeutic administration can be conducted. For unknown drugs, the minimum effective dosage can be measured by multi – administration.

2. Aconitine can also be directly administrated to form continuous ventricular tachycardia, flutter and fibrillation on the surface of atria.

Question

Describe the main similarities and differences between the aconitine – induced arrhythmic model and the ouabain – induced one.

Experiment 5.5   The effect of drug on the threshold of ventricular fibrillation induced by electric stimulation in rabbit

Objective

Learn the *in vivo* experimental method of inducing ventricular fibrillation by electric stimulation. Understand the action of electric simulation – induced arrhythmia in the study of antiarrhythmic drugs.

Principle

During the course of repolarization after depolarization of cardiac muscle there is a vulnerable period indicated by wave T on the electrocardiogram located in relative refractory period. Because the repolarization level is not uniform, strong enough stimulation exerted in the period can cause re-entry activities to induce ventricular fibrillation. When a series of stimulation is adopted, the inhomogeneity of repolarization can be increased so that the stimulation is easy to fall in the vulnerable period to cause ventricular fibrillation.

Most of the ventricular fibrillations occurring on small animals such as rat, rabbit and cat can pause and revert to sinus rhythm, whereas, ventricular fibrillations emerging on large animals such as dog and monkey cannot recover naturally and defibrillator is needed here.

Materials

Animal required: 1 rabbit, 2 – 3kg, male or female.

Apparatus required: pharmaco – physiological electric stimulator, electrocardioscope or electrocardiograph, stimulating electrode, rabbit operation table, surgical instruments, syringe.

Reagent required: 3% sodium pentobarbital, 1% lidocaine, normal saline.

Methods

1. Take one rabbit and weigh it. Inject the animal intravenously with 3% sodium pentobarbital to anesthetize it. Fix it on the back. Cut the hair on the chest.

2. Cut off the skin on the center of the chest. Snip the third and the fourth costal cartilage along the left border of the breast bone. The beating heart inside the pericardium can be seen then.

3. Cut the pericadium open and fix it on the chest wall to raise the heart. Fix the negative electrode on the apex of heart and positive electrode on left and right ventricle junction near the atrioventricular junction. The distance between the two electrodes is about 2cm.

4. Rest for 15 minutes or so. Determine the ventricular fibrillation threshold (VFT) before administration. The stimulating parameters are as follows: width of square wave $0.3 - 0.5$ms, frequency 50Hz; voltage from 1V on, stimulating duration time 10s/time. Exert stimulation every one minute and increase stimulating intensity step by step (0.5V more each time) until ventricular fibrillation appears. Then the voltage value is VFT. If the electrocardiograph is used, don't trace the graph when stimulating. Record the situation immediately after the stimulation stops. Repeat one time after 5 minutes for resting. The average value of the two times is recorded as VFT before administration.

5. Rest for 5 minutes. Then intravenously inject 1% lidocaine (10mg/kg) slowly. Determine VFT at 1, 5, 10, 15, 20, 25 and 30 min after administration.

Results

Based on VFT before administration, calculate the added value of VFT (ΔVFT) of each different time after administration. If possible, utilize the linear regression of ascending and descending phase of ΔVFT to calculate ascending and descending velocity that can indicate the ascending and descending velocity of drug effects. Calculate the area of ΔVFT according to the formula of triangle or trapezoid. If there are relatively many classified groups, a half of the groups can be established as saline – used control groups. Finally compare the results of administration groups with those of control groups and conduct statistical test.

Notes

1. The heart operation can be undertaken without cutting the pleura if enough attention is paid to the operation because the pleura on the chest can be separated from pericardium easily in rabbit. Without a breathing machine, it is required during the operation that the pericardium should be cut from the center and the chest wall pulled by a clasp with suitable strength, ensuring that the pleura is kept intact.

2. The costal cartilage must be snipped very close to the sternum to avoid the internal mammary artery damage by massive hemorrhage.

3. The pericardium is fixed on the chest wall, and forming pericardial swing bed to elevate the heart is conducive to the operation. Be careful that the pericardium of the rabbit is relatively vulnerable and easily lacerated.

4. The electrodes on the heart can be fixed either by suture or by little metal clips. Be sure to prevent short circuit between the two electrodes.

5. The increasing range of the voltage should not vary too much at a time to prevent severe and irreversible ventricular fibrillation. If ventricular fibrillation cannot recover within ten seconds, closed cardiac massage and artificial respiration can be performed for help.

Evaluation

1. The method is one of the commonly used electric stimulation – induced arrhythmic models

due to its convenience.

2. The results are stable and have good ruggedness. They can be used to evaluate the range and duration of VFT increased by drugs.

3. The results are more valuable if program – controlled electric stimulator is used to measure the vulnerable period or single extra – period stimulation is used to cause ventricular tachycardia and fibrillation to determine VFT in the case of pacing.

4. The ventricular fibrillation occurring in rabbit, cat, rat and such small animals is easy to revert to sinus rhythm naturally, so the defibrillator is not needed.

5. Sometimes the result is difficult to evaluate because stimulation is a source of both disturbance and ventricular fibrillation. The arterial cannulation used to measure blood pressure simultaneously is quite helpful to judge whether ventricular fibrillation appears.

6. The alteration of the heart rate can influence VFT, so heart rate should be controlled with pacing if possible.

Questions

1. Review the periodic alteration of excitability in myocardial electric activities.

2. Comprehend the relationship concerning the extent of myocardial repolarization, the conduct of action potential and the formation of reentry.

Experiment 5. 6　The therapeutic effect of lidocaine on arrhythmia induced by barium chloride in rat

Objective

Learn the method of inducing arrhythmia by barium chloride in rat. Observe the antiarrythmic effects of lidocaine.

Principle

Barium chloride can accelerate the inward sodium current of Purkinje fiber and increase the depolarization velocity in the diastolic period to induce ventricular arrhythmia involving ventricular extrasystole, bigeminy, ventricular tachycardia and fibrillation. It is also a kind of model used to screen antiarrhythmic drugs. Quinidine, lidocaine and β – blockers have effect on the model.

Materials

Animal required: 2 rats.

Apparatus required: electrocardiograph, electrocardioscope, surgical scissors, eye forceps, operation table for rat, syringe, intravenous scalp needle, tampon.

Reagent required: 10% chloral hydrate solution, 0.4% barium chloride solution, 0.5% lidocaine solution, normal saline.

Methods

1. Take one rat and weigh it. Anesthetize the animal with 0.3g/kg chloral hydrate by intraperitoneal injection. Fix it on the back on the operation table. Insert the venous cannulation into the external jugular vein to prepare for administration.

2. Insert electrodes of electrocardiograph into subcutaneous part of limbs of the rat to prepare for

扫码"学一学"

tracing the electrocardiogram. Select lead II. Amplitude 1mV = 10mm; paper speed = 50mm/s. After a segment of normal electrocardiogram is traced, inject 4mg/kg barium chloride intravenously and immediately trace electrocardiogram for 20 seconds. Afterwards, trace a potion of electrocardiogram every other minute or use an oscilloscope to monitor the electrocardiogram until sinus rhythm reappears. Record duration time of arrhythmia.

3. Take another rat and anesthetize it by chloral hydrate. Adopt the same method to induce arrhythmia. Immediately inject the animal with 5mg/kg lidocaine hydrochloride from the femoral vein. Trace electrocardiograph according to the above-mentioned requirement or monitor it by an oscilloscope. Based on whether arrhythmia can be stopped right away or the duration time of arrhythmia is reduced, evaluate the therapeutic effects of lidocaine on arrhythmia induced by barium chloride.

Results

Report the administrated drugs, alteration of electrocardiogram and duration time of arrhythmia of the two rats (Table 5 – 1). Clip and paste or copy the typical segments of electrocardiogram. Evaluate the antagonistic effects of lidocaine on arrhythmia induced by barium chloride primarily.

Table 5 – 1   Therapeutic effects of lidocaine on duration time of arrhythmia induced by barium chloride

Drug \ Group	1	2	3	4	5	6	7	8	$\bar{x} \pm SD$
NS									
Lidocaine									

Notes

1. The anesthetic chloral hydrate used in this experiment cannot be replaced by sodium pentobarbital. Otherwise relatively stable arrhythmia is uneasy to be induced. The antagonistic effects of lidocaine on arrhythmia induced by barium chloride act rapidly, so electrocardiogram can be traced during injection of lidocaine in order to observe its alteration (Fig. 5 – 2).

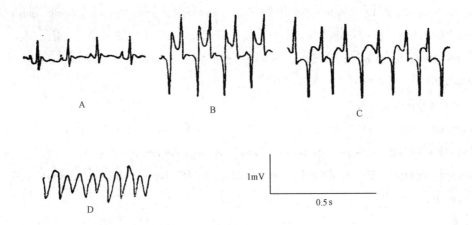

Fig. 5 – 2   The changed elec – trocardiograph (ECG) of rat with intoxication by barium chloride

A. pre – administration; B. 3 minutes after administration; C. 5 minutes after administration; D. 7 minutes after administration. The speed of paper is 50mm/s

2. Mouse, rat, Guinea pig and such small animals are often possible to recover naturally even

if ventricular fibrillation occurs on them. However, large animals such as dog and monkey die finally after ventricular fibrillation emerges.

Experiment 5. 7   The antagonistic effect of lidocaine on arrhythmia induced by ouabain

Objective

Learn the preparation of ouabain – induced arrhythmic model. Observe the therapeutic effects of lidocaine on ouabain – induced arrhythmia. Understand the mechanism of ouabain – induced arrhythmia.

Principle

The poisoning by cardiotonic glycoside, on one hand, can inhibit Na^+/K^+ – ATP enzyme in the myocardial cell membrane to cause intracellular K^+ decrease which results in diminishing maximum diastolic potential and intracellular Na^+ increase which can lead to rising autorhythmicity by yielding oscillating after – potential and trigged activities through $Na^+ - Ca^{2+}$ exchange which increase intracellular Ca^{2+}. On the other hand, cardiotonic glycoside can inhibit the cardiac conduction system directly causing decline of maximum diastolic potential and action potential amplitude, which slows the conduction to make reentry easier.

The poisoning by cardiotonic glycoside can cause various arrhythmia, among which multifocal ventricular extrasystole, tachycardia, fibrillation and conduction block are most frequently seen.

Materials

Animal required: 1 Guinea pig, 300 – 400g, male or female.

Apparatus required: electrocardiograph, electrocardioscope, operation table, surgical instruments, syringe, venous cannulation.

Reagent required: 20% urethane, 0.01% ouabain, 0.5% lidocaine, normal saline.

Methods

1. Weigh the Guinea pig. Inject the animal intraperitonealy with 20% urethane (1.2g/kg) to anesthetize it. Fix it on the back on the operation table. Cut the hair on the neck.

2. Incise the skin along the midline on the neck. Isolate one – side external jugular vein. Insert the venous cannulation filled with saline into the vein 1 – 2cm and fix the cannulation with wires.

3. Link the lead wire of electrocardiogram and record the electrocardiogram of Lead II before administration.

4. Under the monitoring of electrcardioscope, inject intravenously 0.01% ouabain with 90μg/kg for the first time and afterwards 20μg/kg every five minutes until the appearance of continuous ventricular tachycardia. Record the electrocardiogram.

5. Inject 0.5% lidocaine (5mg/kg) from the venous cannulation. Observe and record the time when ventricular tachycardia reverts to sinus rhythm, reappearance of tachycardia and when ventricular tachycardia reverts to ventricular fibrillation (if emerging) and the corresponding electrocardiogram. The observational time limit is 1 hour after lidocaine is administrated. The control group is injected with equivalent saline.

Results

The latent period of the drug is the period from administration to the time when the ventricular tachycardia reverts to sinus rhythm. The duration time of the drug action consists of two parts, the duration of sinus rhythm and the period from sinus rhythm – reverting time point to appearance of ventricular fibrillation. Clip and paste the electrocardiogram and compare it with the control group to evaluate antiarrhythmic effects of the drug.

Notes

1. Ouabain should be administrated when ventricular extrasystole appears. Lidocaine should not be administrated until typical ventricular tachycardia appears.

2. While conducting the venous intubation, it is unnecessary to completely isolate the vein and only the fatty and connective tissues on the vein should be removed clean. The blood vessel should be incised when the vein is full of blood so that the cannulation can be inserted easily.

3. Pay attention to heat preservation of the animal.

Evaluation

1. Cardiotonic glycosides – induced arrhythmic model is frequently used, for the method is stable and the result is reliable.

2. The Guinea pig is very suitable for the model. The reasons are as follows: ①its reaction to cardiovascular drugs is similar to human's. ②it is sensitive to cardiotonic glycosides. ③it is relatively cheap. Another commonly used animal is dog. Rat is insensitive to cardiotonic glycosides, so it is unsuitable for the model.

3. In the experiment therapeutic administration is adopted. If necessary, preventive administration can also be adopted, that is, ouabain is injected intravenously at constant rate after administration of antiarrhythmic drugs, later the dose of ouabain after appearance of ventricular extrasystole, tachycardia, fibrillation and death are calculated

Question

Which drugs have relatively good therapeutic effects on arrhythmia induced by ouabain? Why?

Experiment 5. 8 The inhibitory effects of drugs on arrhythmia caused by ischemia – reperfusion in rat

Objective

Learn the method of causing arrhythmia by ligaturing the coronary artery of rat. Observe the characteristics of arrhythmia caused by ischemia – reperfusion injury. Understand the mechanism of the emergence of ischemia – reperfusion – induced arrhythmia.

Principle

After the coronary artery of the animal is ligated, due to ischemia of cardiac muscle and accumulation of metabolites, the ion permeability of myocardial cell membrane varies, resulting in inhomogeneity of electrophysiological characteristics of ischemic and non – ischemic area. The dysfunction leads to arrhythmia. Ventricular extrasystole, tachycardia and even fibrillation occur several minutes after the coronary artery is ligated, which is similar to the process of incidence of arrhythmia during earlier period of acute myocardial infarction of patients. The reperfusion of ischemic cardiac muscle can cause the generation of oxygen – derived free radicals and Ca^{2+} entry aggravate myocardial injury and electrophysiological disturbance. Therefore, severe ventricular arrhythmia such as ventricular tachycardia and fibrillation can occur more readily.

Materials

Animal required: 1 rat, 180 – 250g, male.

Apparatus required: electrocardiograph, breathing machine for small animals, tracheal cannula, surgical instruments, arteriolar clip, a short segment of silica gel tube (bore 2 – 3mm), syringe.

Reagent required: 0.5% mexiletine, 1.5% sodium pentobarbital, normal saline.

Methods

1. Take one rat and weigh it. Inject the animal intraperitonealy with 1.5% sodium pentobarbital (45mg/kg) to anesthetize it. Fix it on the back on the operation table.

2. Incise the skin along the midline on the neck. Insert the tracheal cannula and link the breathing machine to conduct positive – pressure artificial respiration (frequency: 50times/min; tidal volume: 1000ml/kg/min). Conduct external jugular vein intubation to prepare for administration.

3. Link the electrocardiograph and record the electrocardiogram of standard Lead Ⅱ.

4. Open the chest from intercostal area of the fourth and the fifth costal bone of left chest to expose the heart. Raise the heart out of the chest by squeezing the left thorax with left – hand or by a circular forceps. Put an atraumatic suture thread (5/0) around the coronary artery on the site 2 – 3mm from the root of the left coronary artery. Put the heart back into the thoracic cavity quickly. Draw the suture thrum out through a small segment of silica gel tube to block the coronary artery.

5. After 10 – 15 minutes for stabilization, strain the suture thread and fix it with an arteriolar clip. Be sure that the coronary artery is pressed with the silica gel tube and the blood flow is completely blocked. Observe and record the electrocardiogram. See whether obvious myocardial ischemia (indicated by the elevation of point J) and arrhythmia appear. Once the above phenomena appear, record the situation in time.

6. Loosen the ligature 10 minutes after ischemia to cause reperfusion of ischemic cardiac muscle. Observe and record the electrocardiogram at 0 – 30s, 1min, 1.5min, 2min, 3min, 4min and 5min. In general, arrhythmia including ventricular tachycardia and fibrillation is most likely to occur within 1 minute after reperfusion. If arrhythmia does not emerge within 5 minutes, arrhythmia seldom appears afterwards.

The whole experiment is divided into two groups. One is administrated with mexiletine (5mg/kg) before the blocking of coronary artery. The other is treated with equivalent saline as the control group.

Results

Calculate the incidence rate, duration time and mortality rate of ventricular tachycardia (VT) and ventricular fibrillation (VF) and the times of ventricular extrasystole within 30 seconds during reperfusion according to the results of electrocardiogram. The fraction of severe degree of ventricular arrhythmia can also be determined by rank scoring method. The division of rank can be referred as the following stands.

Grade 0: without ventricular arrhythmia

Grade 1: occasional ventricular extrasystole (<5%)

Grade 2: frequent extrasystole, bigeminy and trigeminy

Grade 3: short – term paroxysmal ventricular tachycardia

Grade 4: continuous ventricular tachycardia

Grade 5: ventricular flutter and fibrillation

Grade 6: death

As to the inter – group significance test of arrhythmia fraction, Ridit test or ranked test can be adopted while parameter statistics cannot be used. Finally evaluate the arrhythmic effects of drugs according to the settled results.

Notes

1. There should be a change caused by ischemia on the electrocardiogram after the blockade of coronary artery, otherwise it is possible that the coronary artery is not ligatured.

2. Reperfusion – induced arrhythmic model must be created successfully just once because arrhythmia is unlikely to occur after ischemia several times.

3. Temperature can affect the incidence rate of arrhythmia of animals obviously, so heat – preservative measures should be taken at relatively low temperature.

4. The pH value of blood also has notable influence on the incidence of arrhythmia, so the tidal volume should be adjusted strictly according to the weight.

5. The suture used for blocking the coronary artery should not be pulled either too loose or too tight as the coronary artery may be broken, which makes reperfusion impossible.

6. The ischemic time ahead of reperfusion affects the incidence rate of reperfusion – induced arrhythmia obviously. The incidence rate of ventricular fibrillation is highest when reperfusion is conducted 5 – 10 minutes after ischemia of anesthetized rat.

7. The site where the coronary artery is ligatured influences the incidence of arrhythmia evidently. It is required that the sites of ligation should be kept with one accord.

Evaluation

1. The method of causing arrhythmia by ligation of coronary artery – reperfusion in rat is one of the commonly used methods of studying anti – arrhythmic drugs. The result is reliable and has good ruggedness. The pathogenesis is almost similar to that of human beings.

2. The ligation of coronary artery demands quick action and accurate site, so the operator should be trained for a certain time.

3. The incidence rate of arrhythmia caused by early ischemia and reperfusion of anesthetized rat is lower than conscious rat, but the latter experiment is more difficult to perform.

Questions

1. The pathogenesis of arrhythmia caused by ischemia and reperfusion.

2. Compare the arrhythmia caused by early ischemia – reperfusion with the arrhythmia induced by the two – stage ligation of coronary artery.

3. The mechanism of antiarrhythmic action of mexiletine.

Experiment 5. 9　The effect of drug on effective refractory period and contractility of *in vitro* atrial muscle

Objective

Grasp the preparation of *in vitro* specimen of atria Guinea pig. Learn the method of determining myocardial effective refractory period by stimulation method and find the effects of drug on myocardial contractility by *in vitro* sample of atria.

Principle

The atria of Guinea pig can survive in vitro and keep systolic range for several hours under fixed electric stimulation if a certain temperature, pH value and nutrient solution with enough oxygen supply are provided. The effects of drugs on myocardial contractility can be indicated by alteration of the atrial systolic range before and after administration. Relatively short – interval coupled square wave stimulation is adopted. When the interval is less than effective refractory period, the cardiac muscle produces one systolic response, and when the interval is more than effective refractory period, the cardiac muscle produce two systolic responses. If the interval of two square waves can just cause two systolic responses, the interval time of the couple square wave is the effective refractory period of atria. The determination of effective refractory period can be used to find out the effects of antiarrhythmic drugs on myocardial electrophysiological characteristics and the mechanism.

Materials

Animal required: 1 Guinea pig, 300 – 400g, male or female.

Apparatus required: experimental devices for *in vitro* organs of warm – blood animals (ultrahermostatic water bath, bath tube, iron stand, oxygen tank), pharmaco – physiological electric stimulator, biological signal acquisition system, oscilloscope, tension transducer, stimulating electrode, surgical instruments, syringe, beaker, plate

Reagent required: Krebs – Henseleit (K – H) solution (components mmol/L: NaCl 118; KCl 14. 7; $CaCl_2$ 1. 25; $MgSO_4$ 1. 2; KH_2PO_4 1. 2; $NaHCO_3$ 25; glucose 11), 10^{-4} mol/L quinidine, 5×10^{-5} mol/L isoproterenol, 10^{-4} mol/L ace tylcholine.

Methods

1. Prepare the *in vitro* specimen of the atria of Guinea pig. Take a Guinea pig. Hit the animal on the head by a mallet to faint. Cut open the thoracic cavity quickly. Take the heart out and immediately place it into the K – H solution that is already warmed and aerated with mixed gas (95% O_2 and 5% CO_2). Now the heart contracts automatically to pump out the blood. Cut off the atria at atrioventricular junction. Change fresh K – H solution. Separate and fit the left atria. Fix its one end on the stimulating electrode and tie the other end with silk thread which is linked with tension transducer after placed in the bath tube. Adjust the resting load to 1. 0g or so. The volume of K – H solution in the bath tube is 20ml. Temperature is 30℃ ±0. 5℃. The mixed gas should be aerated unceasingly. Use electric stimulation to drive atrial systole (stimulating parameters: wave width 2 – 4ms; fre-

quency 1Hz; voltage 120% of threshold value). Commence the experiment after the specimen is stabilized for 30 minutes. Change the nutrient solution 2 – 3 times during stabilization.

Appendix The difference between left and right atrium of Guinea pig: The left atrium, appearing shell – like, is bigger and its edge is relatively neat; the right atrium, with one end pointed and fine, is smaller and its edge is irregular. The right one has higher autorhythmicity because it is connected with sinoatrial node.

2. Record the systolic range and effective refractory period before administration   Under the simulation of basic frequency, record a segment of normal atrial systolic curve on the physiological recorder. Stimulate the specimen by coupled square waves with different interval time (from 200ms on) and determine the effective refractory period before administration based on atrial systolic wave form as the index on the oscilloscope. Adopt stimulation to trigger scanning of the oscilloscope to synchronize the systolic wave. If the interval of coupled stimulation is less than effective refractory period, the systolic wave showed on the oscilloscope is the same as the one produced by single stimulation. If the stimulating interval exceeds effective refractory period, the systolic wave produced by atrium is higher than that caused by single stimulation or can be divided into two waves. The interval time of the coupled stimulation that can just make artial systolic wave alter is the effective refractory period. It is required that the effective refractory periods of successive two measurements should be constant on the whole. The interval time of two measurements is about 10 seconds.

3. 10 minutes after the drug is given, record atrial systolic range and effective refractory period after administration according to Step 2. 20 minutes later, record them again. Then wash off the drug with K – H solution.

The sequence of administration: 10^{-4} mol/L acetylcholine 0. 2ml, 5×10^{-5}mol/L isoproterenol 0. 2ml, 10^{-4}mol/L qunidine 0. 2ml.

4. Wash the specimen 3 – 5 times with K – H solution. After the systolic curve and effective refractory period return on the whole, administer another test drug. Repeat the Step 3. Record the systolic range and effective refractory period.

Results

Clip and paste the curve of systolic range. Convert systolic range into tension (g or mg) and effective refractory period (ms) based on calibration value and record them according to corresponding drug and time. Analyze and discuss the results. In practice, if the systolic tensions of specimen before administration differ greatly, the tension before administration can be deemed as 100%, and inter – group statistical test is done after the tension is converted into percent of that before administration.

Notes

1. The preparation of the specimen should be quick enough to be finished within 2 – 3 minutes.

2. The temperature should be controlled at 30℃ ±1℃ because too high temperature can cause natural attenuation of systolic range and too low one leads to low excitability.

3. The reactivity of the specimen is recommended to examine to prevent false results caused by bad reactivity if the experimental time is more than four hours or several drugs are used.

4. Oscilloscope or bi – channel physiological recorder, but except equilibrium recorder because

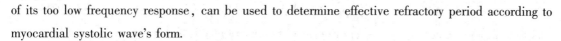

of its too low frequency response, can be used to determine effective refractory period according to myocardial systolic wave's form.

5. The volume of drug solution added into the bath tube should be less than 5 percent of that of the nutrient solution in it so that the influence of the added drug solution can be neglected.

Evaluation

1. The preparation of in-vitro atrial specimen of Guinea pig is easy to be understood. The experimental results are stable. After single systolic wave is recorded by quickly moved paper, the myocardial systolic and diastolic speed can be analyzed (the concrete method referred to experiment of *in vitro* papillary muscle). Besides, the *in vitro* right atrium of Guinea pig can contract and beat spontaneously at about 37 ℃ and the frequency can keep stable for over one hour, so it can be used to observe the direct effects of drugs on sinus heart rate.

2. Because the specimen is atrial muscle possessing irregular direction of muscle fiber, its value is not as important as *in vitro* papillary muscle as to evaluation of the effects of drugs on atrial muscle. The latter one can be used to record myocardial systole and action potential simultaneously. However, the experimental techniques and conditions are to be followed more strictly.

Questions

1. Describe the necessary basic conditions for maintenance of continuous beat of in – vitro atria of warm – blood animals.

2. How to decide effective refractory period if action potential is selected as index?

3. The major mechanism of alteration of effective refractory period of acetylcholine, isoproterenol and quinidine.

Ⅲ. Experiments of anti – myocardial ischemic drugs

The main action mechanisms of anti – myocardial ischemic drugs are: ① to protect ischemic cardiac muscle to reduce the area of myocardial infarction and injured degree. ② to improve coronary circulation. ③ to regulate myocardial metabolism. ④ to regulate cardiac function and hemodynamics and affect hemorheological characteristics such as blood coagulation, platelet aggregation and blood lipid metabolism. Based on these action pathways, various corresponding experimental methods arise. In recent years anti – myocardial ischemic drugs have been developed rapidly in theory, research of new drugs and experimental methods. The resupplying of blood after myocardial ischemia or infarction for some time usually leads to reperfusion – induced injury which aggravates original injury of myocardial ischemia or infarction. The model of injury caused by myocardial ischemia and infarction can be created on different levels including ligation of *in vivo* coronary artery, anoxia of *in vitro* heart or ligation of *in vitro* coronary artery and anoxia of *in vitro* myocardial cell culture.

Myocardial ischemia and infarction induced by the ligation of coronary artery can cause morphological, enzymological and electrophysiological alteration. The direct and reliable method of examining the area of myocardial ischemia and infarction is histological section with light microscope. The reliability of the results concluded by enzymological and electrophysiological methods can only be ascertained after they are compared with those concluded by morphological method. The coronary blood flow is affected by contractive extent of coronary blood vessels, blood pressure and myocardial contractility, so the alteration of blood pressure and myocardial contractility should be noticed when coronary blood flow is determined. In addition, during the course of determination of coronary blood flow, the alteration of partial pressure disparity of oxygen of artery and vein is recommended to determine in order to know whether the increase of myocardial oxygen consumption has caused coronary dilation. The traditional method of screening anti – myocardial ischemic drugs by animal experiment of anoxia tolerance has been superseded due to the poor specificity.

Experiment 5.10 Myocardial infarction caused by ligaturing coronary artery of rabbit

Objective

Learn the method of creating myocardial infarction model by ligating coronary artery. Comprehend the method of estimating the area of myocardial ischemia and infarction and the process of the development of myocardial infarction.

Principle

Coronary heart disease is the common cause of myocardial infarction in clinical practice. Myocardial ischemia or infarction arises when coronary atherosclerosis causes constriction or occlusion of artery. The ligation of coronary artery can cause long – term ischemia of cardiac muscle, resulting in myocardial infarction. The alteration of hemodynamics and myocardial metabolism and the appearance of arrhythmia caused by ligaturing the coronary artery are similar to the situation of myocardial infarction induced by coronary heart disease. The infarction develops quickly and the ischemic area is almost fixed, so indices including tissue section and staining, measurement of ST stage of electrocardiogram and serum enzymological examination can be conducted in order to confirm the area of myocardial ischemia or infraction and injured extent. The determination of the effects of drugs on these indices can be used to evaluate the myocardial ischemia – resistant and infarcted area – reduced actions of drugs. The rabbit's pericardium on the precordial region can be separated from pleura easily, so coronary artery can be ligatured after pericardium is cut without damaging pleura.

Materials

Animal required: 1 rabbit, 2 – 3kg, male or female.

Apparatus required: operation table for rabbit, electrocardiograph, surgical instruments, small chest opener.

Reagent required: 3% sodium pentobarbital, 2% tincture of iodine, 75% alcohol, gentian violet, gentamicin injection.

Methods

1. Take one rabbit and weigh it. Fix it on the back. Inject the animal with 3% sodium pentobarbital (30 – 45mg/kg) intravenously to anesthetize it. Remove the hair before operation. Sterilize the location by 2% tincture of iodine. Then use 75% alcohol for deiodination.

2. Label and measure electrocardiogram   Mark nine points by gentian violet in the area of 1cm up and down away from the center, the fourth intercostal region 1cm beside left border of the breast bone. Record the electrocardiogram of the nine points on the chest before ligation.

3. Cut the skin along the sternal midline to expose the sternum. Snip the costal cartilages from the first to the third along the left border of the sternum. Support the incision of the thoracic cavity gently by a small chest opener. Then the pericardium and the beating heart can be seen clearly

4. Draw up the pericardium and cut the anterior part of the pericardium by eye scissors. Be careful not to break the pericardium. Pull the left auricle gently by hemostatic forceps. Insert thread to ligate the site about 1cm down from the root of the anterior descending branch of the coronary artery by a needle holder with an atraumatic suture needle. In order to reduce collateral circulation and increase the area of myocardial infarction, ligate the coronary artery again about 0.5cm down from the ligature.

5. Close the chest and record the electrocardiogram of the nine labeling points on the chest again. Observe the alteration of ST stage. Inject getamicin 40,000 units to prevent infection.

6. One day later, record the electrocardiogram of the labeling points again. Kill the animal and take out the heart to conduct NBT staining to estimate the infarcted area.

7. If it is required to determine the alteration of serum creatine kinase or its isoenzyme M, take the serum to determine enzyme activity respectively before operation and after infarction.

Results

1. Label and measure ST stage and Q wave of the electrocardiogram. Generally, ST stage of the electrocardiogram with multi – lead labeling on the chest rises obviously two hours after ligation, reaches the peak one day later, ascends continuously within three days and declines spontaneously three days later. The alteration of ST stage of any lead on the chest cannot indicate the area of myocardial infarction quantitatively, but it is generally considered that the total elevation mV ($\sum ST$) of ST stage of multi – lead on the chest can reflect the area of myocardial infarction quantitatively. The lead number of abnormal elevation or declination of ST stage (NST) and the average mV value of displacement of ST stage of each lead (that is, $\sum ST$ divided by all the labeling points) can also be reference for the area of myocardial infarction. Besides, the total mV of the depth of Q wave, the lead number of $\sum Q$ and Q wave emergence (NQ), is also an index reflecting the area of myocardial infarction.

2. Dye the gross specimen by nitro – blue tetrazolium (NBT) staining (referred to NBT staining method) to measure the area of myocardial infarction.

3. Determine CK or LDH. Compare the situation before ligation and 1 hour, 3 hours, 6 hours and 24 hours after ligation (referred to related books).

Notes

1. Be careful to keep the pleura intact when opening the chest and ligaturing the coronary artery in order not to use artificial respiration.

2. The costal cartilage should be snipped close to the border of the sternum to avoid the internal mammary artery injury to cause massive hemorrhage.

3. The anterior descending branch of the coronary artery of rabbit should be ligatured two times

tightly to reduce collateral circulation in order to form relatively large area of infarction that makes observation easy.

4. Notice that the area of myocardial infarction caused by this method is relatively stable within three days and tends to improve spontaneously after three days.

5. The rabbit should be discarded if its anterior descending branch varies greatly with the length less than 1.5cm because the infarcted area is too small after its anterior descending branch is ligatured.

Evaluation

1. The method of ligaturing the coronary artery without breaking the pleura is easy and convenient. Moreover, the success rate is relatively high because rabbit's tolerance is higher than dog's and fatal arrhythmia seldom occurs after the ligation of the coronary artery in rabbit.

2. The area dominated by the anterior descending branch of the coronary artery of rabbit is relatively small, so double ligation should be adopted. Otherwise the infarcted area is too small, which is difficult to evaluate drug effects. The double ligation can block collateral circulation and enhance the infarcted area that is conducive to observation of drug effects, but the mortality rate of the animal increases as well.

3. Rabbit, a kind of animal with a temperate nature, can be used not only to estimate the infarcted area by gross specimen staining or tissue section and enzymological examination but also conduct electrocardiogram labeling and measurement. In addition, rabbit is cheaper than dog.

Questions

1. Describe the sequence of the emergence of the following: myocardial infarction, alteration of electrocardiogram and change of serum enzyme activity. Why?

2. Why does too small infarcted area make difficult evaluation of drug effects?

3. Describe the alteration of myocardial creatine kinase and lactate dehydrogenase in the infarcted area determined after myocardial infarction.

Experiment 5.11   The effects of drugs on myocardial contractility and coronary blood flow of *in vitro* heart of Guinea pig

Objective

Learn the preparation method of Langendorff's heart. Observe the effects of drugs on contractility and coronary blood flow of *in vitro* heart. Understand how to evaluate the effects of drugs on coronary blood flow of *in vitro* heart.

Principle

The heart of warm – blooded animals can contract automatically and survive for a certain time when oxygen supply, heart preservation, a certain ion concentration and energy – supplying substances are provided. The direct effect of drug on coronary blood flow, myocardial contractility and heart rate can be observed through integral *in vitro* heart.

Materials

Animal required: 1 Guinea pig, 350 – 450g, sexuality not limited.

Apparatus required: constant temperature and voltage equipment for *ex vivo* perfusion (perfusion bottle, coil, ultra – thermostatic water bath), thermos cannula for heart, aortic cannlation, oxygen – supplying equipment, crown block, clip for the heart of frog, tension transducer, biological signal acquisition system, surgical instruments, small graduated cylinder, beaker, syringe.

Reagent required: 1% heparin, 10^{-5} mol/L adrenaline, 10^{-5} mol/L isoproterenol, 2.5% aminophylline, 3% sodium pentobarbital, Krebs – Henselit's solution.

Methods

1. Weigh the Guinea pig. Inject the animal intraperitonealy with 3% sodium pentobarbital (30 – 45mg/kg, 1 – 1.5ml) to anesthetize it. Inject 1% heparin (10mg/kg) from external jugular vein for anticoagulation. 1 minute later, open the chest and take out the heart. Place it into the cold K – H solution aerated with mixed gas before and squeeze blood out gently.

2. Insert the aortic cannulation into the aorta and fasten it with silk tread for fixation in the nutrient solution.

3. Connect the aortic cannulation linked with the heart to the outlet of the perfusion equipment. Perfuse the heart with K – H solution (aerated with mixed gas) at 37℃ with 50 – 60cm water pressures. Expel bubbles in the perfusion equipment before handling. Be sure not to allow bubbles enter the heart.

4. Clamp the apex of the heart by a clip and link it with the tension transducer by silk thread that changes the direction of the heart through a crown block. Record the systolic range on the biological signal acquisition system. Enclose the heart with the thermos cannula for heat preservation. Collect the effluent solution by putting a cylinder under the heart and determine the coronary blood flow.

5. After the systole becomes stable, determine the coronary blood flow within 3min twice consecutively. Calculate the average blood flow every minute as the reference value before administration and record myocardial systolic range and heart rate if the values are close to each other.

6. Inject the drug into the perfusion solution from above the aortic cannulation. Then record the coronary blood flow, myocardial systolic range and heart rate 1, 3, 5 and 10min after administration. Render the next drug after the coronary blood flow and systolic range return to base.

The sequence of administration: 10^{-5} mol/L adrenaline 0.5ml, 10^{-5} mol/L isoproterenol 0.5ml, 2.5% aminophylline 0.5ml.

Results

Calculate myocardial contractility and heart rate based on the cardiac systolic curve on the biological signal acquisition system. Calculate the absolute alterative value and relative alterative value (percentage) of coronary blood flow, myocardial contractility and heart rate after administration. List to evaluate and analyze the effects of drugs .

Notes

1. The nutrient solution is required to prepare fresh. Mixed gas should be aerated into K – H solution while pure oxygen can be directly inflated into R – L solution.

2. The operation including isolation of the heart and intubation must be quick. The period from extraction of the heart to commence of perfusion should be less than 2 minutes to avoid the cardiac

muscles injury due to myocardial ischemia and anoxia.

3. The intubation should be conducted inside the liquid. Do not allow air enter coronary artery to prevent embolism. The injection of heparin aims to prevent coagulation inside the microvessels. The step can be skipped if the operation is rapid.

4. When *in vitro* heart is prepared, the aortic cannulation should not be inserted too deeply to prevent blockage of coronary outlet. Be careful not to injure sinoatrial node.

Evaluation

1. The method is a classical one. The equipment requirement is simple and the operation is easy. The cardiac systolic function, heart rate and coronary blood flow can be observed and the biochemical indices in tissues and perfusion solution can be determined at the same time. Some modification of the method can cause *in vitro* arrhythmic model and myocardial ischemic model, used to observe antiarrhythmic or anti – myocardial ischemic effects of drugs.

2. The coronary blood flow is affected not only by systolic and diastolic extent of coronary vessels but by myocardial contractility as well, so the alteration of myocardial contractility should be considered when the effects of drugs on coronary blood flow are analyzed. If necessary, electric stimulation can be adopted to induce ventricular fibrillation to eliminate the influence of myocardial systole.

3. The main energetic source of *in vivo* heart is the fatty acid in the blood, while the energetic source of *in vitro* heart is the glucose in the perfusion solution. Therefore, the maintenance time of systole of *in vitro* heart would not be too long. The operation must be finished in a relatively short time.

4. Langendorff's *in vitro* heart excludes the effects of neuro – humoral regulation, but cannot control preload, after – load and heart rate at the same time. The left ventricular filling pressure (preload) and aortic column height (after – load) of *in vitro* heart can be kept constant, and the heart rate can also be controlled by electrical pacing equipment. Therefore, the three factors can be controlled at the same time according to the requirement to observe the effects of drugs on myocardial contractility, or any two factors are controlled to observe the relationship between myocardial contractility and the rest one.

Questions

1. Describe the difference between the experimental conditions of warm – blooded animal's heart and that of the frog's heart (cold – blooded animal's heart).

2. Judge whether the experiment is a satisfactory method of evaluating the effects of drugs on myocardial contractility or not. Why?

Experiment 5. 12   Measurement of area of myocardial infarction by nitro – blue tetrazolium staining

Two morphological methods are used to measure myocardial ischemic area, one is a histological method and the other is gross specimen staining. As far as quantitative result is concerned, histological section method is accurate and reliable but demands a series of steps that costs time and ener-

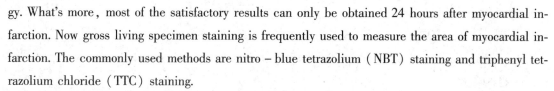

gy. What's more, most of the satisfactory results can only be obtained 24 hours after myocardial infarction. Now gross living specimen staining is frequently used to measure the area of myocardial infarction. The commonly used methods are nitro – blue tetrazolium (NBT) staining and triphenyl tetrazolium chloride (TTC) staining.

Objective

Study NBT staining used to measure the area of myocardial infarction.

Principle

The normal myocardial cells contain dehydrogenase that can reduce colorless dye NBT oxide to blue reductive NBT when NADH exists. The living cardiac muscle can be stained from the principle. Some time after myocardial infarction, dehydrogenase in the cells is released and lost due to cell injury, so NBT can no longer be reduced and stained. That is, the cardiac muscle of infarction cannot be stained. Therefore, the infarcted region that cannot be stained and normal cardiac muscle (that can be stained) can be separated. The area of myocardial infarction can be estimated by weighing method or stereometry of area of plane section.

Materials

Animal required: infarcted heart of rabbit (referred to the method of inducing myocardial infarction by ligaturing the common coronary artery).

Apparatus required: thermostatic water bath box, beaker, plate, surgical scissors

Reagent required: normal saline, 0.5% NBT.

Appendix

Preparation of 0.5% NBT solution: Weigh and take 250mg NBT. Add 80ml potassium phosphate buffer (pH = 7.4). Shake up the solution and then add distilled water to 500ml. 0.5% NBT solution is obtained.

Preparation of potassium phosphate buffer: Weigh and take 4.08g monopotassium phosphate. Add 237ml 0.1% mol/L NaOH solution. After dissolution add distilled water to 600ml.

Methods

1. Take out the heart after the experiment. wash it with saline to eliminate bloodiness. Remove non – myocardial tissues involving blood vessels and fat. Absorb moisture by bibulous paper and weigh the wet weight of the whole heart.

2. Cut off the atria along the coronary sulcus and spare the ventricles to weigh them. Slice the ventricles of the rabbit into parallel myocardial pieces with the thickness of 0.3 – 0.5cm along the coronary sulcus from apex of the heart to floor of the heart and wash them cleanly with saline.

3. Put the myocardial slices into 0.5% NBT solution and incubate them at 37℃ to stain for 10 – 15min. Shake or stir the staining solution some time during the process of staining to let the dye contact cardiac muscle properly.

4. Wash off the extra dye with water immediately after staining. The infarcted region is not stained and the non – infarcted region is stained blue.

5. Cut off the non – infarcted cardiac muscle that is stained of every myocardial slice. Weigh the infarcted cardiac muscle that is not stained.

Results

Calculate the infracted area according to the following formula:

Percentage of area of ventricular infarction = weight of infarcted cardiac muscle/weight of ventricles × 100% ;

Percentage of area of total cardiac infarction = weight of infarcted cardiac muscle/weight of the whole heart × 100% ;

Percentage of area of the left ventricular infarction = weight of infarcted cardiac muscle/weight of the left ventricle × 100%.

Notes

1. Myocardial staining should be conducted immediately after the heart is taken out or after freezing the cardiac muscle, otherwise dehydrogenase of non - infacted region would be released continuously, which affects the staining results. The frozen heart can be stained without complete thaw.

2. The dye NBT solution should be prepared with phosphate buffer just before use and the pH value should be adjusted to 7. 4 – 7. 8.

3. The myocardial slices should be covered by the dye solution. Frequent shake is necessary to allow the dye contact cardiac muscles sufficiently. The staining time should not be too long or too short to avoid the slices get stained too heavy or too light which affects observation.

4. The myocardial slices should not be too thick.

Evaluation

1. The method of measuring the area of myocardial infarction by living staining is a convenient, quick, easily operated, accurate and useful method suitable for the animals bearing relatively large heart such as dog, cat, pig and rabbit. For the heart of rat and such relatively small animals, the method's error is relatively big, but the precision can be enhanced by slice stereometry.

2. 3 – 6 hours after coronary artery is ligated, while only lost glycogen can be and myocardial necrosis cannot be detected by microscopic or electron microscopic examination, NBT staining can be used to measure the infracted area. The infarction can be detected earlier by the method than by microscopic examination, so it has become a generally accepted quantitative method of measuring the area of myocardial infarction internationally. However, it also has disadvantages: the stained cells with residual dehydrogenase are not always living cells, so the infarcted area estimated by this method is lower than histological exam

Questions

1. Describe the experimental factors affecting the measurement of the area of myocardial infarction by nitro - blue tetrazolium (NBT) staining. How to control the effects?

2. Which biochemical indices can be determined when NBT staining is used to measure the area of myocardial infarction?

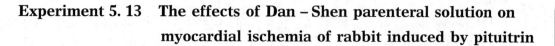

Experiment 5.13 The effects of Dan – Shen parenteral solution on myocardial ischemia of rabbit induced by pituitrin

Objective

1. Study the method of inducing myocardial ischemia by pituitrin.

2. Observe the anti – myocardial ischemic effects of drugs.

Principle

Pituitrin can cause contraction of all the blood vessels including coronary vessels. The effect of puituitrin is ultilized here. Acute myocardial ischemia can be induced on animals after intravenous injection of puituitrin. Based on the alteration of ST stage and T wave in electrocardiogram, the antagonistic effects are observed after administration. All the medicine opposing the vasoconstrictive effects of pituitrin can improve the electrocardiogram of ischemia.

Materials

Animal required: 1 rabbit.

Apparatus required: electronic scale, rabbit operation table, thread, syringes (10ml, 1ml), electrocardiograph, stop watch.

Reagent required: pituitrin injection, den – shen injection, 3% sodium pentobarbital, normal saline.

Methods

Select two rabbits with normal electrocardiogram. Inject the animal intravenously with 3% sodium pentobarbital (24mg/kg) to anesthetize it. Fix it on the operation table. Record the electrocardiogram of lead Ⅱ. (1mV = 10, paper speed = 50mm/s) Inject the rabbit intravenously within 30 seconds with 2.5U/kg pituitrin that is diluted to 3ml by saline. After the injection, record immediately the alteration of the electrocardiogram 30s, 1min, 3min, 5min, 7min, 10min, 15min and 30min later. After the electrocardiogram reverts to normal, inject the animal intravenously with 2ml/kg dan – shen parenteral solution. 5 minutes later, administrate equivalent pituitrin again. Observe the alteration of the electrocardiogram during the above time. The control group is administrated with equivalent amount of saline and the experiment method is as mentioned above. Collect the results in the whole laboratory to compare them.

Results

Fill the blanks in Table 5 – 2.

Table 5 – 2 The antagonistic effects of dan – shen injection on myocardial ischemia of rabbit induced by pituitrin

Group	R – R interval (s)		T wave (mV)		ST stage (mV)		Heart – rate (times/min)	
	before	after	before	after	before	after	before	after
normal saline								
dan – shen								

Notes

1. The animal should be discarded if ischemic alteration of the electrocardiogram (especially ST stage and T wave should be noticed) of the rabbit does not emerge after the first administration of pituitrin.

2. The dosage of pituitrin can be adjusted according to its potency.

3. Ischemic alteration of the electrocardiogram mostly takes places within 15 minutes after the injection of pituitrin.

4. The weight of the rabbit used in the experiment should be about 2kg. Sexuality is not limited, but the female should not be a pregnant one.

5. The rabbit can be replaced by the rat of 200g or so.

6. The data of the time period should be compared and marked on the table, according to the abnormality of the electrocardiogram and the resistant effects of the drug after pituitrin is administered.

7. The animal can revert to normal condition quickly if the dosage of pituitrin is not applied much, so several experiments can be conducted repeatedly on one animal.

Evaluation

1. The method is a frequently used acute experimental method of studying anti – myocardial ischemic drugs. It is convenient and easy to operate. Only electrocardiograph and chronic injection equipment are needed.

2. ST stage alters within 1. 5 minutes, rises within 45 seconds and reverts to normal within 25 – 60 minutes after injection of pituitrin.

Questions

1. Describe the principle and advantages of the method of reproducing pathologic model of myocardial ischemia of animals by pituitrin.

2. Explain the anti – myocardial ischemic action and action mechanism of dan – shen and the relationship between the effective components and its effects.

Experiment 5. 14　Measurement of blood fat

The pathogenesis of atherosclerosis has close relationship to metabolic disturbance of lipid. To measure blood fat level and create pathologic model of atherosclerosis is an important way to screen anti – atherosclerotic drugs.

Objective

Study the measurement of serum total cholesterol and triglyceride. Understand the relationship between atherosclerosis and hyperlipemia.

A. Quantitative Measurement of Total Cholesterol in Serum – iron sesquichloride – acetic acid – sulphuric acid coloring

The cholesterol (CH) in serum is divided into free cholesterol (FC) 25% – 30% and cholesterol ester (CE) 70% – 75%. The generic name of the two parts is total cholesterol (TC).

Principle

Isopropanol is used to extract cholesterol in serum and precipitate proteins, and at the same time the adsorbing agent is added to eliminate phospholipids, bilirubin and other substances affecting coloring reaction of cholesterol.

The content of cholesterol can be obtained by coloring matching of the stable purple red substance produced by reaction of cholesterol, oil of vitriol and trivalent ferric ion with the standard solution treated by the same steps.

Materials

Apparatus required: 1 spectrophotometer 721, desk centrifuge, oscillator, test tubes (coarse orifice), pipette.

Reagents:

1. isopropanol (AR).

2. glacial acetic acid (AR).

3. absorbing agent (aluminium oxide)   Use neutral aluminium oxide (Grade I) for chromatography. Use distilled water four times of the volume to wash for 8 – 9 times until fine granules difficult to sink are completely eliminated. After filtration, dry and activate it in the baker at 110℃ for 10 – 18 hours. Then seal it up or preserve it in a desiccator.

4. 0.1% iron sesquichloride solution (dissolved in glacial acetic acid) (containing $6H_2O$, AR)   The solution can be preserved for a long time.

5. coloring reagent   Mix 0.1% iron sesquichloride solution (dissolved in glacial acetic acid) and oil of vitriol (GR or AR) according to the proportion 1:1. The solution can be kept stable for about two months at room temperature.

6. standard solution of cholesterol (2.0mg/ml)   Weigh 200mg dry and pure cholesterol precisely and dissolve it in isopropanol with the volume 100ml. Store the solution in a refrigerator to stand by.

Methods

1. Take 0.1ml serum and put it into the coarse – orifice test tube having a stopper. Add 2.5ml isopropanol (poured into the tube to granulate serum) and 0.4g aluminium oxide. Put the stopper in and shake up the solution (placed in the water bath at 60℃ for 1 – 2 minutes). Put the solution on the oscillator to oscillate for 10 minutes and then centrifugate it for 10 minutes at 200r/min. In the standard tube serum is replaced by standard solution of cholesterol and the operation steps are the same as the tube for determination.

2. Take three test tubes and operate according the following list.

Added substance (ml)	Blank	Standard	Determination
Supernatant extractive of solution of serum	—	—	1.0
Supernatant extractive of solution of standard solution	—	1.0	—
Isopropanol	1.0	—	—
Put into water bath at 60 ℃ for 5 minutes.			
Coloring agent (added along tube wall in water bath)	3.0	3.0	3.0
Warm it at 60 ℃ for 15 minutes after the solution is mixed up.			

3. Compare the color by spectrophotometer 721 after cooling at room temperature. colorimetric

cylinder：1cm， wave length：530nm.

Results

Calculate according to the following formula：

Total cholesterol in serum （mmol/L） = absorbency of determination tube/ absorbency of standard tube × 200.

Notes

1. Meanwhile If triglyceride is required to be determined, the same extractive solution of isopropanol can be used and cholesterol and triglyceride can be mixed together in the standard solution.

2. The measuring range of total cholesterol in serum can reach 13mmol/L （500mg/dl）. The serum volume should cut down by half if TC content exceeds the value.

Evaluation

The coloring method is stable and has good reproducibility. The recovering rate is close to 100%. The result may be a little lower than other methods because the absorbing agent eliminates the non – specific reactive substances.

B. Quantitative Mensuration of Serum Triglyceride – acetylpropanon coloring

Principle

First of all, isopropanol is used to extract serum lipids and precipitate serum proteins. Then the absorbing agent is used to remove phosphate lipid, glycerine, glucose, bilirubin and such interferential substances. Triglyceride is saponified to glycerine by potassium hydroxide solution. Afterwards, glycerine is oxidized to formaldehyde by sodium sub – periodate. Formaldehyde, acetylpropanone and ammonia can condense into yellow 3, 5 – diacetyl – 1, 4 – dihydrodimethylpyridine （Hantzsch condensation）. Compare the color with the standard solution disposed with the same steps and calculate the content of triglyceride in serum. The reaction equation is as follows：

Formaldehyde + acetylpropanone + ammonia $\longrightarrow$ 3, 5 – diacetyl – 1, 4 – dihydrodimethylpyridine

Materials

1. Equipment   the same as the part of mensuration of cholesterol.

2. Test Solution

1） isopropanol （AR）.

2） absorbing agent （referred to mensuration of cholesterol）.

3） saponifier：Take 10g analytically pure potassium hydroxide and dissolve it in 75ml distilled water. Add 25ml isopropanol. Preserve it in a brown bottle.

4） sodium sub – periodate reagent：Take 7.7g anhydrous acetic acid and dissolve it in 70ml distilled water. Add 6ml glacial acetic acid and 65mg sodium sub – periodate. Again add 100ml distilled water. Put it into a brown bottle at room temperature. It can be preserved for at least six months.

5） acetylpropanon reagent：Extract 0.4 ml acetylpropanon accurately and dilute it to 100ml by isopropanol. Put it into a brown bottle. It can be preserved for six months at room temperature.

6） standard stored solution：Weigh 1.000g triglyceride precisely and dissolve it in isopro-

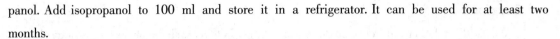

panol. Add isopropanol to 100 ml and store it in a refrigerator. It can be used for at least two months.

7) standard applied solution (100ml/ 200mg)：Extract 2. 0ml stored solution and put it into a volumetric flask of 10ml. Add isoparopanol to the mark. Keep it in a refrigerator. The solution must be prepared every week.

Methods

1. Take three centrifugate tube bearing stppers and operate according to the following list.

Steps	Reagent (ml)	Blank	Standard	Determination
	serum	—	—	0. 1
Extraction	standard applied solution	—	0. 1	—
	distilled water	0. 1	—	—
	isopropanol	3. 0	3. 0	3. 0
	aluminium oxide	0. 4	0. 4	0. 4
Oscillate the solution sufficiently for 10 minutes, centrifugate it for 5 minutes and extract the supernatant clear solution				
Saponification	Supernatant solution	2. 0	2. 0	2. 0
	Saponifier	0. 6	0. 6	0. 6
Shake up the solution and place it in the water bath at 65℃ for five minutes.				
Oxidation	Sodium sub – periodate	1. 5	1. 5	1. 5
Oscillate the solution sufficiently.				
Coloring	Acetylpropanone reagent	1. 5	1. 5	1. 5

2. Shake up each tube and put them into water bath at 65 – 70℃ for at least 15 minutes. Take them out to cool them at room temperature. Compare color with the wave length 420nm. Adjust the nil by the blank tube and record the absorbency of each tube.

Results

Calculate according to the following formula：Total triglyceride (TG) in serum (mmol/L) = absorbency of determination tube/absorbency of standard tube × 200.

Notes

1. Jaundice and hemolytic specimen almost have no effect on the experiment. Anticoagulant heparin, Na_2 – EDTA and sodium oxalate do not disturb the experiment, either. But citric acid can lead to a little lower result at normal concentration.

2. As to the solution with absorbency more than 7. 0, it should be diluted by blank solution or the serum volume is reduced.

Evaluation

In the experiment the color is stable and shows no change within one hour after coloring. The enzyme reagent method developed in the recent years of determining cholesterol and triglyceride in serum, which displays more advantages such as convenience, trace and precision, is the inexorable trend of development, although specific enzyme test kit is needed.

Questions

1. What's the relationship between the several lipid proteins and the diseases, atherosclerosis and coronary heart disease?

2. How to control the affecting factors during the process of determination of total cholesterol and triglyceride in serum?

IV. Experiments of antihypertensives

The preclinical pharmacodynamic research of antihypertensives include three phases:

To observe the acute hypotensive effects on anaesthetized animals, such as cats, rats and dogs etc. To observe the acute hypotensive effects on hypertensive animals.

To conduct the chronic experimental treatment in hypertensive animals. The hypertensive models involve high renin hypertension rats, spontaneously hypertensive rat strain, DOCA – salt hypertensive rat etc.

To study the hypotensive mechanisms of the potent drugs.

It will take a long time to estimate the hypotensive efficacy of drugs, which mainly depends on experimental therapy. The test drug generally will be administered consecutively daily for 1 – 2 weeks following the development of hypertensive model. The trial drug will be invalid as if it has no significant hypotensive efficacy for 1 – month therapy. The blood pressure will be measured until it returned to the level before administration. Because antihypertensives need to be administered for a long time, they are required to be given orally.

There are two methods to survey the blood pressure, one is direct manometry and the other is indirect one. The direct method is also called intubation. The procedures are performed as follows: Insert the heart catheters or polyethylene catheter into artery to survey the blood pressure or measure the blood pressure with arteriopuncture. The encheiresis is performed on general or local anesthetized animals, which often hurts the animals so the method is only for acute trial. The blood pressure of the catheter is transmitted to the baroceptor through liquid, the signals of blood pressure can be received accurately, and the change of the blood pressure also can be acquired by receiver pressure.

If we want to conduct the chronic experiment, the animals need to be implanted with a chronic use and high quality catheters. The chronic catheters should be filled with heparinized saline every day to keep the catheters unobstructed.

When we study the mechanisms responsible for the physiopathologic development of experimental hypertension, we always adopt the indirect method which is non – traumatic and reproducible. The indirect manometry refers to: press an artery by aerated compression, interrupt the blood stream and reduce pressure. The volumetric change or pulsation occurrence is the index of the blood pressure. The methods involve plethysmography in rats, sphygmography in rats, paw manometry in rats, carotid artery vagina manometry in dogs, and ear manometry in rabbits.

In 1934, Goldblatt confirmed that constricting the renal artery in dogs can produce continuous hypertension and carried out a new stage of experimental hypertensive research. Experimental hypertensive animal models such as neurogenic hypertension, renal hypertension, endocrine hypertension and alimentary hypertension, are always established via surgery and disposed by drugs or other factors. Although there are some differences between these models and human hypertension, they are still very important ways to screen the effective antihypertensives and research the pathological mechanisms of hypertension. Monkey and cats are difficult to gain, and the blood pressure can't be raised to high level and is unstable in rabbits, so dogs and rats are the common animals for antihypertensive experiments.

Smirk reported a genetically spontaneously hypertensive rat strain in 1955, then many hereditary hypertensive rat strains are developed in Japan and USA, they are spontaneously hypertensive rat strain (SHR), SHR – stroke proce strain (SHRSP), Dahl salt – sensitive strain (DS), Milan hypertensive strain (MHS) etc. The SHR and SHRPS are the most extensive models in the world, whose features are as follows:

1. SHR is similar to human hypertension and is the ideal animal model for studying hypertensive pathological mechanism and screening the antihypretensives. The similarities between SHR and human hypertension are:

1) Genetic factor dominate over others. Ion transportation of cytomembrane of erythrocytes is normal.

2) There is no obvious organic alteration at early stage of hypertension.

3) They have similar course. The blood pressure is increased with the age, and reaches the maximal level at 6 – month old in rats.

4) They have similar alterations in hemodynamics, the vascular peripheral resistance increased obviously.

5) With the development of hypertension, the angiocardiopathies will occur, such as cardiac, cerebral and renal complication. Antihypertensives or other remedies can prevent and abate the development and occurrence of complications.

6) Some experimental factors such as stress or excessive salt – uptake can accelerate the development of hypertension and aggregate the complication.

2. SHR is different from the human hypertension as follows:

1) SHR is acquired from genetic selective reproduction, and it is different from the occurence of hypertension.

2) There are some abnormalities in thyroid and immunologic function.

For the above reasons, we should be careful in deriving the research from SHR to human hypertension. But SHR and SHRPS are the best animal models for studying the hypertensive mechanisms and seeking the prophylactico – therapeutic measures.

Antihypertensives can affect the central nervous systems, autonomic ganglia, sympathetic nerve terminals, sympathetic nerve transmitter's receptors, vascular smooth muscle, humoral regulation factors and blood volume etc. Most ganglion blockers that historically are used in the treatment of hypertension are no longer available in clinic, because of the intolerable adverse effects. The drugs that act on sympathetic nerve terminals are used less and less. The antihypertensives that act on vascular smooth muscle, sympathetic nerve transmitter receptors and humoral regulation factors are the major research orientations, such as calcium channel blockers, α – receptor blockers, β – receptor antagonists, angiotensin – converting enzyme inhibitors etc. We designed different experiments according to different mechanisms of antihypertensives. Conversely, we can infer the mechanism of action by the corresponding experiments.

Experiment 5. 15　Analysis of the mechanism of hypotensive action of hexamethonium

Objective

Study the methods of researching the acute hypotensive effect of antihypertensives and analyze the mechanisms of hypotensive action of hexamethonium.

Principle

Both the sympathetic and the parasympathetic divisions of the autonomic nervous systems have preganglionic fibers originating from the CNS that synapse outside the CNS in autonomic ganglia. The postganglionic fibers leave the ganglia and innervate the effector organs. Postganglionic sympathetic fibers secrete norepinephrine (NE) from their terminals while postganglionic parasympathetic fibers secret acetylcholine (Ach) from their terminals. NE and Ach activate corresponding receptors present on the heart and vasculature, which cause the change of blood pressure. Under normal circumstances, the innervation of vascular smooth muscle is dominated by the sympathetic regulation, and ganglion blockers competitively block the ganglionic transmission to produce pharmacological action. If the agent can block the change of blood pressure caused by stimulating preganglionic sympathetic or parasympathetic fibers and administering neurotransmitter, the agent can be concluded to be a ganglion blocker.

Materials

Animal required: 1 rabbit, 2 – 3kg.

Apparatus required: physio – pharmacological universal instrument, surgical instruments needed, manometer, arterial catheter, arterial clip, pediatric scalp needle, stimulating electrode syringes.

Reagent required: hexamethonium bromide 2. 5% solution (W/V), urethane 20% solution (W/V), noradrenaline bitartrate 0. 01% solution (W/V), acetylcholine chloride 0. 001% solution (W/V), heparin 0. 2% solution or sodium citrate 5% solution, Saline.

Methods

1. Anesthetization　The rabbit with body weight about 2 – 3kg is anesthetized by 20% urethane (1g/kg), through the vein on the edge of the ear.

2. Operation　The anesthetized animal is securely fastened on the operating table. The cervical fur is removed and a median incision is made on the skin. Blunt dissection is used to divide muscles between the sternocleidomastoid muscle and the trachea to separate the common carotid artery on both sides and right vagus nerve. Lay a line under the common carotid artery to block the blood stream later. Put two ligatures under the right vagus nerve, tie the ligature near the proximal cephalic end, and reserve the ligature near the cardiac end to prepare for electric stimulation.

3. Insert the arterial cannula that is already filled with anticoagulant into left common carotid artery, and connect the cannula with force – displacement transducer and the pressure detector for

recording blood pressure.

4. Insert the pediatric scalp needle filled with Saline into the marginal vein of ear, fix the needle with adhesive tape, prepare to inject drugs.

5. After the blood pressure stabilizes, record the normal blood pressure for several minutes. Do the experiment following the steps showed below:

1) Draw up the ligature under right carotid artery to occlude blood flow for 15 seconds, observe the change of blood pressure.

2) Cut off right vagus between two ligatures, stimulate the peripheral end of the vagus with current induced by the electronic stimulator according to following stimulating parameters: rectangular pulse, frequency 8Hz, wave width 2ms, output of voltage about 3 – 4V (120% threshold voltage), time 15 seconds.

Find the lowest stimulative strength, and observe the change of blood pressure.

3) Inject intravenously 10μg/kg of noradrenaline bitartrate (0. 1ml of 0. 01% solution), observe the change of blood pressure.

4) Inject intravenously 1μg/kg of acetylcholine chloride (0. 1ml of 0. 001% solution), observe the change of blood pressure.

5) Inject intravenously 0. 1μg/kg of hexamethonium bromide (0. 4ml of 2. 5% solution), observe the change of blood pressure.

6) After the blood pressure attains the lowest point, repeat steps 1, 2, 3, 4 and observe the reaction of blood pressure.

Results

Measure and calculate the change of blood pressure, mark the names and dosages of drugs administered or stimulating condition, and analyze the results of experiment.

Notes

1. Don't anesthetize the rabbit too deep otherwise the blood pressure will decline excessively.

2. Pay attention to the arterial catheter and scalp needle, and don't let blood coagulate in them.

3. Don't damage the vagus while separating it, and moisten it in the experiment.

Evaluation

The rabbit is easily obtained, docile and of medium size, which is suitable for doing some general experiment and basic operational practice. But the blood pressure of the rabbit isn't stable enough, thus it is not used to screen antihypertensives. Cats, dogs and rats are usually selected. The nictitating membrane of the cat is dominated by superior cervical postganglionic sympathetic fibers, so we can realize the action of drugs that block the sympathetic ganglion by observing the constriction of the nictitating membrane.

Questions

1. What's the mechanism of causing the change of blood pressure in each experimental step?

2. How do you explain the effect of hexamethonium bromide on the change of blood pressure?

3. What happens if hexamethonium bromide is converted into central antihypertensives?

Experiment 5. 16　Vascular perfusion of isolated ear of rabbit

Objective

Study the pharmacological experimental methods of vascular perfusion of isolated rabbit ear. Observe the effects of isoprenaline and noradrenaline on isolated vascular smooth muscles.

Principle

$R \propto P/Q$, where R is vascular resistance, Q is volume of flow, P is perfusion pressure. The eye of the rabbit is dissected free, the auricular artery is perfused with prewarmed (37℃) and oxygenated Krebs solution from proximal cardiac end with the constant pressure. After perfusion, the perfusion solution flow from auricular vein. The volume of flow is diminished after drug is given, the resistance of blood vessel is increased and blood vessel is contracted by drug. Observe the change of the volume of flow between pre − and post − treatment to know the effects of drug on blood vessels.

Materials

Animal required: 1 rabbit, 2 – 3kg.

Apparatus required: circulating and thermostat water bath, surgical instruments, mixed gas (5% carbon dioxide in oxygen) provided device, arterial catheter for auricular artery, syringes, volumetric cylinders, beakers, fixed device for rabbit ear.

Krebs solution of the following composition (g/L) NaCl 9. 2, KCl 0. 42, $CaCl_2$ 0. 24, $NaHCO_3$ 0. 15, glucose 1. 0), urethane 20% solution, noradrenaline 10^{-5} solution, isoprenaline 8×10^{-5} solution.

Methods

1. Weigh the rabbit with the infant scale, inject 20% urethane (1 – 1. 2g/kg) into the femoral vein slowly, fix the animal on the table on its abdominal position, and clip the fur on the root of the ear.

2. Incise the skin about 2cm along the blood vessel on the dorsal root of the ear. Find and separate the posterior auricular artery between the underside of central vein and nervus auricularis magnus. This artery runs parallel to the vein, but locates too deep to be touched. Place two ligatures under the artery. Use the operating lamp to locate the position of the artery.

3. Tie the centripetal ligatures, insert arterial catheter into the centifugal end of artery. Inject oxygenated Krebs solution into the artery rapidly, clean up the blood of the vessel until the vein of ear is filled with colourless solution. Cut off the ear quickly, and irrigate the blood vessel to remove the surviving blood until the colourless solution flows from the vein. Fix the ear on the glass or plastic plate leaned at 45^{β} with gummy mud. Put the tip upward and the root downward, so the fluid from vein can flow from the inferior horn of plate. Connect the arterial catheter to the emulsive tube which convey the prewarmed (37℃) and oxygenated Krebs solution. The bottle filled with Krebs solution is about 60cm high above the arterial catheter. Regulate the flow rate of perfusion to 30 – 40 drops per minute. When the flowing rate is steady, record the volume of flow for 3min. Select the mean value as referrence data before administration.

4. The drugs are added into perfusion slowly from the emulsive tube where arterial catheter is

connected. Observe and record the flow rate of perfusion. The drugs need to be added with uniform speed and volume, the speed of administering is no more than 1ml per minute. The order of drugs is as follows: (a) 0.5ml of 8×10^{-5} isoprenaline (injecting within 30 seconds). (b) 0.5ml of 10^{-5} noradrenaline (injecting within 30 seconds).

Results

Record the data of experiment as the table shown below and compare the results.

Table 5 – 3　Effects of drugs on the perfusion flow of isolated rabbit ear

Drugs	Dosage	Perfusion flow rate (ml/min)						
		Pretreatment	Time after administering (min)					
			1	2	3	5	10	15

Notes

1. The experiment must be done at constant temperature and pressure. No air bubble is allowed to be in the constant pressure perfusion device. The bubble must be removed immediately in order to avoid clogging the vessel and influencing the results.

2. Cut off the ear rapidly or else the catheter will be slid from the artery. Douche the vessels clearly with perfusate to prevent blood coagulation.

3. The position between the catheter and ear must be maintained uniformly from beginning to end, or the artery will be twisted owing to the movement of catheter. Therefore the perfuse speed will be lower.

4. Don't give next drug until the former drug is washed thoroughly and the flow returns back to the initial level.

5. Arrange the experiment indirectly, do it as soon as possible because the ear edema will affect the results.

Evaluation

1. The method is easy to be used to evaluate the direct effects of the drugs on vessel smooth muscle, and it can reflect the influence of drugs on the resistance of the small – medium sized arteries and veins.

2. Because there is no central nerve which controls the isolated ear, angiohypotonia appears, so the vessel is sensitive to vasoconstrictive drugs and insensitive to vasodilators.

3. The vascular resistance of isolated rabbit ear is influenced by the room temperature, stretching and the position of catheter. So we must control the condition of experiment strictly to get good results.

4. We can test several drugs by injecting it into perfusate in a short time. It is a routine method of observing the pharmacologic effects of drugs on the blood vessels.

Questions

1. What kind of drugs are suitable for the isolated otic vascular perfusion in rabbit?

2. Which factors can affect the isolated otic vascular perfusion of the rabbit?

V. Diuretics and dehydrating agents

Experimental methods of diuretics in animals have two classes, acute animal test and chronic animal test. In the former one, we usually collect urine form urethra or urinary bladder directly. It is applicable to bigger animals such as dog, cat, rabbit, etc. The test can be completed in a relatively brief time and can be little affected by external environment. But the disadvantage of acute animal test is that the animal should be in a non - physiological state which may be anesthetized or be operated, so that it is not the same with normal ones. If to carry out the operation in conscious state animals, urethra fistula method or bladder fistula method can be adopted to avoid the effects of anesthesia on urine volume. But the test is relatively complex and is seldom used in screening experiments. In the latter one, metabolism cage is used to collect urine of small animals for several hours. we call it "metabolism cage experimental method", and it is suitable for rat and mice. In order to reduce urinary evaporation and excremental pollution, urine can be weighed with particular urine collecting device or filter paper. To this method, animals are in a physiology state or approaching physiology state so that the result is reliable. But the experiment is greatly affected by the experimental environments and the experimental time is oppositely long.

Rat and dog are commonly used in screening experiments of diuretics. Rabbit and mice are second to them. Most effective diuretics used in human have better diuretic effect in rat test. Therefore, rat is mostly adopted. If necessary, dog is used for the further verification or deep study. Dog can be replaced by rabbit in some primary screening experiment because rabbit is cheap and easily obtained.

Various diuretics not only promote water excretion but also affect salt excretion. Therefore, ion (Na^+, K^+, Cl^-, HCO_3^-) quantity in urine should be analyzed as index beside urine volume. Drugs can be classified into several kinds by determining ions in urine, such as sodium drained - potassium protected diuretic etc. As concerning action mechanism research of urine drugs, other analyzes method should be used as subsidiary method, for example, free water clearance method can be used to judge the nephric ability to concentrate and to dilute urine, and to analyze the effect of diuretics on concentrating or diluting urine; stop - blow method can be used to analyze transportation function of uriniferous tubules and to locate action site of diuretics primarily; Micropuncture technology can be used to locate action site of diuretics more accurately and more directly.

Experiment 5. 17   The diuretic effect of furosemide and hypertonic glucose on anesthetized rabbit

Objective

1. Study the acute animal test for diuretic action.

2. Observe the diuretic action of furosemide and Hypertonic glucose on anesthetized rabbit.

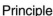

Principle

Furosemide is a very potent loop diuretic. It mainly acts on epithelial cell of thick ascending loop of Henle's loop; it inhibits the coupled $Na^+ - K^+ - 2\ Cl^-$ symport system in the tubular membrane. It inhibits active transport of Cl^- and thus reduces reabsorption of Na^+, which result in increasing of Na^+, Cl^- in tube and reduction of the kidney function of diluting urine. At the same time, Na^+, Cl^- reabsorption decreases from ascending loop of Henle's loop to medulla internal fluid prevents the formation of hyperosmolality and thus reduces the kidney function of concentrating urine. Therefore, the reabsorption of Na^+, Cl^- in the renal tubule is decreased, and so is the reabsorption of bivalent cation such as Mg^{2+} and Ca^{2+} etc. A large number of Na^+ transport into the distal convoluted tubule and collecting duct, which promotes $Na^+ - K^+$ exchange and makes K^+ excretion increase. But because Cl^- is not affected by ion exchange, Cl^- is more than Na^+ in urine. Therefore, the excretion of large quantities of electrolytes and water can cause great diuretic action. Hypertonic glucose is an "osmotic diuretic" that inhibits reabsorption of spare glucose in the proximal convoluted tubule. Reabsorption of glucose in the proximal convoluted tubule is limited. And the limitation is called renal glucose threshold. High osmotic pressure will form in the tubular fluid when large quantity of 50% glucose is given by injection of vein at a time that exceeds the limitation of absorption, and spare glucose is excreted by urine, meanwhile, plenty of water is carried out, so diuretic action is produced. Since the moiety glucose can diffuse from vessels to tissues and can be metabolized and used easily, so its effect is weak and short. By collecting urine volume in unit time before administration and after administration, increased urine volume in unit time can be calculated to analyze latent time, intensity and duration of action of each drug.

Materials

Animal required: 1 rabbit, 2 – 3kg, female or male.

Apparatus required: rabbit box, operating table, mouth – gag for rabbit, catheter (for oral injection), infant scale, cylinder, beaker, syringe, polyethylene tube, operating knife, tissue scissors, eye scissors, vascular forceps.

Reagent required: urethan 20% *W/V* solution; glucose 50% *W/V* solution; furosemide 1% *W/V* solution; normal saline.

Methods

1. Pretreatment   take a rabbit, weigh it and place it into a rabbit box and then give the rabbit warm water 40 ml/kg by oral injection.

2. Anesthetization   20min later, anesthetize the rabbit by injecting urethane 20% *W/V* solution (1g/kg) slowly into marginal vein of the ear.

3. Operation   Fix the rabbit on the operating table. Cut off the fur on the lower abdomen. Open the skin for about 4 – 5cm above the pubic symphysis, then cut the muscle and the peritoneum along the Linea alba abdominis to expose the urinary bladder. Lift up the bladder, find out and separate the bilateral ureters. Pick up the ureters and place in each a ureteral cannula. Record urine volume excretion with a graduated cylinder (ml/5min), Fig. 5 – 3.

4. Administration   Inject intravenously hypertonic glucose 2.5g/kg body weight into the marginal vein of the ear. Observe the effect on urine flow and record the urine volume at 5, 10, 15, 20, 25, and

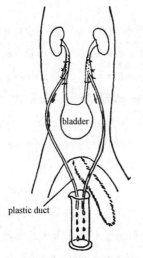

Fig. 5 – 3　Cannula and urine collection in acute diuretic experiment

plastic duct

bladder

30min after administration.

Give enough saline to replenish body fluid.

After the urine volume recovers, inject intravenously 1% Furosemide solution (4mg/kg), observe the effect on urine flow and record increase of urine volume at 5, 10, 15, 20, 25, and 30min after administration.

5. Calculate urine volume (ml) increased in unit time　The millilitre value of urine volume increased = millilitre value of urine volume in unit time after administration-millilitre value of urine volume in unit time before administration.

Results

1. Report the kind, sex, weight of the test animal, and the process of giving load – water, and the name and the dosage of the drug given, and the route of administration.

2. Collect the data of the whole class. Calculate the mean (x) and the standard deviation (SD) of the increased urine volume in each unit time. Make a chart by using increased milliliter value of urine volume as ordinate and each time after administration as abscissa. Compare the peak time and duration of furosemide and hypertomic glucose on the anesthetized rabbit.

Notes

Slowly inject urethane at the same time, observe the case of cornea reflecting, respiring and muscle relax.

Be careful when cutting open abdominal cavity. Don't damage the viscera in the abdominal cavity; Pay attention to avoid the blood vessel and make a blunt dissection

The ureters of rabbit are very thin and weak. So to be careful when inserting urethral cannula to avoid injuring ureters.

Diuretic action takes place in 1 – 2min and 3min after injecting intravenously hypertomic glucose and furosemide. If there is no urine flow out, check the ureteral cannula whether it is blocked by blunt dissection or the ureters are distorted.

The later drug should be injected after the action of former drug disappear and the normal urine excretion recovery.

During the test, operating part of the body should be covered with the gauze containing mild warm Saline in order to keep the temperature and the humidity of animal's abdominal cavity.

Evaluation

Ureters inserting cannula method is perfect for the acute diuretic test. The test can be completed successfully in a short time. The result is more precise, it is not relate with the spared urine in urinary bladder, and it is little affected by the environment. But the condition of anesthetized animals is different from conscious animals. Bladder inserting cannula method is similar to the former. In this method, the operation process is the same with our experiment. After finding out the urinary bladder, turn it over and reveal abdomen side. Avoid vessels and make a purse – string suture on the ventral side,

cut a small opening, insert a bladder canula (fill the canula with water and remove the air). The o-
pening of the cannula should aim at the opening of both ureters. Tighten up the small bag.

Bladder fistula – making method, which is done beforehand, can be used in the diuretic test
on Conscious animals. After 2 weeks, the wound may heal. Fix the animal on a special trestle, collect the urine and test. The method can avoid interference of anesthetic drugs. But the test process is
more complex.

In addition, urine conduct method can be often used. The method is simple. It can avoid surgical trauma in experimental animal, It is easy to insert the tube into uterine cavity of female animal
and to result in the failure of the experiment. Now the method is introduced in brief as follows:
Choice male animals. Lubricate the top of urethral catheter by liquid wax. Insert urethral catheter into ureter slowly and lightly. The urine will pour out along the urethral catheter after urethral catheter
is inserted into bladder through vesical sphincter.   Then put it further to $1-2$cm again. Inserting total depth is determined by the size of the animal. Usually, it is about $8-12$cm for rabbit, $22-$
26cm for dog. At last, fix the urethral catheter and the animal with some rubberized fab-
rics. Abandon the urine flow out for the first 5 minutes. Wait for the urine drop numbers steadily. Put
a graduated cylinder under the urine conduit. Collect and record the urine volume.

Besides, counting the urine volume, the urine drop numbers of unit time also can be recorded
by the drop recorder.

Questions

What is the definition of diuretics and dehydration separately? Can you tell the difference between the two drugs after the experiment? What experiment should be replenished, if you can not
find out the difference?

The sequence of the drug given in this test is administering glucose before furosemide. If to give
furosemide before glucose, is it rational? Why?

Experiment 5. 18   The diuretic action of hydrochlorothiazide on rat

Objective

1. Study the chronic animal test for diuretic action.

2. Observe the effect of hydrochlorothiazide on urine volume of the rat.

Principle

Hydrochlorothiazide is a medium efficient diuretic whose action site is located on the anteri-
or part of distal convoluted tubule. It inhibits $Na^+ - Cl^-$ symport system and then reduces the
reabsorption of Na^+, Cl^-. So the thiazides are also named $Na^+ - Cl^-$ Inhibitors. Inhibiting
active transport of Cl^- can reduce absorption of Na^+, which lead to the osmotic pressure increase in tubule cavity. Large quantity of NaCl is expelled from the body with water. Because the
quantity of Na^+ and Cl^- excreted is almost equal, it can't effects the acid – base balance of
the body fluid. But the agent may make the body lose more K^+.

The experiment is a chronic diuretic test in which urine is collected in some metabolic cages after administering drug intrperitoneally. Diuretic action of drugs can be observed by comparing with

the control group.

Materials

Animal required: 2 male rats, 180 – 220g each.

Apparatus required: metabolic cage for rat, balance, graduated cylinder, Syringe.

Reagent required: 5% hydrochlorothiazide solution, normal saline.

Methods

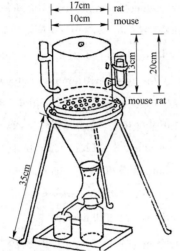

Fig. 5 – 4 Abirdged general view of acute diuresis cannula and urine collection

1. Fit the metabolism cage device to collect the urine The device is composed of a circular cover, circular chassis with some holes, a device used to supply water and food, a conical funnel collecting urine and a feces separating instrument. There is a 150 – 200ml graduated cylinder or beaker at the side opening of the feces – urine separating instrument to collect urine (Fig. 5 – 4). Put the animal on the circular chassis. Then the urine can be separated from the feces with the feces – urine separating instrument in the bottom of the cage. And the urine can be collected.

2. Give water load Weigh the two rats, and give them Saline 5ml/100g orally.

3. Administration 30 minutes later, press lower abdomen of the rats to empty the bladder. Inject 5% hydrochlorothiazide solution (25mg/kg) for the test group, and inject normal saline (5ml/100g) for the control group.

4. Urine collection After administration, place the rats into two metabolism cages separately. Record the time, and begin to collect urine. Measure the urine volume of each rat every 30 minutes until 120 minutes after administration.

Results

1. Report the kind, sex, weight of the test animals, the process of giving load – water, the name and the dosage of the drugs, and the route of the administration.

2. Collect the data of the whole class. Calculate the mean (x) and the standard deviation (SD) of urine volume of two groups in unit time. Do the significance test among groups by t – test. Fill the results into the following table (Table 5 – 4).

3. Take the urine volume of control group as 100. Calculate the increasing percent of urine volume of given group, use it as the ordinat. Use the time after giving drug as abscissa. Make a chart to show the strength of diuretic action at different time intervals.

Table 5 – 4 Effect of urine volume on hydrochlorothiazide solution in rats

Rat numbers	Weight (g)	Drug dose (mg/kg)	Urine volume (ml) in different time after the administration			
			0 – 30 minutes	30 – 60 minutes	60 – 90 minutes	90 – 120 minutes
1						
2						

continue

Rat numbers	Weight (g)	Drug dose (mg/kg)	Urine volume (ml) in different time after the administration			
			0 – 30 minutes	30 – 60 minutes	60 – 90 minutes	90 – 120 minutes
3						
4						
5						
..						
$\bar{x}$ + SD						

Notes

Ensure the urine is separated from the feces by the use of metabolism cage. Prevent the urine being polluted. The device is made of glass or Plexiglas except the bracket, so it is easy to clean. Be sure not to use a metabolism cage, which is made of metal material, when you analyze the metal ions in the urine.

There is little body fluid of the normal unloaded – water rat; it is easy to get dehydration phenomenon under the action of powerful diuretic, so the normal action of the drugs given may not take place. At the same time, the urinary output is very little (about 0.5ml/100g per hour), some operating mistake may take place, the urine may evaporate, and the discharging urine from bladder in rats is not identical. All that can lead to error. So the loaded water is necessary before the test. It is better to use 5% glucose Saline as the loaded water.

Press the lower abdomen of the rat with hand lightly in order to remove the remaining urine before collecting every time.

Choose the rats, which have the similar weight (about 200g each) and the same sex (the male first) in order to reduce the individual difference. Adapt the animal to the environment of the metabolic cage for 1 – 2 days before test. Observe whether the urinary output is steady under free drinking water, then give the rats Saline by oral injection, if the urinary output in 2 hours is more than 40% water loaded, the animals are ideal.

If the urine volume of one rat is too little, 2 or 3 rats in the same group can be placed in the same metabolism cage.

Evaluation

Metabolism cage method of collecting urine is applied to chronic tests of small animals (such as mice and rat). The urine can be collected continuously for several hours, several days or at some special time. Operation of the test is simple and safe. The result is reliable because the test is done under the physiological state. But the effect of the environment (air temperature, humidity) is relatively great. So control the experiment condition, and make the room temperature at about 20℃.

If there are no rats or rat metabolism cages, the mice of body weight 20 – 25g can be used to observe the action of the diuretic. Simple mouse – metabolism cage is showed in picture. In the left picture, the device is made of conical funnel, copper gauze, plastic lid, graduated centrifuge tube, etc. Conical funnel is covered by copper gauze to prevent the feces leakage. The mouse is placed on copper gauze. Copper gauze is covered by a plastic lid with some ventilative holes whose diameters are about 3 – 4 mm. The lid is fixed with the collar of the conical funnel and the rubber band and the metallic hooklet. The urine of mouse flows into the graduated centrifugal tube along the funnel. In the right picture, it is a simple metabolism cage that has a good effect. It is made of a big beaker, an Aluminum gauze and an Aluminum holder. Several sheet of filter paper weighed is placed on the Aluminum wire and the mouse is placed on the filter paper. There is 1 cm deep water on the bottom, which can reduce the volatilization of the urine. Change the filter paper regularly. Record the increased weight of the filter paper to show the urinary output.

Food should be withheld to the mice for 12 hours before test. After weighing, give the mice Saline (0.3ml/10g) by oral injection. Then give the mouse of administrated group 0.5% hydrochlorothiazide (5mg/10g) by oral injection, give the mouse of control group Saline (0.2ml/10g) by oral injection. Compare the urinary output of the two groups.

Questions

1. Diuretics are divided into three kinds depending on the strong, medium and weak effect, what are their differences in clinical application?

2. What is the difference between side effects of furosemide and hydrochlorothiazide?

VI. Experiments of antitussive, expectorant and antiasthmatic agents

Antitussive, expectorant and antiasthmatic agents are widely used in treating bronchial inflammation and asthma.

1. Antitussive agents   There are two groups of antitussive agents: drugs acting on the central and drugs acting on end – brush. The former directly inhibit the medullar cough center and the latter mainly suppress the recepter or one point of the coughing reflex arc (coughing reflex arc consists of receptor, afferent nerve, cough center, efferent nerve and effector). The kinds of cough may be different, if different irritants are given. We always choose chemical irritation, mechanical irritation and electric irritation to cause cough.

1) Chemical irritation: The aerosol or gas of ammonia water, sulfur dioxide, sulfuric acid, acid citric and acetic acid can irritate the receptors under the respiratory epithelia to cause cough. Coughing induced by this way is similar to physiological cough and we can detect the intensity of cough primarily, but the animals can't be reused in a short period.

2) Mechanical irritation: Insert a feather in the trachea by some special tracheal cannula, and pull the feather come – and – on. This method is easy to operate without any special device and the animal can be reused in a short period, but we cannot control the intensity of irritation exactly and make quantitative comparison.

3) Electric irritation: Stimulating any point of afferent nervous pathway of coughing reflex arc can induce coughing. We always choose two places to stimulate: ①superior laryngeal nerve (we always chose cat or Guinea pig). ②tracheal mucosa (we always chose Guinea pig or dog). This method can be reused in a short period without passivation, and we can quantify the intensity precisely and evaluate the antitussive action of drugs by detecting the liminal value of current that can

cause cough . If we need to make a judgement whether the antitussive action belongs to central, stimulate the medullar cough center.

Cats' coughing reflex is the most sensitive in animals, but it is expensive. Guinea pig is sensitive to chemical irritation and mechanical stimulation. Stimulate the guinea pig's superior laryngeal nerve can give rise to cough, and it is easy to accomplish in a common lab. Therefore, we always choose guinea pigs to be our experimental animals. Rabbits are seldom used due to its lack of sensitivity to chemical stimulation and electric stimulation.   Mice and rats can be induced to cough with chemical stimulation. We always use mice, rats and guinea pigs to do preliminary screen, and then use cats or dogs to rescreen and to analyse the action mechanism.

Anesthetic agents can restrain cough reflex and therefore have an influence on experimental result. So if the animals are to be anaesthetized, we had better choose Urethan and α-chloralose instead of inhalation anesthetics, to make sure that the condition of test is relatively stable.

2. Expectorant agents   Expectorants are claimed to increase the quantity of excretion of the respiratory tract to make the sputum less viscous, and therefore the sputum is more easily cleared. Collecting tracheal secretory fluid directly and detecting the phenolsulfonphthalein excreted by the trachea are two ways to screen the expectorant. In addition, ciliary movement of respiratory mucosa plays an important role in clearing sputum away, therefore detecting ciliary movement has some benefits to our study and evaluation to the action of Expectorant agents.

1) The method of collecting excretive fluid of the trachea: Animals like cats and dogs are the best choice for the experiment . We can also use superficial anesthesia to the rat. Put a slim glass – tube in its trachea, and collect the excretion which flow in the glass – tube by capillary action and finally evaluate the action of the agents by the quantity of liquid collected.

2) phenolsulfonphthalein excretion determination: It is easy to operate, but it is not accurate, so it is often used in primary screening.

3. Antiasthmatic agents   Bronchial spasm is the most direct reason of asthma, so most anti – asthma agents can relax the bronchial smooth muscle. There are obvious differences among different kinds of animals when their bronchial smooth muscle response to the same drug. The smooth muscle of guinea pigs is the most sensitive and is always used. We can use the *in vitro* trachea or *in vivo* animal in the experiment.

1) *In vitro* trachea test: We always use tracheal volume method, tracheal strand method, bronchial perfusion method and so on. *In vitro* experiments can be used to observe the effect of drugs on tracheal smooth muscle directly, but they have some limitations and therefore are just used in the first screening.

2) *In vivo* animal tests: Inhale the air of histamine or acetylcholine, which is anaphylactins, the animals will have asthma. By this way we can observe the protection eff- ects of drugs. Somatic animal can reflect the anti – asthmatic effects of drugs in clinical standard.

Asthma is a symptom of allergic reaction. So we should take use of some immunological methods when we study anti – asthmatic agents.

Experiment 5. 19　The antitussive effect of codeine on mice coughing induced by ammonia water

Objective

Study the way to test antitussive effect of agents by ammonia water spraying method. Observe the antitussive effect of codeine.

Principle

Link the air compressor with the vitreous nebulizer, then the ammonia water will be sprayed well – distributed into a sealed container. After inhaling ammonia, which is irritative, the mice cough. We can evaluate the antitussive effects of drugs by counting the times of cough in unit time.

Materials

Animal required: 2 mice, 18 – 22g, male or female.

Apparatus required: vitreous nebulizer、air compressor、mercury manometer、vitreous te、stopwatch, vitreous bell jar (with volume of 500ml), stethoscope for child.

Reagent required: Codeine phosphate, 0.2% solution *W/V*. Saline. Strong ammonia water (25% – 27% NH_4OH solution).

Methods

Weigh and mark two mice, put them in the bell jar and then observe their normal activity as well as the features of breath. Inject intraperitoneally 0.2% codeine phosphate (40mg/kg) into one mouse and inject intraperitoneally Saline with equal volume as comparison into the other.

Put the two mice into the bell jars separately 20 minutes after injection. Link the outfa of air compressor with the vitreous tc (Fig. 5 – 5) and regulate atmospheric pressure to around 27 kPa. Open the stopcock of nebulizer and spray the ammonia water into vitreous bell jar well – distributed for 10 seconds. Allow the mice to stay in the bell jar for 2 minutes and then take the mice out of the jar.

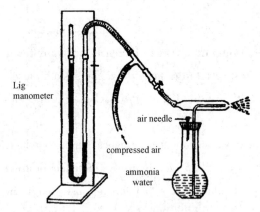

Lig manometer

air needle

compressed air

ammonia water

Fig. 5 – 5　The spray assembly　of ammonia water inducing coughing

Put the mice into another bell jar immediately and observe their cough voice from the neck of the bell jar by stethoscope for child. Record the latent period of each mouse (period from beginning spraying to the first voice of cough) and count the number each mouse coughs in three minutes.

Results

Collect all experiment results in your laboratory and calculate the mean and standard deviation of times of coughing in 3 minutes ($\bar{x} \pm s$). Then do significance t test in groups and fill the result in Table 5 – 5.

Table 5 – 5 The antitussive effect of codeine on cough induced by ammonia water of mice

Number	Weight (g)	Drugs and dose (mg/kg)	The latent period of cough (minute)	Times of cough in 3 minutes

Notes

1. If there is no special vitreous nebulizer, you can use bottle of chromatography reagent instead. If there is no air compressor or spraying equipment, you can use other equipment instead, such as evaporating equipment made by self which is put 1 ml strong ammonia water in boiling water bath. Let the ammonia vapor stimulate mice for 45 seconds, then bring the mice out and observe.

2. You can observe cough of mice carefully by naked eyes, If there is no stethoscape for child. They should show contraction of abdominal muscle and at the same time open their mouth.

3. If you need to evaluate quantitatively the antitussive value of the drugs, you can use the prolongation of EDT_{50} (the time that half of mice are induced coughing) as an index. Measure the latent period time of every mouse and calculate the EDT_{50} of the whole group by sequential method.

Questions

How many kind of models of cough do we use? What are their benefits and limitations?

Appendix The determination of EDT_{50}: You should prepare Table 5 – 6 before experiment and formulate a series of spraying time arranged by geometric progression (the logarithmic interval of time is 0.7 – 0.8). The logarithmic difference of two close time is invariable.

Table 5 – 6 The sequential method used in detecting EDT_{50} of antitussive agents

Group	Time second	Time lg(x)	1	2	3	4	5	6	7	8	9	10	11	12	r	Rx	Count
Control group	15.9	1.2															
	20.0	1.3		−											1	1.3	$n = 12$ $c = \sum rx = 17.4$
	25.1	1.4	+		−		−			−		−		Z	5	7.0	$EDT_{50} = lg^{-1}\frac{c}{n}$
	31.6	1.5				+		−	+		+		+		5	7.5	
	39.8	1.6						+							1	1.6	$= lg^{-1}\frac{17.4}{12} = 28.2$ (s)
	50.1	1.7													add	12	17.4	
															↑ n	↑ c	
codeine group	20.0	1.3															$n = 12$ $c = \sum rx = 19.4$
	25.1	1.4															
	31.6	1.5		−				−							2	3.0	$EDT_{50} = lg^{-1}\frac{c}{n}$
	39.8	1.6	+		−		−		+		−		−	Z	6	9.6	
	50.1	1.7				+		+				+		+	4	6.8	$= lg^{-1}\frac{19.4}{12} = 41.4$ (s)
	63.1	1.8													add	12	19.4	
															↑ n	↑ c	

Notes: "+"——cough "−"——not cough; "X"——the logarithm of time; "r"——the sum of animals in each group of mist spray time (include positive and negative reaction). The EDT_{50} of controlled group is 25 – 25 seconds.

This case : $R = \dfrac{41.4}{28.2} \times 100\% = 147\%$

Conclusion: Codeine have antitussive effect.

The equipment and ways of cough induced is written above.

When the former mouse presents coughing response (three times typical coughing per min), the later will be administrated within longer time, that is responsing to change time and observe in turn, 10 – 20 mice each group is better. After determination, calculate EDT_{50} and R value according to the method of table and formula.

$$R = （treating\ group\ EDT_{50}/controlling\ group\ EDT_{50}）\times 100\%$$

If R > 130% we can conclude that the agents have antitussive effect and if R > 150%, we can say its effect is obvious.

later will be administrated within longer time, that is responding to change time and observe in turn, 10 – 20 mice each group is better. After determination, calculate EDT_{50} and R value according to the method of table and formula.

$$R = （treating\ group\ EDT_{50}/controlling\ group\ EDT_{50}）\times 100\%$$

If R > 130% we can conclude that the agents have antitussive effect and if R > 150% we can say its effect is obvious.

Experiment 5. 20   The antitussive effect of codeine on coughing induced by electric stimulation on superior laryngeal nerve of cat

Objective

Study ways to test antitussive effect of agents by cough induced method of electric stimulation on superior laryngeal nerve of cat and observe antitussive effect of codeine.

Principle

Sensory nerve ending in larynx is dominated by superior laryngeal nerve which is an important afferent nerve in cough reflex arc. Irritation of superior laryngeal nerve with current can induce cough. We can evaluate the antitussive effects of drugs by detecting the threshold of inducing cough.

Materials

Animal required: 1 cat, 2kg, male or female.

Equipment required: operating table, scissors, surgical scissors, surgical knife, hemostat, muscular tension transverter, balancing recorder, YSD – 4 pharmacological and physiological experiment meter, stopwatch, protective electrode, venous infusion equipment, gauze, absorbent cotton, silk suture, needle, syringe.

Reagent required: codeine phosphate 0.3% solution, 3% pentobarbital sodium, liquid paraffin.

Methods

1. Anesthesia   Take a cat, weigh it and then give 0.3% pentobarbital sodium (30mg/kg) by intraperitoneal injection.

2. Operation   After anesthetization, fix the cat on operating table supinely. Shear its hair on the neck, incise the skin along the median line of neck, and separate the subcutaneous tissue, expose its thyroid cartilage, we can see unilateral vagus nerve. Separate the skin along the vagus nerve to the head till the knuckle. There is a branch divided from the ganglia, which is perpendicular to muscle fiber, point to the thyroid cartilage aslant, It is the superior laryngeal nerve. Separate nerve can make good connect with the electrode, drop a little liquid paraffin at the connection. Then cover the operation field with wet gauze. Seam a suture in the skin under xiphoid

process of epigastrium. Link one side of the suture to the muscular tension transverter and the other side to the balancing recorder. When the cat coughs, its diaphragm will contract and therefore affect its abdominal wall move, the times and the amplitude of cough will be recorded by the recording device. Separate the femoral vein of one side and insert venous infusion equipment into the vein for administration.

3. Detect the threshold of inducing cough of cat   After operation, irritate the superior laryngeal nerve and detect the threshold of inducing cough. Adjust the stimulative way of the meter (YSD – 4) to "continue B" with its frequency of 10 Hz and wave – length of 10 ms. The time of stimulation persists for 5 seconds and the interval of two consecutive stimulations is 5 minutes. The intensity of voltage increases from 0. 5 V to an intensity that can first induce coughing, it is commonly not more than 5 V. The minimum of the intensity of voltage, which can induce coughing, is its threshold. Repeat it for three times and count the average of three times as a control before administration.

4. Administration   Infuse the animal with codeine phosphate 0. 3 percent solution (3 mg/kg). Irritate the superior laryngeal nerve with the threshold every 5 minutes after administration and observe the change of times and intensity of voltage and then find out the threshold after administration. Record the period of inducing cough, the multiple the threshold improves and the time it persists of codeine phosphate solution.

Results

Record the results according to Table 5 – 7.

Notes

1. Depth of anesthesia influences intensely the effect on inducing cough, and the excessive anesthesia will inhibit cough reaction obviously. It is better to anesthetize with alphachloralose (dissolved in propylene Glycerin, i. p 80 mg/kg), which doesn't influence cough reflection. When more drugs need to be supplied in the experiment, don't determine threshold until animal is stable.

Table 5 – 7   The antitussive effect of codeine on cough induced
by electric stimulation on superior laryngeal nerve of cat

Number	Drugs and dosage	Inducing cough threshold before administration (V)				Inducing cough threshold after administration (V)						
		1	2	3	average	15	30	45	60	90	120	(min)

2. Guinea pigs can replace the cats when cats are absent. Anesthetize it with urethane by intraperitoneal injection. Incise the skin of its neck, separate its vagus nerve, cut it down and then stimulate its middle site to induce cough.

3. Expect codeine phosphate, morphine hydrochloride and antess citrate can be used as positive drugs. The former dosage is 0. 6 mg/kg, and the latter is 10 mg/kg.

Evaluation

Stimulating the superior laryngeal nerve of cat with electricity to induce cough is the most common method. Definite stimulative frequency and intensity can cause reliable cough. Quantity comparison can be made before and after administration, which is accurate and reliable. It is one of the important methods to find antitussives. However, the quality of cough induced by the above method is different from physiological cough, so definite condition and definite capacity is needed in the operation.

Questions

1. What are the screening methods for antitussives? What are experimental animals often used? And what are the advantages and disadvantages of each method?

2. What should be paid attention during experiment, especially during operation?

Experiment 5. 21　The effect of Siberian milkwort root decoction on phenolsulfonphthalein secretion of mice's bronchus

Objective

Study the method of phenolsulfonphthalein secretion test to screen expectorant agents and observe the effect on phenolsulfonphthalein secretion of mice's respiratory tract.

Principle

Phenolsulfonphthalein indicator is injected into mice's abdominal cavity and it can be partly secreted by bronchi. The expectorant agents can increase the secretion in bronchi as well as phenolsulfonphthalein secretion in mucosa of respiratory tract. So we can indirectly deduce expectorant function of the sample from the effect on phenolsulfonphthalein secretion. Phenolsulfonphthalein show red in alkali solution and phenolsulfonphthalein in respiratory tract can be rinsed out by Na_2CO_3 solution and quantified by colorimetric method.

Materials

Animal required: 2 mice, weight: 18 – 24g, male or female.

Equipment required: syringes, mice perfusing stomach implement, surgical scissors, ophthalmologic forceps, test tubes, 721 – spectrophotometer, pins, cotton thread.

Reagent required: 100% Siberian milkwort root decoction (get 200g Siberian milkwort root in pieces and add 200ml alcohol in it, reflux for 2h in water bath.) Saline, 5% Na_2CO_3 solution, 0.25% phenolsulfonphthalein solution (precisely take phenolsulfonphthalein 0.25g, dissolve it with 2.5ml 1mol/L NaOH solution, then add saline to the volume of 100ml. Shake it to be homogenous).

Methods

1. Get 2 mice fasted about 8 – 12h before experiment, weigh and mark them. Give one mice 100% Siberian milkwort root decoction [0.25ml/10g (25g/kg)] by oral injection, give the other mice Saline in equivalent volume by the same way.

2. Inject 0.25% phenolsulfonphthalein solution of 0.25ml into two mice's abdominal cavity 30 minutes later. After another 30 minutes, kill the mice by detaching cervical vertebra. Fix the mice supinely on a wood broad with pins, stretch its neck, incise its skin from the middle of its neck, i-

solate its bronchus and then put a cotton thread around the bronchus for fixing the needle.

3. Suck up 5 percent baking soda of 0.5ml with a 1ml syringe and attach a dull needle of size 7 on it. Prick the needle into the bronchus for approximately 0.3 – 0.5cm from thyroid cartilage and fasten the needle with cotton thread. Rinse for 3 times, then take down the syringe, put the flushing fluid into a test tube. Repeat the method mentioned above for 2 times. Mix the flushing fluid together and detect its absorption at 558nm with 721 – spectrophotometer.

Results

Collect all the data in the class and figure out the mean and standard deviation of the administered group and the control group respectively. Then make a significant t test between two teams and fill the result in Table 5 – 8.

Table 5 – 8   The effect of siberian milkwort root decoction on phenolsulfonphthalein secretion of mice's bronchus

Number		Weight	Dosage	A value	Significant t test
administration	1				
	2				
	3				
	4				
	$\bar{x} \pm SD$				
control group	1				
	2				
	3				
	4				
	$\bar{x} \pm SD$				

Notes

1. Isolate the bronchus gently to avoid damaging thyroid and blood vessels nearby, because bleeding will contaminate the flushing fluid and affect the result.

2. Don't prick the needle into bronchus with 5% sodium hydroxide solution, its quantity must be accurate and the velocity must be slow enough or the bronchus may be damaged. Draw out the fluid to make the bronchus dry as much as possible, and avoid blowing air into the bronchus.

Question

What are the Principles of the expectorant to spit out sputum? Do the expectorants have antitussive effect?

Experiment 5.22   The antiasthmatic effect of aminophylline on asthma stimulated by histamine – acetycholine

Objective

Study the way of inducing asthma in Guinea pigs by spraying acetylcholine and histamine, observe the antiasthmatic effect of aminophylline.

Principle

Acetylcholine and histamine given by spraying can cause Guinea pig's bronchus to spasm, asphyxia, resulting in its ticing and stumbling. This animal experimental model can be used to observe the function of bronchus smooth muscle relaxing drugs.

Materials

Animal required: 2 guinea pigs, weight: 150 – 200g; male or female.

Equipment required: spraying assembly, air compressor, vitreous bell jar (volume 2L), syringe, stopwatch.

Reagent required: 2% acecoline solution, 0.4% histamine phosphate solution, 12.5% aminophylline solution, Saline.

Methods

1. The day before the experiment, put guinea pigs into bell jars. Spray the solution mixed by 2% acecoline and 0.4% histamine phosphate solution (2 : 1) into the jar for 8 – 15 seconds at a stable pressure of 53 – 67kPa and then observe the reaction of animals carefully. Usually, the animal breathe deeper and faster, and then it gets dyspnoea, finally it tic and stumble. Take the guinea pig out of the jar immediately if you see it stumble, or it will die. Record the latend period of inducing asthma (time from beginning spray to tic and stumble). In general, the latent period is no more than 150s. If the period exceeds 150s, the animal is not qualified for the experiment for it is not sensitive to the stimulation.

2. On the second day, take 2 guinea pigs which have passed the preliminary experiment. One is injected 12.5% Aminophylline intraperitoneally (125mg/kg), and the other is injected Saline with equivalent volume. 30min later, put 2 guinea pigs into bell jars respectively and do as the above – mentioned step and them record the latent period. If the period exceeds 6min, take it as 6min.

Results

Record the results according to Table 5 – 9.

Gather the results of all class, calculate the average and standard deviation of stimulating asthma latent period before and after administration ($\bar{x} \pm s$). Make a significant t test of before administration and after administration. Show that whether it has significant deviation before and after administration by P (It can be compare between groups either).

Notes

1. Young guinea pigs should be chosen, whose weight are no more than 250g, and the latent period of inducing asthma is not more than 150 seconds.

2. Latent period of asthma is obviously extended, and the experimental animals don't stumble after administration because of dyspnoea and smother. Generally speaking, observe for 6 minutes and the latent period of animals that don't stumble are calculated as 6m.

Table 5 – 9 Antiasthmatic influences of aminophylline on guinea pigs

Number	Drugs	Dosage and gateway	Reaction after inducing asthma withsprayer	Latent period of inducing asthma	
				Before administration	After administration
1					
2					

3. Antihistamine agents have no direct relaxant effect on bronchus smooth muscle. However,

expected results can be gotten while using in this kind of animal model. So we should discard false positive findings when analyzing experimental results.

4. Some guinea pigs may tolerant to histamine if they contact histamine for several times. So be careful to make guinea pigs sprayed equally when arranging experiment. In general, each guinea pig can only be used one time a day.

Evaluation

Drugs inducing asthma by sprayer are inhaled through respiratory tract, so inhaled quantity is influenced by respiration quantity. Stimulative test drugs are given by i. p , the pain may possibly inhibit breathing and make inhaled quantity of the drugs inducing asthma (acetylcholine and histamine) descend, which will cause false positive results of lengthening latent period. In addition, it is also affected by concentration of inducing asthma solution, sprayer pressure, structure of sprayer etc. Particles whose diameter are shorter then $5\mu m$ will be inhaled into pulmonary alveolar, the process is quick and intense. The bigger ones will be absorbed in bronchus and the much bigger ones will accumulate in trachea or in upper respiratory tract, the process is slow and weak.

Some people judge asthma degree according to the action asthma attacks. Ⅰ: respiratory is deeper and faster; Ⅱ: dyspnoea; Ⅲ: convulsion; Ⅳ: stumble. There is no obvious limitation among Ⅰ、Ⅱ、Ⅲ, so it is hard to judge accurately sometimes. Majority of effective drugs can postpone or inhibit attack of Ⅲ or Ⅳ. Furthermore, latent period of inducing asthma is lengthened or the phenomenon of dyspnoea, asphyxia and stumble is disappear after administration.

Questions

How many kinds of common – used antiasthmatic drugs? What characteristics do each kind of antiasthmatic drug? And what clinical values do they have?

Experiment 5. 23　Effect of drugs on isolated Guinea pig trachea

Objective

Study the method of making in – vitro tracheal chain of guinea pig and observe the contractile or relaxant effects evoked by drugs and the relationship between them.

Principle

There are β_2 – receptor, M – receptor, and H_1 – receptor on the *in vitro* tracheal smooth muscle. Evoked β_2 – receptors can have relaxant responses on tracheal smooth muscle and evoked M – receptor and H_1 – receptor can make it contract. Isoproterenol is β_2 – receptor agonist and makes tracheal smooth muscle relax, while acetylcholme and histamine are respectively M – receptor agonist and H_1 – receptor agonist, they make tracheal smooth contract.

Materials

Animal required: 1 guinea pig, weight $400 - 500g$, male or female.

Apparatus required: Mayer's bath groove, homoiothermy bath, thermometer, force displacement transducer, automatic balance recorder, inflated ball, scissors, ophthalmological forceps, Petri dish, iron cage, di – pit clip, cotton thread, and syringe

Reagent required: 0. 2% histamine phosphate solution, 0. 05% acetylcholine chloride,

2.5% aminophylline, 0.1% isoprenaline sulfate, 0.5% atropine sulfate, Krebs – Henseleit solution (NaCl 8.0g, MgCl₂ 0.42g, CaCl₂ 0.4g, all these are dissolved in deionized water and added to the bath to 1000ml and needed to be added to glucose 1.0g before using).

Methods

1. Apparatus adjustment　Turn on balance recorder and recording pen and adjust recording pen to a suitable site. Then add preload of 0.5 – 1g, turn the switch to 20mv and paper rate to 4mm (4mm/min).

2. Tracheal tract making　Kill the guinea pig by a blow on the head, incise the skin of neck and then shear the integral tracheal from thyroid cartilage to tracheal crotch. Immense it in Krebs – Henseleit solution, the trachea is cut into 5 – 6 tracheal cartilage circles of 3 – 4mm. Cut each tracheal circle in the midpoint of cartilage to produce tracheal slices whose edges are connected with cartilage and middle parts are glossy (flat) sarcolemma. 5 – 6 sliced trachea is linked to a tracheal chain by cotton thread (Fig. 5 – 6), whose length depends on the volume of bath groove. If the volume is 30ml, the length should be 3 – 4cm; if 10ml, it should be 1.5 – 2cm.

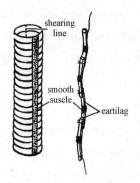

Fig 5 – 6　The method of installing tracheal chain

3. Tracheal chain installation　Put finished tracheal chain in Mayer's bath groove with Krebs – Henseleit solution at 37℃, make one side in the bottom of the bath groove and the other side in a hook of the transducer which links to the automatic balance recorder. Put the breather into tracheal chain and make bubbles (one by one) out of ball by supplying oxygen to the trachea. Make tracheal chain adapt to Krebs – Henseleit solution for 10 minutes. Finally, record a part of formal curve as base line.

4. Administration　Administrate and observe the responses of tracheal chain after the base line gets stable (the bath capacity is 30ml). When the responses evoked by one drug are observed, wash and don't give another drug until the base line restores. The order of drugs given is：①0.1% isoprenaline sulfate solution 0.1ml. ②2.5% aminophylline solution 0.1ml. ③0.2% histamine phosphate solution 0.1ml, added to 0.1% isoprenaline sulfate 0.1ml when it reaches its effective acme. ④0.2% histamine phosphate solution 0.1ml, added to 2.5% aminophylline solution 0.1ml when it reaches its effective acme. ⑤0.05% acetylcholine chloride 0.1ml , added to 0.1% isoprenaline sulfate solution 0.1ml when it reaches its effective acme. ⑥0.05% acetylcholine chloride 0.1ml, added to 2.5% aminophylline solution 0.1ml when it reaches its effective acme. ⑦0.05% acetylcholine chloride 0.1ml, added to 0.1% atropine sulfate 0.1ml when it reaches its effective acme.

Results

Copy curve of tracheal chain and illustrate it.

Notes

1. In order to avoid injuring tracheal smooth muscle, be sure to separate and ligate tracheal slices softly.

2. Unlike intestinal vessel, tracheal smooth muscle hasn't spontaneous rhythmic contraction before administration. Administrate as soon as the base line is stable.

3. Recording drum can replace force displacement transducer and automatic balance recorder. Because tracheal smooth muscle is relatively fragile, the load of recording lever should be light and amplification may be increased properly.

4. After adding one kind of drug to tracheal chain, observe it for 5min to make sure its effect, then change solution. wash used drug away completely (3times as usual) and don't add another drug until base line restores. Turn down the switch to avoid making recording pen away from right site when solution in bath groove is changed.

5. Supply oxygen abundantly when conducting the experiment. If base line rises, or it is away from original site, supply oxygen enough to restore it.

Evaluation

Isolated trachea method is one of the common experimental methods to screen antiasthmatic drugs. It is effective, convenient and economical, and it needs little test substance (TS). In addition, the contractive and relaxant effects evoked by drugs can be observed without the aid of any apparatus. Among ordinary experimental animals, guinea pig is sensitive to drugs, and its bronchi is similar to that of human. So we always make it as the first choice.

According to different sectioning methods, there are tracheal circles method, tracheal spirals method and tracheal chain method used in this experiment. Its operating procedures are as followed: Separate trachea, cut it transversely into 5 – 6 pieces of circles with similar width along cartilage and link them to a tracheal chain (Fig. 5 – 7). The *in vitro* trachea made by this method doesn't response intensely to bronchoconstrictor agents or bronchodilator agents, the extent is 1/3 of that of tracheal chain method. Method of tracheal spirals can exempt the disadvantage of little breath response caused by tracheal circles method. So it is able to research bronchoconstrictor agents or bronchodilator agents. Its operating procedures are as followed: Incise the trachea into spirals (the width is 2 – 3mm and the length is 3 – 4cm) from one edge to another. (Fig. 5 –8). In addition, we can also use integral trachea. Because of tracheal smooth muscle is distributed annularly (sometimes obliquely or longitudinally). The contractile and relaxant effects of annular muscle may induce constriction or expansion of tracheal radius correspondingly, which can be reflected by solution height of baresthesiometer attached on trachea. That's called volume – detecting method.

What are the differences among the mechanisms of isoprenaline, aminophylline, histamine phosphate and atropine sulfate on guinea pig tracheal chain? And what clinical values do they have?

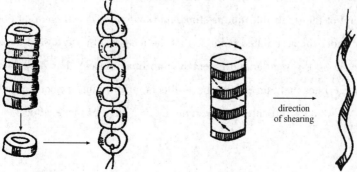

direction of shearing

Fig 5 –7　Method of make tracheal circle　　　Fig 5 –8　Method of make tracheal spirals

Ⅶ. Experiments of drugs affecting digestive system

The effect of the drugs on the digestive system is usually studied through their influence on gastrointestinal smooth muscle, prevention and treatment of ulcer, and the choleretic function and so on.

There are many methods applied to measure the effects of drugs on the functions of the gastrointestinal smooth muscle such as method of recording movement of in vitro gastrointestinal smooth muscle of guinea pigs and rabbits, experimental method of gastric emptying and intestinal vermiculation, method of studying the movement of digestive organs through pressure – sensitivity sensor, method of study the moving of digestion organs through bioelectricity and so on.

The models of experimental peptic ulcer are classified into four kinds according to the methods of experiments on therapeutic effectiveness: ① method of surgical operation, way of ligaturing pylorus can be adopted to rats and dogs. ② administration method, it can be administrated by aspirin, indomethacin, and resperpine, etc. ③ Stress method, there are methods of bound stress, bound infusion stress and so on. ④ artificial injury in digestive tract mucosa such as thermal method and glacial acetic acid method etc. the evaluation of the operation, and the reappearance of results, the sensitivity of the drugs, the relation to the causes of diseases are concerned, all that have their merits.

The effect of drug on bile excretion: Dogs, cats and rabbits are usually used. After anesthesia, use in common bile duct intubation to drain, observe the effect of drugs on bile excretion. It also can be perfused from the direction of common bile duct to intestinal to observe the effects of drugs on the ejection movement of oddi's sphincter. It is convenient to use rats to gather bile quantitatively in common bile duct because the animal is lack of bile – cyst.

Experiment 5. 24   The effect of drugs on gastrointestinal movement

Objective

To determine the rate of mobility of anthracotic in gastrointestinal and observe the effects on gastrointestinal movements.

Principle

The animals' intestinal smooth muscles consist of thick circular muscular and slight vertical muscles. The contraction of circular muscles mainly predominates the intestinal contents propeling to anus. When any point of the small intestine is stimulated by foods, it will contract above the stimulated point and relax under the stimulated point so that the foods can move toward the anus to form the intestinal movement. It is the regular movement of intestinal muscle that propels the chyme from small intestine to large intestine. Some drugs have effects on intestinal smooth muscles, which contribute to enhance or weaken the intestinal vermiculation, so they have effects on the peristaltic movements.

Materials

Animal required: 6 mice, all of the same sex, which are 20 – 24g each.

扫码"学一学"

Apparatus required: syringe, infusion syringe needle for mice, scissor, forceps, ruler.

Reagent required: morphine hydrochloride, 0. 01% solution W/V; 0. 01% neostigmine methyl sulfate; normal saline; anthracitic suspension, 5% solution W/V (contended with Acacia, 10% solution W/V).

Methods

Mark and weigh 6 mice which are fasting for 24 hours and divide them into 3 groups.

All the mice are treated by oral injection. Group A: morphine hydrochloride 0. 01% solution (0. 2mg/10g); group B: clear $1 : 10^4$ solution of neostigmine methyl sulfate (20μg/10g); group C receive normal saline 0. 2ml/10g.

Each mouse is given anthracitic suspension 5% solution (0. 1/20g) by oral administration after 15 minutes.

Kill the animals by vertebrate dislocation 15 minutes after they are administrated anthracitic and then incise their abdominal cavities. Free the whole digestive tract from cardia to the end of rectal tube and pave it nicely without traction. Detect the whole length of the distance from the front edge of anthracitic to cardia and compute the percentage of the distance that the anthracitic moved corresponding to the whole length of gastrointestinal tract.

Results

Calculate according to the following formula and collect the results of the whole class. Get the mean and standard deviation and compare them.

The percentage of anthracitic moving distance to whole length of GI tract =

$$\text{anthracitic moving distance} / \text{whole length of GI tract } 100\%$$

Notes

The animals must fast for one day before experiment.

The time of infusing charcoal powder to the animals and the time of killing them must be exact, or else it will change the result of experiment dramatically.

Avoid of traction when cutting the stomach tract, or else the accuracy of detection will be affected much.

Evaluation

People often put a kind of tracing substance in stomach cavity and catch up with its moving and observe its distance propeled in stomach in exact time.

The method is easy and safe, but it only detects the general crossing condition in stomach and does not tell the contraction form in detail and the animal in experiment must be killed after experiment.

Currently, there is an active research method in which people study electronic activities of smooth muscle of gastrointestinal tract by using electricity of gastrointestinal muscle as an index to show the smooth muscle activity.

Question

What are the differences in the effects of morphine hydrochloride and neostigmine methylsulfate on gastrointestinal tract? What is the clinical significance?

Experiment 5. 25　Prevention and treatment function of drugs　on experimental gastric ulcer

Objective

Learn the experimental method of inducing gastric ulcer by ligating rats' pylorus and observe the prevention and treatment of drug on experimental gastric ulcer.

Principle

The retention of gastric juice which comes after ligating of rats' pylorus makes the stomach wall digested, so that the gastric ulcer appears. In addition, fasting for 48 hours is a significant factor which leads to gastric ulcer. The method was first reported by Shay et al. In 1945 and later adopted in screening antiulcer drug universally.

Materials

Animal required: 6 rats, weight 200 – 500g, of the same sex.

Apparatus required: mouse cage, operation plate of rats, surgical knife, surgical scissors, forceps, surgical pin, yarn, carbasus, bullet of infusing to rats' stomach, injection syringe, measuring cylinder, litmus paper, drainage and Microscope.

Reagent required: 1% aluminum hydroxide gel, 2% Cimetidine, normal saline.

Methods

1. Mark six rats, and feed them only water for 48h. Then conduct the operation.

2. Anesthetize the rat superficially with diethyl ether and fix it on the operation plate supinely. Cut off the hair on abdomen and disinfect the skin with 2% tincture iodine and 75% alcohol. Incise the abdominal wall for 1.5cm from xiphoid, draw out the stomach from abdominal cavity by blunt forceps without hurting the blood vessels on the mesentary and then Ligate at the meeting of pylorus and dodecadactylon. Put its stomach to the former position and suture the abdominal wall. And put the rat into mouse cage without giving food and water.

3. The rats are divided into three groups (three rats/group). Each rat in group 1 is infused with 5ml of 1% aluminum hydroxide gel; each rat in Group 2 is subcutaneous injected with 2% Cimetidine per 6mg; each rat in Group 3 is infused with 5ml of normal saline.

4. 18 hours after operation, kill all the rats by cutting down their heads. Incise the abdominal wall and ligate at the cardia. Take out the stomach and immediately put it into 1% formaldehyde for 5 minutes. Bring it out and absorb the solution from it by filter paper. Cut a bouche at the big curvature and take out the content of stomach into measuring cylinder via a funnel. Cut stomach along the big curvature and rinse stomach softly with water. Tile it on the glass plate, then observe and calculate ulcer area and the area of the whole stomach under the microscope. Measure the volume of gastric juice and get the acidity of gastric juice by litmus paper.

Results

Calculate the area of gastric ulcer, and measure the volume and pH of gastric juice. Gather the results of all class and compare the indexes of the three different administration groups.

Notes

1. Absolute hunger before operation is necessary to cause the ulcer. We should close the rats into the proper mouse cage to prevent them from eating the discharge and underlay.

2. Dodge the blood vessels when ligating the pylorus in case of not obstructing the blood circulation of gastrointeslinal tract.

3. The stomach should be taken out very softly by forceps to avoid injury of the tissue and organ.

Evaluation

The incidence of gastric ulcer induced by pylorus ligation is from 85% to 100% and this method is always applied with water – dipped restrain method.

The degree of gastromucosa injuring induced by pylorus ligation is related to the fast condition before and the lasting time after pylorus ligation. The volume of stagnated gastric juice, the acidity of gastric juice, the general acidity and the pepsin activity also can be got by analysing the stagnated gastric juice to observe the effect of drugs on the former index.

Questions

1. What are the factors which cause the gastric ulcer by pylorus ligation?

2. What are the functions of Aluminum hydroxide gel and Cimetidine separately on gastric ulcer?

Experiment 5.26　The cholagogic function of dehydrocholic acid on rat

Objective

Study the method of detecting the quantity of the excreted bile of rat, and observe the cholagogic function of drug.

Principle

In the experiment, the cholagogic function of cholagogue drugs on rat can be observed using the dehydrocholic acid to increase the excretion of bile which can make cholerythrin and the other components of bile thinner and increase the water in bile .

Materials

Animal required: 2 rats, weight about 300g, the same sex.

Apparatus required: syringes, slim plastic tube (diameter 1 – 2mm), surgical scissors, eye forceps, test tube clamp, homeostatic forceps, surgery knife, operating table of rat, the marked suction tube, beaker, ganze, silk thread, iron stand, cylinder, and ophthalmology scissors.

Reagent required: 3% sodium pentobarbita, 2.5% dehydrocholic acid, Saline.

Methods

1. After fasting rats for 12 hours , weigh and mark them, and then divide them into two groups.

2. Anesthetize the rats by intrperitoneal injection of 3% sodium pentobarbita, and fix it supinely. Cut off the fur along the midline on the abdomen and incise the skin and peritoneum about 2cm. Take the pylorus as standard, turn over the dodecadactylon and the papilla of dodecadactylon

will be seen so that the general bile duct can be tracted from the papilla. At about 3 – 5mm above the papilla, strip the capsule covering on the papilla with the forceps for about 5 – 10mm continuously to expose the common bile duct completely.

3. Put 2 silk threads through the end of the bile duct near the papilla and the above. Knot firmly the thread near papilla, incise a notch on the bile duct by a eye scissor, insert the Polyethylene plastic tube from the notch to the liver and fix the tube with the thread prepared after making sure the bile can flow out. At last close the abdominal cavity temporarily with hemostatic forceps.

4. After collecting the bile for one hour in a cylinder, calculate the volume and take it as the normal value of bile before administration.

5. Give Saline (0. 4ml/100g) to each rat in group 1 from dodecadactylon; give 2. 5% dehydrocholic acid (100mg/kg) to each rat group 2 from dodecadactylon. Collect the bile at the first and second hour separately after administration and compare the data after administration with that before administration.

Results

Collect the results of all the class and compare them.

Addition of bile = excretion of bile in one hour after administration − excretion of bile in one hour before administration

Compare the data of two groups to match.

Notes

1. The wound should be as small as possible and be careful not to hurt liver and dodecadactylon in the operation.

2. Keep the animals warm, especially in winter.

3. The drug should not be used until it is prewarmed to 38℃.

Evaluation

The effect of cholagogue agents varies according to different species of animals. Hence, it is perfect to evaluate the effects by clinical results. However, it is difficult to collect the bile of patients in clinical trials. As a result, we often take the results of animal experiment as reference in evaluation.

When evaluating cholagogic agents and especially cholagogue drugs, the species of animal in experiment, the method of bile collection, anesthetizing or not, the way of anesthesia, the dosage of cholagogic agent, the ways of administration of cholagogic agent and the time of collection must be recorded clearly. In addition, water, cholerythrin, bile acid, cholesterol concentration in bile, excretion of these substances in a given time, the appearance, density, and the change of deposit of bile must also be recorded. These factors are necessary to evaluate the effect of drugs.

Questions

1. Is it feasible if other animals are taken as the object in the experiment? What is the difference in methods?

2. What is the function of dehydrocholic acid in clinical use? And what diseases are treated by the dehydrocholic acid clinically?

VIII . The experiments of coagulants and anticoagulants

Under the physiological state, blood flowing in the blood vessel neither flow out of vessel to cause bleeding nor form thrombus in blood vessel. This is because there are the complex blood coagulation system and the anticoagulative fibrinolytic system in the body, both of which cooperate to maintain dynamic balance. If the balance is broken, hemorrhagic diseases or thrombotic diseases may occur.

Blood turning from the flow state into the gel state is named blood coagulation. Relation factors attending blood coagulation process are known together as blood coagulation factor. According to International Blood Coagulation Factor Nominate Committee, 12 blood coagulation factors are coded by Rome number based on the subsequenceof their finding. When the factors are turned into active blood coagulation factor, "a" is added at the right lower corner of the code numbers. Prekallikrein (PK), Kallikrein (K_a), High molecular weight kininogen (KMWK), Thrombocyte phospholipin (PL or PF_3), Plasminogen, Plasmin also participate in the chain reaction of blood coagulation and fibrinologsis.

The process of blood coagulation and fibrinologsis can be divided into 4 steps:

1. Formation of prothrombin activator   According to the water – fall theory of blood coagulation, blood coagulation process is composed of endogenous pathway (all participating composition are in the blood), exogenous pathway (besides competent in the blood, there are some cellular protein under endothelium which is tissue factors to participate in the action) and common pathway. It is a chain reaction which is strengthed and amplied by many kinds of preenzyme activated subsequently. In endogenous pathway , at first, contact factors that is factor XII, Kallikrein (Ka) and High molecular weight kiniogen (KMWK) are exposed on surface with negative charge to activated XII to XIIa, which lead to the activation of factor IX, and then the factor is activated to IX a, factor X is activated by X enzyme complex formed by factor IXa, cofactor VIIIa, phospholipin and Calcium. In exogenous pathway, firstly, plasma factor VII is exposed to tissue factor, and then both, together, form a complex that activates factor X directly. When blood coagulation process develop to the stage that factor X is activated. Both pathways are joined together to make the factor X activated to factor Va. Then Va and V link at surface of phospholipin by Calcium to form a complex. The complex is named as prothrombin activator.

2. Formation of thrombase   Thrombogen is changed into thrombase by prothrombin activator.

3. Formation of fibrin   Fibrinogen in colloidal sol is changed into fibrin gel state (clot) by thrombase.

4. Dissolution of fibrin   Fibrin is liquified, dissolved and changed into degradation product of soluble fibrin.

Coagulants are drugs that can stop bleeding by accelerating blood coagulation process or prohibiting fibrinolysis; anticoagulants are drugs that can delay blood coagulation or accelerate fibrinolysis. The drug is useful in prevention and treatment of thrombosis.

In vitro method is a method that can be used to obtain effect of drugs on clotting time and fibrinolytic time *in vitro*. The method is simple and can be used to screen drugs primarily without any special device.

Pathological pattern method is creating a pathological bleeding or clotting state which is similar to human on experimental animals and curing them with coagulant or anticoagulant. The method can be used to observe and analyze the action of drugs or screen new drugs. It is easy to form these pathological patterns, for example, the pathological pattern of hypoprothrombinemia is formed by forcing mouse to take dicoumarin.

Experiment 5. 27　Anticoagulant action of drugs *in vitro*

Objective

1. Study test tube method *in vitro*.

2. Observe anticoagulant action of sodium citrate and heparin.

Principle

Heparin has strong and quick anticoagulant action *in vitro* and *vivo*. As the cofactor of AT – Ⅲ, after binding with AT – Ⅲ, it combine rapidly with thrombase, Ⅸa, Ⅹa, Ⅺa, and Ⅻa, which result in their inactivation. Heparin has the greatest Inhibiting action on thrombase and blood coagulation factors Ⅹ, Both of which are essential in endogenous and exogenous coagulation pathway. And heparin, too, inhibit the action of factor Ⅸ, Ⅺ, Ⅻ. So it can inhibit almost all steps of blood coagulation process to cause the strong anticoagulatant effect.

Sodium citrate, which can reduce Calcium ion in blood to block blood coagulation process, is often used as an extracorporeal anticoagulant.

Materials

Animal required: rabbit, 2 – 3kg, female or male.

Apparatus required: test tube (diameter 8 mm), test tube rack, graduated test tube, injector, stop watch, constant thermostat water, small glass rod.

Reagent required: 4% sodium citrate solution, Saline, 4U/ml heparin solution, 3% calcium chlorine solution.

Methods

1. Take five test tubes. One is dripped 0.1ml of Saline, two are dripped in 4% sodium citrate solution 0.1ml separately, and two are dripped in 4U/ml heparin solution 0.1ml separately. (Referring follow table)

2. Take about 5ml blood with 9[#] needle from the heart of rabbit. Drip 0.9ml of blood in each test tube quickly. Mix them to homogeneity. Place the tubes in constant thermostat water of 37℃ ± 0.5℃.

3. Incline the tubes one time per 30 seconds. Observe fluidity of blood till the blood does not flow when tubes being inverted slowly. Compare the clotting time of 5 tubes.

4. If coagulation phenomenon does not appear in later 4 tubes, drip 2 – 3 drops of 3% calcium chlorine solution in the second and the third tubes separately and mix them to homogeneity. Observe coagulation phenomenon again. Compare the clotting time.

Results

Observe condition of blood coagulation in each tube. Record and compare clotting time (Table 5 – 10) .

Notes

1. Caliber of test tubes should be well – distributed and suitable. Generally speaking, blood clotting time is shorter in the small caliber tube than in the big one.

2. Taking blood by puncture in hearts of rabbits should be done quickly and accurately to avoiding blood coagulated in the injector. Reduce tissue fluid and bubble being mixed into blood as possible.

3. When the blood of rabbits is dripped into tube, mix them homogenized with small glass rod immediately, or the accuracy of determination can't be assured. Bubble formation should be avoided while mixing.

4. Interval time from taking blood of animal to placing tubes into thermostat should not overpass 1 min.

5. Temperature of constant thermostat should be controlled well. Clotting time may be lengthened due to high or low temperature.

6. Action of inclining tubes should be done gently. Inclination should be small (<30°) to reduce the contact of blood and tube wall .

7. Injectors and test tubes should be dry, clean. Otherwise blood coagulation will be accelerated or hemolysis can take place.

Table 5 – 10   Effect of drugs on clotting time

Drugs/tube	1	2	3	4	5
Saline solution	0. 1	—	—	—	—
Drugs/tube	1	2	3	4	5
4% sodium citrate solution	—	0. 1	—	0. 1	—
4U/ml heparin solution	—	—	0. 1	—	0. 1
Blood of rabbit	0. 9	0. 9	0. 9	0. 9	0. 9
constant thermostat water 37℃ ±0. 5℃					
Clotting time					
3% calcium chlorine solution	—	2 – 3 drops	—	2 – 3 drops	—
Clotting time					

Evaluation

The method is used to observe the effect of drugs on clotting time in vitro. The method is easy and needs no special equipment. It can be used for first screening of drugs. But there are many factors affecting the method. The accuracy of results is easily affected by the factors. So identical operation of control group and treat group should be emphasized in the first screening of drugs to keep the continuity of effect factors to the utmost.

The test tube method *in vitro* can be used to evaluate the conditions of blood coagulation of volunteers or patients. Prolongation of clotting time is usually seen in situations as follows: ①Factor Ⅷ, Ⅸ, Ⅺ decrease remarkably, such as hemophilia A, B, C. ②Thrombogen decreases seriously, such as hepatopathy, obstruative jaundice, hemorrhagic disease of newborn. ③Fibrinogen decreases seriously, such as hypofibrinogenemia, serious hepatopathy. ④Anticoagulant is used such as heparin. ⑤Heperibrinolysis, such as later period of disseminated intravascular coagulation product (DIC), and when there are a lot of fibrin degradation product (FDP). Shortening of clotting time is seen in the situations as follows: ①Blood assumes hypercoagulability, such as early stage of DIC. ②Hyperglycemia and hyperlipidemia.

Activated clotting time (ACT), plasma recover calcium time (RT), serum prothrobin time (SPT), activated part thrombokinase time (APTT) can also be assayed by similar methods.

Questions

1. Please compare the similarities and differences of anticoagulation action of sodium citrate and heparin?

2. What is the effect of protamine on anticoagulant action of heparin? What is the mechanism of their interaction? What is their clinical significance?

Experiment 5.28　Action of drug on promoting coagulation

Objective

Study the method of establishing the animal pattern of action of drugs on promoting coagulation. Observe action of drug on promoting coagulation.

Principle

Prepare hypoprothrombinemia pathological pattern by taking dicoumarin orally and observe coagulant action of vitamin K_1.

Materials

Animal required: 3 mice, 18 – 22g, female or male.

Apparatus required: capillary glass tube (diameter 1 mm, length 10 cm)、slide glass、stopwatch.

Reagent required: distilled water, Saline, 0.25 % dicoumarin suspended solution, 1% vitamin K_1 solution.

Methods

1. Weigh and mark all the mice .

2. Force mouse A to take distilled water 0.2ml/10g orally, mouse B and C to take 0.25% dicoumarin suspended solution 0.2ml /10g orally.

3. 16 hours later, inject Saline 0.2ml/10g introperitoneally to mouse A, B separately, inject vitamin K_1 solution 0.2ml/ 10g introperitoneally to mouse C.

4. 24 hours after forcing mice to take dicounarin, determinate clotting time with capillary glass tube or slide method.

5. Clotting time test

1) Capillary glass tube method: Insert capillary glass tube of diameter 1mm into venous plexus at the back of eyeball of mouse about 4 – 5mm. Rotate gently and then retract. Record time at the beginning of blood flowing into capillary glass tube. Take and place capillary glass tube on the table

flat when capillary glass tube is full with blood. Snap capillary glass tube 3 – 5mm from end to end of capillary glass tube every 30 second and pull slowly. Observe until clotting strands appear. Count time from taking blood with capillary glass tube to clotting strands appearing, that is clotting time. Take average value of two end data of capillary glass tube as clotting time of the mouse.

2) Slide method: Extract one eyeball of mouse with crooked tweezers of ophthalmology, and blood flow out at once. Drip a drop of blood on two sides of slide glass separately. Diameter of drop is about 5mm. Count time at once with stopwatch, raise the blood drop with clean pin from edge to inside every 30 second. Observe if clotting strands up. Time from taking blood to clotting strands appearance is clotting time. Another drop is used to recheck. Take average value of two side data as clotting time of the mouse.

Results

Collect all experimental results. Count average value of clotting time of mice in 3 groups. Do significance testing of different averages. The drug actions can be judged by the clotting time.

Notes

1. Clotting time can be affected by room temperature. The lower the temperature is, the longer the clotting time is. It is better that room temperature is about 15℃.

2. Mice should be prohibited to feed before 2 hours of oral administration. Dicoumarin suspension should be swayed to be homogeneous in order to avoid being heterogeneous.

3. It is better that diameter of glass tube is 1 mm and homogeneous. Capillary glass tube can not be taken in hand for long time after taking blood as clotting time is affected by body temperature.

4. Blood drop should not be stirred up from different directions as it can affect fibrin's formation time.

Evaluation

The method is to establish the pathological pattern similar to human body after disturbing coagulation in experiment animal, then to take experimental therapy with coagulant. It is used to observe and analyze actions of drugs or screening new drugs. The model is formed easily and operated simply, mice is conveniently used in this experiment. It can also be used to screen drugs.

The interval time between giving drugs and determining coagulation time is determined by different drugs and the way of giving drug. If the drug is injected, then 30min after giving drug, several point of time can be chosen to observe time – effect relationship of drug.

Questions

1. What are the methods used as screening coagulant and anticoagulant drugs?

2. What are the effects of dicoumarin and vitamin K_1 on clotting time separately? How about their action mechanisms? What is their clinical significance?

IX. Platelet inhibitors

Normally, platelets move in blood vessels dispersedly. When blood vessels are injured, blood flow is changed or the body is stimulated by chemical material. Relational change of platelet take place they are morphological change、adhesiveness、aggregation and releasing action.

Hemorrhage can be caused by reduction of platelet number, adhesiveness, aggregations and releasing action. But too much platelet and too strong aggregation may strengthen blood coagulation and lead to thrombus formation as well. Adhesiveness, aggregations and releasing action of platelet is not only the basic condition of hemostatic function in normal physiology but also the main factor of forming thrombus in pathological condition.

When blood vessels are injured, platelets contact with collagen fibers of broken endothelium, aggregate and form firm platelet thrombus. Blood coagulation system is activated, because coagulation factors release after blood platelet aggregating and blood vessels wall injured. Then the formation of fibrous protein is accelerated, which lead to the formation of blood platelet fibril thrombus.

There are many factors of adjusting blood platelet function. they are arachidonic acid (AA) system、cyclic nucleotide system including cyclic adenosine monophosphate (cAMP) and cyclic guanosine nucleotide monophosphate (cGAP) system, phosphatidylinositol (PI) system and Ca^{2+}. With developing of biology and medicine, study of platelet action in physiological and pathological state has been further done. The method of studying blood platelet has also been developed quickly.

Anti – platelet drugs are a kind of new drugs. At present, anti – platelet drugs are mainly used to treat diseases of cardiovascular system such as ischemic heart disease and thrombotic disease etc. Now we will introduce anti – platelet test from the effect of drugs on platelet adhesiveness、aggregation and releasing action of reactive product.

Experiment 5.29 Determining method of platelet adhesiveness

Objective

Study experimental principle and operation of platelet adhesiveness.

Principle

The characteristic of platelet adhesion on the surface of injured vessels is named as platelet adhesiveness. Under normal circumstances, surface of platelets and vessel's endothelial cells carry negative charges, so platelets can not be adhered on the vessel's endothelium because the things having the same charge repel each other. When vessel's endothelium is injured, collagen under endothelium is exposed. Platelets with negative charges adhere with collagen with positive charge.

According to the platelet adhesiveness, platelets adhere on the surface of foreign matter after blood touches the foreign matte for a period of time. Platelet numbers in blood are reduced. Determining difference of platelet numbers before and after touching with foreign matter can be calculated. Platelet adhesion rate can be calculated. Two main kinds of improved rotating glass ball methods are introduced as follow.

Materials

Animal required: 1 rabbit, 3kg, male.

Apparatus required: Platelet adhesion apparatus, siliciferous injector, siliciferous graduated test tube, 1ml siliciferous graduated pipette, spherical glass bottle, blood cell counting plate, sharp dropper, microscope.

Reagent required: 3.8 % sodium citrate solution, 1% ether meth – silicon oil solution (1ml silicon oil, ether added to 100ml).

Methods

1. Take a rabbit. Draw blood with siliciferous injector from the heart of the rabbit.

2. Determination methods of platelet adhesiveness.

1) method: Place 2.7ml blood into siliciferous graduated test tube containing 0.3ml 3.8 % sodium citrate solution and shake it lightly. Take 1.5ml anti – coagulated blood and put it in 12ml spherical glass bottle. Fix spherical glass bottle on the rotating device of platelet adhesion apparatus. Rotate 15min with 3r/min. Let blood contact with bottle wall completely. Draw 1ml blood from spherical glass bottle (after adhesion) and test tube (before adhesion) separately after rotation and drip them in siliciferous graduated test tube containing 19ml 3.8% sodium citrate solution. Cover the opening of test tube with plastic film. Topple over 3 times. Make it homogenous. Place 2 hours at room temperature without moving. Wait red cell sinking. Take supernatant of test tube to count platelet numbers of adhesion before and after. Each sample is done twice. Take average of platelet numbers.

2) method: Take 1.8ml blood and place it into siliciferous graduated test tube containing 0.2ml 3.8% sodium citrate solution. Mix it to be hemogenous. Take 1ml anticoagulation blood with 1 ml siliciferous graduated pipette. Put blood into 8 ml spherical glass bottle with long neck. Fix spherical glass bottle on the rotating device of platelet adhesion apparatus. Rotate 15min with 3r/min at 37℃ constant thermostat. Determinate platelet numbers before and after adhesion. Count twice. Calculate average of platelet numbers.

Result

Calculate platelet numbers rate according to the following formula:

Platelet numbers rate (%) = (platelet numbers of adhesion front – platelet numbers of adhesion later) /platelet numbers of adhesion front ×100%

Notes

1. The glass instruments and injector needles of test used should be washed with 1% ether meth – silicon oil solution to be silicified except spherical glass bottle.

2. The volume of spherical glass bottle with long neck should be same in order to reduce effect of platelet adhesion rate due to the change of contacting area.

3. It is better to use sodium citrate solution、EDTA as anticoagulant. Proportion of anticoagulant and blood should be accurate.

4. Blood taking from vein and heart should not contain bubble and clot. After taking blood, the determination should be finished in 15 – 25min. Blood sample can not be placed for long time.

5. The counting of platelet should be accurate.

Evaluation

There are many determining methods of platelet adhesiveness. But the basic Principle is similar. Perfusion chamber method is advocated overseas, which is pumping blood into chamber of aoral wall without endothelium. Platelet adhesiveness is calculated according to numbers of platelet adhering with endothelium. The conditions of above method are similar with physiological or pathological state. But the method needs 50ml blood one time and its operation is complex. Rotating glass ball method、glass fiber method、glass fulcrum method and glass ball method are used in Chi-

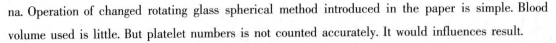
na. Operation of changed rotating glass spherical method introduced in the paper is simple. Blood volume used is little. But platelet numbers is not counted accurately. It would influences result.

Questions

1. Why do the glass ware used in test need to be silicified?

2. What is the basic Principle of determining platelet adhesiveness?

Experiment 5. 30　Determining method of platelet aggregation

Objective

Study experimental Principle and operation of platelet aggregation.

Principle

Adhering and aggregating interaction of platelets after endothelial injury is called platelet aggregation. Platelets usually are stimulated by inductions and then the aggregation takes place in vitro. There are many inducements of platelet aggregation such as ADP, collagen, thrombase, adrenaline and arachidonic acid. When activated degree of platelet increases, spontaneous aggregation may take place. Platelet aggregation has two phases. First phase represent forms of platelet aggregation. Second phase represent releasing reaction.

There are many kinds of determining methods of platelet aggregation such as ratio method, turbidimetric method and blood coagulation method. The turbidimetric method is commonly used. Its basic Principle is showed as follows:

Platelet rich plasma (PRP) is colloid. While Platelet is dispersing and turbid lightly in nature. Its concentration is relative to its platelet numbers. Accompanying stirring, put inducement (ADP、collagen、adrenaline) in, then platelets aggregate. Scattered platelet numbers and the concentration decrease, transmittance increases. So the concentration change of PRP show the degree of platelet aggregation. The concentration change of PRP can be transformed into photoelectric signal by photoelectric system of platelet aggregation apparatus and be recorded by record apparatus. Degree of platelet aggregation can be calculated by recording curve.

Materials

Animal required: 1 rat, 250 – 300g, male.

Equipment required: operating table and apparatus, platelet aggregation apparatus, steel or copper core glass stir rod. Centrifuge machine, siliciferous injector and graduated centrifugate tube.

Adenosion diphosphate (ADP): sodium ADP is mixed into 1mol/L ADP with 0. 1mol/L phosphate buffer solution (pH 7. 2) and pentobarbital sodium solution.

Methods

1. Weigh the rat. Anesthetize the rat with pentobarbital sodium solution. Fix the rat and separate its abdomen aorta. Take 5. 4ml blood from abdomen aorta with silicidized injector (9[#]number) and place it into test tube containing 0. 5ml 3. 8 % sodium citrate solution. Mix it lightly, Centrifuge it 5min with 1000r/min, draw 1ml supernatant, that is PRP, the rest is centrifuged 10min with 4000r/min again. The supernatant is PPP.

2. Count platelet numbers in PRP. If platelet numbers is too much, dilute PRP with PPP.

3. Preheat aggregation apparatus 15min before beginning. Take some PRP and PPP into turbidimetric tubes separately. Place turbidimetric tubes containing PPP into assay hole of aggregation apparatus. Adjust transmittance to 10. Repeat again until base line becomes steady. Place stir rod into PRP tube otherwise platelet will not aggregate. You may put Drugs or control solution in PRP tube.

4. Record a length of base line. Fill ADP into PRP tube. Observe the biggest aggregation degree of PRP within 5min. Calculate aggregation percent or drug inhibition percent.

Results

Calculate aggregation percent or drug inhibition percent according to the following formula.

The biggest aggregation percent = distance between the biggest aggregation of PRP and base line/90 × 100%

Platelet aggregation inhibition percent = (platelet aggregation of control tube % - platelet aggregation of drug tube %) / platelet aggregation of control tube % × 100%

Notes

1. Taking blood　Patient or volunteer tested should avoid using platelet function inhibitors such as aspirin before taking blood two weeks. Prohibit drinking milk, soybean milk that can affect transmittance at the same day of taking blood. Take blood quickly and accurately. Avoid repeating puncturing in order to mix tissue fluid into blood and activating platelet. It is better to take blood from abdomen aorta of rat or heart of rabbit. Internal time of taking blood and test should not be too long. Test after 2 hours blood taking is best. Should not surpass 4 hours or results would be affected.

2. Silicification　Silicidize all the glassware that touch blood, including injector, test tube, turbidimetric tube and stir rod.

3. Anticoagulant　Common anticoagulants used are sodium citrate, heparin and EDTA. But different anticoagulants affect differently on platelet aggregation. Comparing with sodium citrate, first phase reaction of PRP anti - coagulated and separated by heparin on ADP or adrenaline inducing aggregation is stronger. On the contrary, the second phase reaction of heparin PRP induced by adrenaline and aggregation induced by collagen is weaker than sodium citrate PRP. That may be because heparin inhibit releasing mechanism. EDTA has strong chelation, so it can combine with whole Calcium and magnesium ion in serum. Besides ristocetin leading to EDTA PRP aggregation, the other methods of induction can't lead to platelet aggregation without extra Calcium.

4. Temperature　Sample should be placed at room temperature of 15 - 25℃. Platelets will spontaneously aggregate under lower temperature. Temperature of aggregation apparatus should be controlled in 37℃ ±0. 1℃. If temperature is lower than 30℃, ADP and adrenaline can not induce second phase aggregation, that is called releasing reaction.

5. pH value　Suitable pH value is usually about 7. 5. It is better to have reaction in between pH 6. 8 - 8. 5. For example, ADP can induce shape change of platelet but can't induce aggregation when pH is lower than 6. 4 or higher than 10. 0. So change of pH value should be noticed when effect of drug on platelet aggregation is determined.

6. Platelet counting　Numbers of platelet counting affect the aggregation. The lower platelet counting is , the slower aggregation speed is, the biggest aggregation degree is also lower. For example, it is better that platelet counting scope of human, rabbit and rat PRP should be 20 - 25, 40 -

45 and 60 – 75 ten thousand/ ul respectively.

7. Inducer   ADP solution should be stored at – 20℃ in order to prevent spontaneous decomposition. Collagen solution is stored at 4℃. Adrenaline, nor – adrenaline and 5 – hydroxytryptamine can induce platelet aggregation of human, but they can't induce platelet aggregation of animals (rat, rabbit, guinea – pig and dog). The action mechanism of platelet induction differs. So it is better to take more than two kinds of inductions.

8. Drug color   For reducing the effect of drug color, relevant volume drug should be filled into blank tube as blank contrast.

Evaluation

Platelet aggregation is an important function of platelet. Many hereditary diseases cause unusual platelet aggregation. Increase of platelet aggregation can be taken as reference index of hypercoagulability diagnosing. Ratio method can be used to determine function of platelet aggregation in quantitative analysis. Its operation is simple. But the test method can't responses platelet aggregation state in body completely. There are many effects. Response degree of induction in " normal crowd" is different. Generally speaking, platelet aggregation rate reducing on diagnosing some diseases has significance. But platelet aggregation rate increasing has only reference value in clinic.

If the method is used as drug test in vitro, drug or control solution should be hatched for certain time with PRP at 37℃, contrary, test cab be made directly *in vivo*.

Questions

1. Do you use other instrument to replace platelet apparatus according to experimental Principle?

2. In the course of separating PRP, which effect will take place when red cells are drawn in?

Experiment 5. 31   Thrombus formation with arteriovenous shunt in rat

Objective

Study the method of thrombus formation with arteriovenous shunt in rat.

Principle

Blood platelets are not ordinarily adhesive in nature. However, vascular injury or exposure to rough surface which results in platelet clumping.

Link up the arteria vein with polyethylene tube, to produce bypass circulation. As the blood platelets touch the rough surface of thread, they will adhere the thread, then the thrombus is formed.

Platelet activation is an important step in the pathophysiology of acute arterial thrombosis and emboli. The anti – platelet effect of drug is useful for the prevention of strokes and myocardial infarction, as well as for the prevention of thrombus episodes.

Materials

Animal required: 1 rat, 250 – 300g, male.

Apparatus required: operating table, surgical instrument needed, arterial clip, polyethylene tube, surgical thread (No. 4).

Reagent required: 3% pentobarbital sodium solution, 50U/ml heparin, normal saline.

Methods

1. Intravenously inject pentobarbital sodium 30 – 40mg/kg into a raty. Fix the animal on the operating table, cut off the fur on the front of neck and open the skin along midline. Isolate and open the trachea and insert the tracheal cannula. Separate right common carotid artery and left external jugular vein. Clamp the right carotid artery with arterial clip.

2. Weigh a 7cm – length No. 4 surgical thread, put it into the middle part of 3 – segment polyethylene tube. Let 6cm – length thread in the tube, let 1cm – length be revealed from artery end of the tube.

3. Insert the venous end of the tube into the left external jugular vein, fill the tube with 50u/ml heparin Saline. Then insert the artery end of the tube into the right common carotid artery after injecting 1ml/kg heparin Saline for anticoagulative action.

4. Remove the arterial clip, make the blood move from the right common carotid artery to the polyethylene tube, and then flow into the left external jugular vein. 15 min later, stop the movement and take out the thread from the tube to weigh.

Results

Compare the thrombus weights of drug treatment group and control group.

Thrombus weight = total weight thread weight

Calculate the inhibitory rate:

Inhibitory rate (%) = (thrombus weight of control group – thrombus weight of administrated group) /thrombus weight of control group ×100%

Notes

1. Make sure the weight of animal of control group and that of administrated group is strictly same.

2. Size of polyethylene tube caliber should be identical and be closed joint part between 3 – segment polyethylene tubes to prevent leakage of blood.

3. Depth of anesthesia of each animal should be identical.

4. Operation process should be quick and skillful. The operation should be completed in 15 min.

5. Secretion of organ should be sucked in time to keep respiratory system unblocked.

6. Do not touch the vessel wall while taking thrombus out of the tube.

Evaluation

The method responds well to the function of platelet adhesion and aggregation in the animal body. Thrombus structure is similar to white thrombus in the artery. Which is similar to physiological and pathological conditions. The method is simple and convenient. Many kinds of animals can be used in the test. It can respond to inhibiting action of drug on blood platelet aggregation. If drug is given by Intravenous injection after thrombus formation, thrombus dissolution action of drug can be observed.

The formation of platelet is relative to velocity of blood flowing and platelet numbers, which should be taken care of in pharmaceutical analysis. The blood thrombus in the test is mixed thrombus. Besides anti – platelet drugs, anticoagulant can also inhibit thrombus formation.

Questions

1. Why should the animal weight of control group and that of administrated group be identical?

2. Why should the depth of anesthesia be identical?

Experiment 5. 32   The competitive antagonistic effect of diphenhydramine on histamine and the measurement of pA_2

Objective

1. Observe the competitive antagonistic effect of diphenhydramine on histamine in the isolated ileum preparation of Guinea pig.

2. Study the measurement and significance of pA_2.

Principle

An antagonist is a drug which can combine with the receptor reversibly, but it has no intrinsic activity. When the antagonist is present, the log dose – response curve is shifted to the right, but the E_{max} is unchanged, indicating that a higher concentration of agonist is necessary to achieve the same response when the antagonist is absent. In the presence of the antagonist, if enough agonist is given, the E_{max} can be achieved, indicating that the action of the antagonist has been overcome. This results in a parallel shift of the dose – response curve.

PA_2 is a index of the antagonist, which indicates the intensity of the anagonist. Two times concentration of agonist should be given to achive the active effect as before once given the antagonist. The negative logarithm of the mol concentration is PA_2.

PA_2 is not changed in different species or in different organs. The bigger PA_2 is, the more affintty with the receptor is. Different isoforms have different PA_2. So we use it to study the characterization of the isoforms.

The equilibria of the free receptor [R] with an agonist [A] and competitive antagonist [B] can be described by the reaction.

$$[R] + [A] \xrightleftharpoons{K_A} [AR]$$

$$K_A = \frac{[A] \cdot [R]}{[AR]} \tag{1}$$

$$[R] + [B] \xrightleftharpoons{K_B} [BR]$$

$$K_B = \frac{[B] \cdot [R]}{[BR]} \tag{2}$$

Where K_A and K_B are respectively equilibrium dissociation constants for complex formed between the receptor and agonist or antagonist, respectively. The total receptor population R_T is given by the sum of the free [R] and complex receptor.

Therefore $R_T = [R] + [AR] + [BR]$

$$\frac{R_T}{[AR]} = 1 + \frac{[BR]}{[AR]} + \frac{[R]}{[AR]} \tag{3}$$

From Eq. （1）and （2）

$$\frac{[BR]}{[AR]} = \frac{K_A}{K_B}\frac{[B]}{[A]}$$

$$\frac{[R]}{[AR]} = \frac{K_A}{[A]}$$

Substituting to Eq. （3）

$$\frac{[AR]}{R_T} = \frac{K_B[A]_B}{K_A K_B + K_A[B] + K_B[A]_B}$$

Assuming that　$[AR]/R_T$ is equal to E/E_{max}, then

$$\frac{E}{E_{max}} = \frac{[AR]}{R_T} = \frac{K_B[A]_B}{K_A K_B + K_A[B] + K_B[A]_B} \tag{4}$$

When the antagonist concentration is zero（$[B] = 0$）

$$\frac{E}{E_{max}} = \frac{[A]_0}{K_A[A]_0} \tag{5}$$

The value of the antagonist equilibrium dissociation constant can be determined from the concentrations of agonist producing equal responses in the absence （$[A]_0$）and presence （$[A]_B$）of antagonist.

$$\frac{[A]_0}{[A]_0 + K_A} = \frac{K_B[A]_B}{K_A K_B + K_A[B] + K_B[A]_B}$$

Which can be rearranged and reduced to

$[A]_B/[A]_0 - 1 = [B]/K_B$

If $[A]_B/[A]_0 = dr$ （dose ratio）$= 2$, then $1 = [B]/K_B$ $[B] = K_B$lg$[B] = lgK_B$

so $pA_2 = -$lgK_B and $pA_2 = -$lg$[B]$

Materials

Animal required: 1 guinea pig, 250 – 300g.

Equipment required: magrus glass organ-bath; force-displacement transducer. Recorder.

Reagent required: Tyrode's solution Histamine 3×10^{-5}M, 3×10^{-6}M in 5% NaH_2PO_4 solution.

Diphenhydramine Hydrochloride　6.85×10^{-5}M.

Methods

1. Kill the animal by a knock on the head. Then open the abdomen. A length of ileum is removed and placed in a dish containing Tyrode's solution. The length of the piece of ileum should be 1. 5 – 2 cm. A thread is attached to each end by inserting a needle from the inside of the gut outwards. The piece of ileum is tied in the organ bath and the load should be about 0. 5g.

2. Fill 10ml Tyrode's solution into the bath and mark the level. The organ – bath is heated to constant temperature of 37 ± 0.5℃. Connect the aerator to blow the air. Turn on the recorder and record a length of base line until the base line become steady.

3. Observe contraction of guinea – pig ileum up to maximal response by adding 3×10^{-6}mol/L

histamine solution using cumulative means, 0. 1ml each time. Add next dose of drug at once when the contraction plateau appears.

4. Wash histamine three times to allow the base line to become steady. Add 0. 02ml $6. 85 \times 10^{-5}$ mol/L diphenhydramine. 5 minutes later, repeat step 4 with 3×10^{-5} mol/L histamine solution. Thus, obtain the Dose – response curve in the presence of antagonist $[A]_B$.

Results

Record the strength of contraction to calculate the fractions of the maximal responses at different doses of histamine. Results are listed in following table (Table 5 – 11).

Plot log dose – response curve. Compare the slops and maximal responses to determine whether or not the action of antagonist is competitive.

Calculate pA_2 value in "three points" assay.

Pick out two points, r_1 and r_2, between 25 and 75 percent of maximal response in dose – response curve of agonist, and the corresponding doses are a_1 and a_2 respectively.

Select one point R between r_1 and in the dose – response curve in the presence of antagonist. The dose of agonist required to induce R in absence of antagonist is assumed to be A_0.

Table 5 – 11   The effect of drug on the isolated ileum of Guinea pig

Diphenhydramine (0)				Diphenhydramine ($1. 37 \times 10^{-7}$ mol/L)			
Histamine		Effect		Histamine		Effect	
C	$\lg C$	E	E/E_{max}	C	$\lg C$	E	E/E_{max}

Notes

Keep the volume of Tyrode's solution in organ – bath constant to avoid alteration of drug concentration.

Add next dose of drug at once when the contraction pleateu appears.

Evaluation

Cumulative dose method is used to give drugs in the test. Dose is increased from lower to higher. Dose-response curve can be obtained in short time. The method can be grasped easily. Two dose-response curves are needed in "three points". Although the method is a coarse one and the accuracy is inferior, the method is still widely used in calculation of pA_2.

Questions

Try to describe the definition and significance of pA_2.

Are there effects on pA_2 with changing of Tyrode's solution volume in Magrus glass organ – bath?

Chapter 6   Experiments of anti-inflammatory drugs

Inflammation is a common clinical symptom. In the pharmacological research, some factitious interference (such as physical irritation, chemical irritation and biological irritations etc) is done on laboratory animals to simulate the occurrence, development and treatment of inflammation in humans. However, it is very difficult to make a perfect animal inflammatory model because inflammation is a quite complicated pathological and physiological process. At present an anti – inflammatory drug is screened mainly according to its effects on many models by overall observation, analysis and evaluation.

Making inflammatory models needs considering many factors related to experimental requirements such as choice of animal species, that of inflammatory factors, that of the marker and the control of observation and environment etc. In general, mammals are often used in experiments and animal species are chosen according to different models. For instance, rats are chosen for the model of tumescence of the foot and guinea pigs are usually chosen for the allergic inflammation. Various irritants have different mechanisms; however, these irritants are approximately divided into the physical, the chemical and the biological ones. The ideal stimulating factor should be precisely quantified, it should be reliable, it should act unvaryingly, it should have few interindividual variations of animals, and it should have a long action duration. The factors, which should be chosen objectively and are easily used in the statistics, mainly include the magnitude of tumescence, capillary permeability, leukocyte migration, granuloma formation etc. This chapter will briefly introduce the common experimental methods of anti – inflammatory drugs based on the research of primary pharmacodynamics, the discussion of general mechanism and the explanation of molecular mechanism.

Experiment 6. 1   Effect on intraabdominal capillary permeability of mouse by injection of hydrocortisone

Objective

Observe the effect on intraabdominal capillary permeability of mouse by injection of glucocorticoids

Principle

Glucocorticoids at pharmacological dosage have the anti – inflammatory effect, antitoxic effect, anti – shock and anti – immune actions. To observe the hormonal anti – inflammatory action, the method is taken as follows: induce the topical inflammation at the skin of back or belly, at eye or peritoneal cavity with the appropriate irritants, then inject intravenously Evan's blue dye, observe how the glucocorticoids inhibit the dye effusing, and determine quantitatively the dye exuding from the inflamed tissues by colorimetry.

Materials

Animal required: 10 mice, 18 − 22g, male or female.

Apparatus required: centrifuge, spectrophotometer.

Reagent required: 0.5% Evan's blue dye (dissolved in normal saline), 0.5% hydrocortisone, 0.6% acetic acid solution, normal saline.

Methods

1. Ten mice are weighed and divided into two groups randomly (control and treatment group). Hydrocortisone (0.5%, 20mg/kg) is subcutaneously injected in the treatment group and the same volume of the normal saline to the control group.

2. 30 minutes later, 0.5% Evan's blue (10ml/kg) is intravenously injected into the mice's tail, then 0.6% solution of acetic acid per mice 0.2ml is injected into the peritoneal cavity of two groups.

3. 30 minutes later, the mice are killed with the dislocation of cervical vertebra and their peritoneal cavity is opened.

4. The mice's abdominal cavities are repeatedly washed and the washing liquid is collected to 5ml and centrifuged at 3000rpm for 5min.

5. The absorbance of extract of the supernatant liquid is measured at the maximum of 590nm. Content of Evan's blue dye of the solution each ml in peritoneal cavity is calculated with the standard curve.

6. Calculate the average of each group and carry out T test. Normalize the dye permeability of the control group as one hundred percent, calculate the inhibitory rate of the exudates in the treating group.

Results

Calculate the inhibition percentage according to subsequent equation and fill in the table

Inhibition rate = (dye permeability of control group − dye permeability of treating group) / dye permeability of control group

Table 6 − 1   Effect on capillary permeability by injection of hydrocortisone

group	animal number	dosage (mg/kg)	dye permeability (μg/ml)	(inhibition rate)%
Hydrocortisone				
Control				

Notes

1. The injection site of acetic acid in the peritoneal cavity should be the same and pay attention to injecting into the peritoneal cavity or false − negative results will be obtained.

2. When the mouse peritoneal cavity is opened, the hemorrhage resulted from the lesion of blood vessels should be avoided, otherwise the result will be affected by amount of the exudates of the dye in the peritoneal cavity.

3. The eluant should be discarded if it is a turbid gel.

Evaluation

1. According to the same principle, the capillary permeability of the skin back or belly of the mouse can be observed. Although it is a little complicated, it has the same significance with current experiment.

2. Because any substance able to damage tissues can become an inflammatory factor, the actions of inhibitors are nonspecific.

Question

What are the characteristics and mechanism of the anti – inflammatory action of glucocorticoids?

Experiment 6. 2　Effect of indomethacin on auricular tumescence induced by croton oil in mice

Objective

Grasp the fundamental method of anti – inflammatory experiments.

Principle

Indomethacin can dramatically inhibit the prostaglandin synthesis and release of prostaglandin synthetase, thus it has a good therapeutic effect on the nonspecific inflammation induced by many factors.

Materials

Animal required: 4 mice, 18 – 22g, male or female.

Apparatus required: 8mm pin – hole plotter, torsion balance.

Reagent required: 0. 5% indomethacin, 1% CMC suspension, 2% croton oil mixture (2% corton oil, 2% anhydrous ethanol, 73% ethyl ether, 5% distilled water) .

Methods

1. Four mice are weighed and divided into two groups randomly (control and treatment group). Give 0. 5% indomethacin (50mg/kg) for the control group by intraperitoneal injection and the same volume of CMC (10ml/kg) for the treating group.

2. 30 minutes later, two groups are induced inflammation at the bilateral of the auricle of the right ears by the steady application of 2% croton oil mixture 0. 05ml with microsyringe, let the left ears be control.

3. 30 minutes later, kill the mice and take the ears along the auricled basic line. Take a piece of ear from the same location of each ear respectively by the pin – hole plotter and weigh them.

4. The magnitude of ear tumescence is defined as that the difference between the weight of the control side and that of the inflamed side.

Results

According to the requirements, collect the data of each group to take statistics　(referred to experiment 6 – 1) .

Notes

1. The environmental temperature should be over 15℃. It should be higher if the irritant is xy-

lene.

2. Collect the materials from the same location as far as possible.

3. The hole – digger should be sharp.

Evaluation

The method is easy and feasible without special instruments, and it is sensitive to two kinds of anti – inflammatory drugs and suitable for screening drugs at the same time.

Questions

1. What are the two kinds of anti – inflammatory drugs?

2. What are the functional characteristics of indomethacin?

Experiment 6. 3　Effect of indomethacin on tumescence produced in the hind paw of the rat by injecting carragheenin

Objective

To study the usual method of estimating tumescence in the hind paw of the rat

Principle

Among the many methods used for screening and evaluation of anti – inflammatory drugs, one the of the most commonly employed techniques is based upon the ability of such reagents, which inhibit the tumescence produced in the hind paw of the rat by injecting a phlogistic reagent. The most frequently used phlogistic reagents include brewer's yeast, formalin, dextran, egg albumin and carragheen. For the inflammation caused by local use of carragheen, the synthesis of prostaglandin is apparently increased, together with histamine and bradykinin, which deteriorate the tumescence of inflammatory tissues. Phlogistic reaction mainly mediated by prostaglandin is obviously inhibited by indomethacin.

Materials

Animal required: 4 rats, 120 – 150g, male.

Apparatus required: outside micrometer.

Reagent required: 0. 2% indomethacin (suspended in 1% CMC), 1% carragheen (dissolved in sterilized normal saline, stored at 4℃).

Methods

1. Divide four rats into two groups. the control group and the treatment one. Indomethacin 0. 1ml (0. 2%, 20mg/kg) is intraperitoneally given to the latter and the same volume of CMC to the former.

2. 30 minutes later, measure the thickness of rat's right hind paw with the outside micrometer. Then give 1% carragheenin 0. 1ml by subcutaneous injection to induce inflammation.

3. Measure swollen paw respectively at 30, 60, 120, 180 and 240min after the administration of carrragheenin (Fig. 6 – 1).

Results

The swollen degree is the difference between the thickness of rat hind paw with inflammation and before treatment. Calculate the means and the standard deviation of the swollen degree and carry

扫码"学一学"

out statistical analysis. Chart a time – response, which is figured with time as abscissa and swelling as ordinat.

Notes

1. 1% carragheenin should be prepared the day before use and be put into the refrigerator over night.

2. The site for measuring swollen thickness and the use of outside micrometer should be kept ‐ constant.

3. Rats with body weight of 120 – 150g are sensitive to phlogistic materials, its tumescence is significant, and the difference is little.

Evaluation

It is the most extensive inflammatory tumescence model with the advantages of little difference, high sensitivity and repeatability etc. But owing to its low specificity, the method is effective on many non – anti – inflammatory drugs. Besides outsider micrometer, special soft ruler can also be used to measure the circumference of tumescence region and the volume of paw. Those methods possess respective merits, so no uniform method is available at present. The titer of some anti – inflammatory drugs acquired with the model are basically consistent with clinical experiments, thus primary positive results of drugs can be further measured with this model.

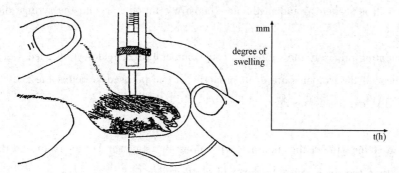

Fig. 6 – 1　Measure of tumescence magnitude of rat's paw with an outside micrometer

Question

1. Discuss the different anti – inflammatory actions between the indomethacin and hydrocortisol.

2. What should be noticed in the experiment?

3. The tumescence induced by carragheenin has two – phase process, what substance is released mainly in each phase?

Experiment 6. 4　Effect of drugs on the experimental pleuritis

Objective

Use *in vivo* method to observe the effect of drugs on leukocyte migration.

Principle

The injection of carragheenin into the rat's pleural cavity will cause serious inflammatory exude from the pleural cavity in which a lot of leukocytes aggregate. Because the exudate of pleural cavity can be easily collected with little contamination, it can be used for further study of the anti – inflammatory drugs.

Materials

Animal required: 4 rats, 180 – 220g, male.

Reagent required: 0. 5% carragheen, 0. 2% pentobarbital sodium.

Methods

1. Four rats are taken and divided into treatment and control group.

2. To grasp the skin of the nape of the conscious rat with the back fixed on the palm and the chest upword. Sterilize the right side chest wall with 75% ethonal, inject the anti – inflammatory drugs (such as above – mentioned indomethacin or cortisol) in the midclavicular line, which is the location of breast. After 30min, inject 0. 5% carragheen in the pleural cavity to inflame. Administrating every 4h or only once in whole process is determined by the potency of drug and duration time.

3. After 8 – 12h (a large amount of exudates aggregating in the pleural cavity) of the inflammation, anesthetiz the rat by injecting 0. 2% pentobarbital sodium (40mg/kg) in the peritoneal cavity, and then kill the rat by cutting the abdominal aorta.

4. Open the pleural cavity, get the exudates from the bilateral pleural cavity with the pipette whose inside – wall is soaked by indomethacin – heparin solution (or with the syringe directly).

Results

After calculating precisely the exudates, count numeration of leukocyt at once. Get the exudates to stain and smear. If the exudates are dealt properly, it can be used to detect the activity of β – glycuronidase, TXB_2 and 6 – keto – PGF.

Notes

1. When injecting, inject the pleural cavity along the superior border of the costa, and inject slightly deeper than the thick muscular layer of chest wall.

2. The exudates containing blood should be discarded.

Evaluation

1. The two kinds of anti – inflammatory drugs are both effective on the inflammatory exudation.

2. The steroids have more intensive inhibition of cell migration.

3. The method requires accurate and skilled operations.

4. The method is mainly used to further study the drugs effective in the primary screening.

Question

Compare the different effects of the two kinds of anti – inflammatory drugs on inflammatory exudation.

Chapter 7　Experiments of chemotherapeutic drugs

The concept of chemotherapy was firstly introduced by Ehrlich in 1908. The drugs that can kill pathogen and parasite or inhibit their growth and breeding either *in vivo* or *in vitro* all belong to the category of chemotherapy. But only those drugs, which merely exert effects on pathogen or parasite without notable toxicity on the human body, can be used as general chemotherapeutic drugs in clinical practice.

Prontosil has no anti – streptococcus effect in the test tube, but it can decompose to sulfanilamide in the body, which has the antibacterial activity. Enlightened by that, a series of sulfanilamide derivatives are synthesized one after another, by which many systemic infections can be controlled, and it also opens up many new fields in the pharmacology. As early as 1929, Fleming reported that contamination of penicillium can inhibit the growth of staphylococcus, which leads to the discovery of penicillin. Because penicillin has high effect and low toxicity, many researchers transfer their attention to the research of antibiotics. Now, antibiotics play an important role in the prevention and cure of infectious diseases. Synthesis of sulfanilamide by Domagk, discovery of penicillin by Fleming and successful separation of streptomycin by Waksman started the golden period of drug development history. Because of their prominent contribution, the three people were awarded Nobel Prize respectively in 1939, 1945, and 1952.

Malignant tumor is one of the most health – threatening diseases at present. More than 6,000,000 people are killed by cancer every year in the world. It has taken half the century and lots of resources to investigate anticancer drugs. Now, the number of confirmable anticancer drugs is over 310. Tumor treatment is changing from palliative treatment to permanent control. But the most protrudent problem is the severe toxicity and poor selectivity. Tumor is still one of the most intractable diseases. Conquering tumor has become a common wish of all people and a hard task for drug researchers.

I . Antibacterial experiment

To observe whether a substance has the antibacterial effect, we screen *in vitro* firstly, then verify *in vivo* on the positive findings.

【*In vitro* test】

The common methods to assay bacteriostasis of drugs are agar osmotic method and tube dilution method.

1. Agar osmotic method　In agar osmotic method, the trial strain is mixed with agar culture medium and decanted into plates; or spread trial strain on the surface of agar plates; then put drugs on the agar plate containing the trial strain by various methods. Because drugs can permeate into agar culture medium, we can observe and judge whether drugs have an effect on the trial strain

after cultivating in optimal temperature. We can also blend drugs into agar culture medium then inoculate the trial strain.

It includes filter paper method, digging hole method, slip of paper method, trenching method, channel& saucer method and plate dilution method, according to different ways to add drugs. Among them, filter paper method, paper slip method, trenching method are used for qualitative assay, channel& saucer method, plate dilution method are used for quantitative assay, and digging hole method can be used for either of them according to specific situations.

(1) Qualitative assay

1) Filter paper method: Add molten broth agar culture medium into a sterile plate, use it as bottom layer after its coagulation. Cool proper molten broth agar culture medium to about 50℃, then add certain amount of the trial bacterium solution to it, shake evenly and take 4 – 5ml as superior layer on the bottom layer, put till its coagulation. Moisten sterile filter paper with the drug solution and paste it on the surface of the culture medium; cultivate it in a proper temperature for a certain time. Get it out and observe results (Fig. 7 – 1).

The most marked character of this method is that it is convenient and quick for test, and can test many exponents at one plate. This method is suitable for initial screening of drugs, that is, one bacterium for many drugs.

Note: the bacterium selected as the trail strain should be susceptible to the exponent. Control the concentration of the trail strain and the temperature of the agar, when preparing the plat containing the bacterium.

2) Trenching method and slip of paper method: Prepare the sterile agar plate first, then trench in the centre of the plate, inoculate various trail strains apart at both sides of the trough, distance some space between every two strains. Add exponent to the trough, cultivate at 37℃ for 18 – 24h, then take out and observe the result (Fig. 7 – 2). Slip of paper method is similar to trenching method; just change the trough to the paper slip containing the drug solution.

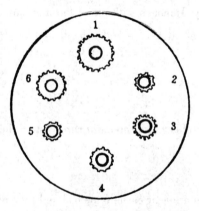

Fig. 7 – 1 Screen antibacterials by cup&channel in plat method, holing method or slipping of paper method

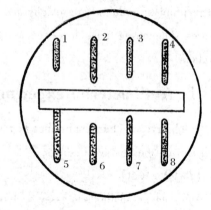

Fig. 7 – 2 Screen antibacterials by trenching method or slip of paper method

The most marked character of this method is that it can detect the antimicrobial spectrum of drugs quickly, that is, one drug for many strains.

Inter ring is cup & channel, hole, or slip of paper, extra ring is bacteriostasis ring.

(2) Quantitative assay   Use plate dilution method: dilute drug to a series of concentrations according to ratio dilution method, that is 1 : 2、1 : 4、1 : 8···, then add these drug solutions (2ml/plate) into sterile plates, add MH culture medium cooling to about 50℃ (18ml/plate), shake to homogeneity, and cool for reserve. The final dilution concentration of drug is 1 : 20, 1 : 40, 1 : 80···

Preparation of the trial bacteria solution : Inoculate various trial bacteria at MH broth culture media packed with the fixed quantity (except special bacterium, such as pneumonia diplococcus, Streptococcus, etc), cultivate them at a proper temperature for 8 – 10h, then take them out and dilute them in certain ratios (between 1 : 100 to 1 : 1000). Compare the turbidity with turbidimetry before diluting, the concentration of bacterium should be 10^8 – 10^9 CFU, then dilute them for use. Special bacterium should be added with a small quantity of serum (rabbit serum or caprine serum) when cultivated.

Inoculate 2μl of the diluted bacterium solution on plates containing drugs. At this time the final quantity of live bacteria is 10^3 – 10^4 CFU. After cultivating at 37℃ for 18 – 24h, these plates should be taken out and observe the growth state of bacterium one by one. Record the highest dilution degree with no bacterium, which is the test drug's minimal inhibitory concentration (MIC) to the trial strain.

The result of the plate dilution method is of the high accuracy and doesn't need a lot of time, with low rate of pseudo – positive, and what's more, it is not easily to appear the leaping tube phenomena. This method can show the growth state of bacterium and the effect of drugs directly. And it can test one drug with many bacteria, save drugs and culture media. According to the present request for the antibiotic application, this method is very suitable and convenient. So it is widely used in assaying the antibacterial activity *in vitro* of antibiotics at present.

In the middle is the trough or paper slipping with drug, at the two sides are the growth state 8 bacterium inoculated with streaking method

Now, the examination and approval of new chemotheraputic drugs is much more strict. Trial strain used must be detached in clinical, and is ruled clearly in number and species. For the new drug in class I, the number of trial strains must be above 1000, and over 20 species are required; For class II, the number of trial strains must be above 500, and also over 20 species are required; for class III and IV, the number of trial strains must be above 200, and over 20 species are required. Thus, the plate dilution method shows its superiority. This method is a specified pharmacodynamic method of assaying the antibacterial activity in vitro for the examination and approval of new drugs. The strain used in this experiment must be in the logarithmic growth period, because in this period bacteria are the most sensitive to drugs. The concentration of the trial strains must be properly controlled, or the results will be affected.

[Attached] MH culture medium, that is hydrolytic casein agar culture medium, is in common use internationally.

2. Tube dilution method   Dilute drug with broth culture medium to a series of concentration according to ratio dilution method, that is 1 : 2、1 : 4、1 : 8···, put 2ml of each concentration of the drug – containing culture medium into sterile test tubes, in each tube add 0. 1ml 1 : 1000 dilution of the sensitive bacterium in logarithm growth period and mix it to homogeneity.

A tube with no drugs is a positive controlling group, a tube with no drugs or bacterium dilution is negative controlling (objective: check if culture medium was contaminated by bacterium). Put them in 37℃ incubator to culture for 24 hours, then observe the result, record the bacterium growth state of each tube. The value of the highest dilution degree of no bacterium clarification is the minimal inhibitory concentration (MIC) (Fig. 7 – 3).

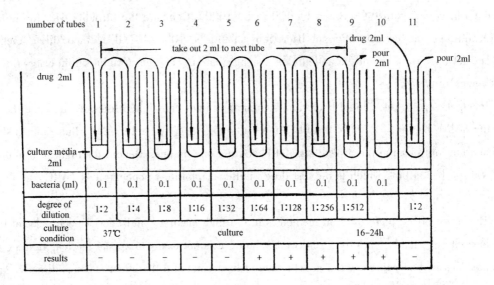

number of tubes	1	2	3	4	5	6	7	8	9	10	11
bacteria (ml)	0.1	0.1	0.1	0.1	0.1	0.1	0.1	0.1	0.1	0.1	
degree of dilution	1:2	1:4	1:8	1:16	1:32	1:64	1:128	1:256	1:512		1:2
culture condition	37℃				culture				16–24h		
results	–	–	–	–	–	+	+	+	+	+	–

Fig. 7 – 3   This method operates tediously, needs much work and culture medium is easy to present pseudo – positive, and appear leaping tube phenomena, which influence the accuracy of results.

[Attached]   the method to prepare the common culture medium

1) Meat dip solution: Take fresh beef, remove muscle tendon and fat, smash it into mince and add 3000ml water per1000g, mix it to make it full even. Soak at 2 – 10℃ for 20 – 24h, then boil for 1h, filter, squeeze the meat dregs, and complement the volume of the solution. Process with 15pound autoclaving for 20 minutes, and then put it in cold storage for use. Beef extract 3g, added water 1000ml and dispensed to solution can also be used as the substitution.

2) Broth culture medium: Take peptone 10g, NaCl 5g, add them into 1000ml of the meat dip solution. Adjust PH to 7. 6 with 0. 1mol/L NaOH, after thawing. Then boil it for 10 minutes, filter after cooling.   And then process with 15pound autoclaving for 20 minutes.

3) Broth agar culture medium: Take peptone 10g, NaCl 5g, agar 20g, add them into 1000ml of the meat dip solution. Filter after thawing, adjust pH to 7. 6, then process with 15pound autoclaving for 20 minutes.

【*In vivo* test】

The drugs showing antibacterial effects *in vitro* perhaps have no effects in vivo because of toxicity, binding to proteins, or biotransformation. So, to the drugs which have effects *in vitro*, we should test whether they have effects on infected animals. Only when a drug also has effect *in vivo* with little toxicity, can it be tested in clinical trials.

1) Preparation of bacterium solution: Select the strain of high virulence and sensitivity to certain drugs in the preserved typical strains or clinical detached pathogenic bacteria, transferring it into liquid medium, and cultivate it at 37℃ for infecting animals.

2) Infecting animals: Select the animal according to the pathogenicity of the strain. Mice of 20g are commonly used. Infect animals by bacterial solution ip. , the dose of which should kill over 90% of mice. Mice are not sensitive to staphylococcus aureus and dysentery bacillus, so add proper quantity of gastric mucosin to raise the pathogenicity.

3) Grouping and administration: Divide the infected mice into several groups, treat every group with the test drug, except one control group. The dose of drug should not exceed the maximum tolerance dose of mice. In general, at 1, 6 and 12 hours after infection, the drug should be given orally or in injection seperately, or pre – administrate before infective inoculation.

4) Result judgment: Usually count the number of dead mice in each group at 72 hours after infective inoculation and make statistics. If the death rate of treatment group is notably lower than that of the control group, it shows the drug's utility. We can verify results with other animals and take other relational pharmacological experiments.

Experiment 7. 1　Assay the antibacterial activity *in vitro* of norfloxacin, ofloxacin and cinrofloxacin

Objective

Comprehend the procedure of plate dilution method and slip of paper method in testing the antibacterial effects of drugs. Observe the influence of different drug concentrations on the antibacterial effects. Comprehend the operation process and the evaluation of the result.

Principle

Norfloxacin, ofloxacin, and cinrofloxacin belong to the third generation of quinolone synthetic antibacterials, which has wide antimicrobial spectra, high efficacy, and little adverse effects, especially, it has great antibacterial effects on pseudomonas pyocyanea and other anaerobes. These drugs can mainly combine to subunit A of DNA spiral enzyme, accordingly inhibit the cutting and connecting function of enzyme, restrain the replication of DNA, and present their antibacterial effects.

Materials

Bacterium required: Bacterium solution of staphylococcus aureus (or Escherichia coli) after cultivating for 16 – 18h.

Apparatus required: MH agar culture medium, sterile plat, sterile filter paper (diameter 0. 5cm), forceps, sterile saline, sterile test tube, sterile straws (5ml), micropipette, broth culture medium, and slide gauge.

Reagent required: 80μg/ml solution of norfloxacin, ofloxacin, and cinrofloxacin.

1. Slip of paper method

Methods

1. Put the sterile plate base upward, draw three radial lines on the base and divide it into 6 parts, mark 1 – 6 on each part.

2. Take test bacterium solution 0.1ml quantitatively with sterile straws, add it to 100ml agar culture medium, which has been kept at 45℃ temperature, shake to even, then decant it into sterile plate, cool it for use.

3. Dilute drug to a series of concentration with sterile saline, according to ratio dilution method, and lay it up for use.

4. Take sterile filter paper slips by forceps, moisten them apartly with drug solution of different concentrations, and then paste them on the surface of culture medium according to certain places marked in advance.

5. Cultivate the Petri dishes in incubator at 37℃ for 24h, then observe the results. Measure the diameter (mm) of bacteriostatic ring in each slip.

Results

Record the result in Table 7 – 1.

Table 7 – 1　The result of assaying the *in vitro* antibacterial activity（slip of paper method）

No. of slip	1	2	3	4	5	6
Drug solutions and their concentration						
Diameter of bacteriostasis ring（mm）						

Notes

1. When preparing the plate containing bacterium, agar must be kept at proper temperature and the quick operation is needed to get uniform coagulating.

2. Keep proper distance between the slips, when pasting them on the culture medium. And note numbers at proper place on the bottom of the plates, previously.

3. Make the volume of drug solution coincident as possible as you can, otherwise the test results will be erroneous.

Evaluation

The biggest advantage of this method is that it is convenient, quick and a great quantity of agents at one time. We can test norfloxacin, ofloxacin, cinrofloxacin and even more exponents in a staphylococcus aureus plate at the same time. Work as one bacterium to screen many drugs.

Question

1. In which conditions, the filter slip method can be used?

2. According to the result, compare the effect of several Quinolone drugs.

2. Plate dilution method

Methods

1. Dilute the bacterium solution (1 : 100), after culturing for 12h, and shake evenly for use.

2. Dilute drug to a series of concentrations with sterile saline, according to ratio dilution meth-

od, that is 1 : 1, 1 : 2, 1 : 4, 1 : 8···

3. Add drugs of various concentrations to sterile plates (2ml/plat), then decant MH culture medium (18ml/plat), which has been cooled to about 50℃, shake evenly, and the final concentrations are 1 : 10, 1 : 20, 1 : 40, 1 : 80. Lay it up for coagulation.

4. Add 2µl bacteria solutions with micropipette to the plate, lay it up for flowing evenly After 20 minutes, incubate in incubator at 37℃ for 18 – 24h. Then take it out and observe the result, record the highest dilution degree with no bacterium as the MIC.

Results

Record the result in Table 7 – 2.

Table 7 – 2   The result of assaying the in vitro antibacterial activity (Plate dilution method)

Drug \ Concentration	1	2	3	4	5	6	7	control
1								
2								
3								

Notes

1. Must shake quickly when add MH culture medium into plats, otherwise it will be coagulated to cause drug divergence uneven.

2. The test bacteria solution must be sensitive bacteria in logarithm growth period.

3. The control group is required.

4. The surface of desk to place the plate must be flat.

Evaluation

Plate dilution method is widely used in assaying the in vitro antibacterial activity of antibiotics at present. The method is convenient, reasonable, accurate, rapid and causes less false – positive. It can show directly the bacterial growth condition and drug action.

Question

Discuss the anti – bacterial Principle of Norfloxacin.

Experiment 7. 2   The protective test of norfloxacin on *in vivo* infcction of mice

Objective

Comprehend the basic procedure of the treatment of the bacterial infection test, and the basic method of *in vivo* test of pharmacodynamics. Observe the effects of Norfloxacin (Quinolone drug) on infected mice.

Materials

Animal required: mice 12, 18 – 20g, male or female would all be used.

Apparatus required: syringe, scale, mouse cage, sterile cotton.

Reagent required: bitter acid, bacterium solution, saline, Norfloxacin (3mg/kg), 2.5% iodine tincture, 70% alcohol, Escherichia coli solution diluted with 5% gastric mucin.

Methods

1. Take 12 mice, mark, weigh them and divide them into 6 groups (2 mice/group, 5 group are administered and 1 group is control).

2. Decide the concentration of drug: make the concentration of given drug as medium dose and set 2 doses upward and 2 doses downward with ratio of 1 : 0.7, to form 5 dose groups. Control group is administered with saline. Inject every mouse with 0.5ml bacterium solution by ip., according to weight, administer the drug once by ig. at right. Then observe and record the death state of mice during 72h.

Results

Calculate the mortality and get ED_{50} by statistics.

Notes

1. The concentration of drugs must be pretested, and proceed with the experiment after finding out the proper concentration. The trial strain must be detached in clinical trials and with strong toxicity.

2. The trial strain must be protected with gastric mucin otherwise the test result will be affected.

3. The drug concentration must be strictly controlled, and should not be change it abruptly The dose administered must be enough, or the result will be affected.

4. The weight of animals should be controlled, otherwise the result will be affected.

5. Manage the bacteria-carrying animals carefully, and prohibit their escaping. Incinerate cadavers of animals or put them into the jar containing 5% carbonic acid after experiment. The live animal should be killed immediately and disposed properly. Wipe to dry with tincture of iodine or alcohol, and wash hands with soap, after experiment, in order to prevent disseminating disease. Sterilize all the equipment and supplies contacted with bacteria.

Evaluation

Having effects *in vitro* is the premise of *in vivo* test, and having effects *in vivo* in the base of clinical experiment. If the drug has apparent effects on infected mice, verify it with other animals, and make further tests of pharmacology and toxicology to prove that it has apparent effects and little toxicity. In this way, we can possibly prepare a new antibacterial drug. So the protective test of infection is a key point. This method is reliable, with high repetition, and can reflect the effect of the drug objectively.

Question

1. What is the fundamental mechanism of therapeutics in experimental bacterial infection?

2. Can we confirm that norfloxacin has effects on escherichia coli infection of mice in this experiment? Based on what?

II. Experiments of antitumor drugs

The screening methods of antitumor drugs are various and can be divided into *in vivo* methods and *in vitro* methods. Each method has its advantages and disadvantages, so it's hard to confirm the anticancer effect of a drug by only one of them. If the sample is small, we can screen with the inhibitory effect on external cultivated cell strains. It is possible to find if the drugs have effects on a certain cancers, when choosing this human cancer strain as screening sample. *In vitro* test can only be used in initial screening, and the anticancer effect of one drug can only be judged by *in vivo* test.

1. *In vivo* test Up to now, animal graft tumor test is a commonly used method, which is more feasible than spontaneous or induced animal tumor test. In this method, mass steady tumor can be obtained simultaneously, which can be used in the treatment and the control. But animal graft tumor has much difference in biological behavior with human tumor. It has higher malignancy, grow rapidly, and has much higher drug susceptibility than the human tumor. This method has low percentage of hits.

At present, commonly used experimental animal tumor strains can be divided into ascites cancer, sarcoma, and leukemia. From domestic viewpoint, we ever used S_{180} (mice sarcoma 180), ascites cancer, and L_{615} leukemia. American National Cancer Institute (NCI) has recommended to use P_{388} (leukemia), L_{1210} (leukemia), W_{256} (rat carcinosarcoma), B_{16} (melanoma), and 3LL (Lewis pulmonary carcinoma), several years ago.

It is obviously unsuitable to screen all types of new drugs with one model, because the sensitivity of drug to various animal graft tumors are different. When screening alkylating agent, we can use W_{256}, or sarcoma; when screening antimetabolites, we can use S_{180}, L_{615}, or L_{1210}; when searching for new anticancer drugs from natural products, we can use P_{388}, L_{615}, ascites cancer, or U_{14}, etc.

2. *In vitro* test Making short or long terms culture of human or animals' tumor cells as screening system to observe the anti - tumor effect of drugs is the methods with many advantages such as convenience, little dosage, getting result quickly and massive screening etc. But the method is different from the *in vivo* test, so it can't show the relations of effects, toxicity and metabolism. It shows false - positive and false - negative errors usually. Thus *in vitro* test must be taken with *in vivo* test. The main methods of in vitro test comprise:

1) Contact staining: After adding the drug to the animal's ascites cancer cells diluted solution, the dead cancer cells can be stained by trypan blue at 37℃ in 24h because of the change of membrane permeability, While the vital cells can't be stained. We can identify and count with microscope, regard more than 50% staining rate as effective initial screening.

2) Methylene blue reduction method: Cancer cells contain dehydrognase that can transmit hydrogen from substrate to methylene blue, which reduce Methylene blue to fade. If tumor cells are killed by drugs, the activity of dehydrognase disappears, so methylene blue can't fade. The method is convenient but non - specific because common cells also have dehydrognase.

3) Respiratory depression method: Determine the aerobic metabolism inhibitory rate of drugs on tumor cells by tissue respiration meter, and regard more than 50% rate as effective initial screening.

4) Tissue culture method: Add drugs to artificial cultured animal's cancer cells, especially the human's, in order to observe the effect on cells, the number of cells and the morphologic change.

In addition, the non - tumor system such as spermatogenous cell, bacteriophage can be used for anti - tumor drug screening.

Experiment 7. 3　Methylene blue tube method of screening anti – tumor drug primarily

Objective

Understand an *in vitro* test method for anti – tumor drugs——methylene blue tube method.

Principle

The activity of dehydrognase is related to the function of cancer cells. The anti – cancer drugs, when inhibiting or killing cancer cells, usually cause the decrease and disappearance of the activity of dehydrognase, which can be showed by methylene blue indicator. Living cancer cells' dehydrogenase can convert hydrogen to methylene blue to make it fade, while dead cancer cells' dehydrogenase is inactive and can't reduce methylene blue. Judging by the aforementioned Principle, we can primarily verdict whether a drug has anticancer effects.

Materials

Animal required: Anshi Ascites cancer (EAC) mice 1 – 2, weight, male or female.

Apparatus required: sterile tube, sterile straw, incubator.

Reagent required: 1% and 10% 5 – FU solution, 0. 05% methylene blue, test drug solution. Tumor cells culture solution (contain 0. 8% NaCl, 0. 02% KCl, 0. 02% CaCl$_2$, 0. 01 MgCl$_2$, 0. 05% NaHCO$_3$, 0. 005% NaH$_2$PO$_4$, 0. 1% glucose, pH 7. 0 – 7. 5). The solutions are sterilized.

Methods

1. Take the EAC mice which have been inoculated 8 – 10 days ago, draw ascites by aseptic manipulation, and dilute it with tumor cells nutrient solutions at ratio of 1∶2.

2. Take 8 sterile test tubes, add tumor cells nutrient solutions 0. 75ml and 1∶2 ascites diluted solutions 0. 25ml in each tube. Then add substances mentioned below respectively: 0. 1ml of tumor cells nutrient solution into two tubes (control), 1% and 10% 5 – FU solutions each into two tubes, the test drug into two tubes. Keep temperature at 37℃ in constant temperature oven for 4h, add 0. 05% methylene blue solutions 0. 2ml in each tube, and then go on to keep temperature at 37℃. Observe and record the color of each tube at the time interval of 2h, 4h, 8h, 12h, and 24h.

Results

Record the substances added into each tube, and the color at every time point. Draw a conclusion with the effect of drug according to the result.

Notes

1. If no EAC mice available, it can be substituted by any sterile fresh tumor cells' suspension of human or animals.

2. Don't shake the tube when check the degree of color, *in order* to prevent methylene blue molecule from being oxidized and presenting color.

3. The color of EAC ascites should be ivory. If it presents pink, it shows that there are many erythrocytes in it, bloody, and not suitable to use. To draw the ascites conveniently, inject sterile diluted solutions into abdominal cavity, flush and draw it. The ascites suspension drawn from several

mice can be mixed for use.

Evaluation

1. Methylene blue tube method has the advantages of convenience and quickness, but it is only used in initial screening. We must proceed doing *in vivo* test, such as animal graft tumor method, to decide the anti – tumor effect of the drug.

2. This method is easily influenced by oxidants and reluctants to present false – positive or false – negative results, so the control group is needed.

Question

1. How to proceed doing the experiment if the drugs for screening are oxidants or reductants?

2. What is the difference between methylene blue reduction method and trypan blue contact staining? What are the advantages and disadvantages of them?

Experiment 7. 4   Therapeutic effect of 5 – Fu on mice sarcoma S_{180}

Objective

Comprehend the *in vivo* screening method of anti – tumor drugs. Initially understand the anti-cancer activity of 5 – Fu (5 – fluorouracil).

Principle

Make the mice sarcoma S_{180} as experimental model, and treat it with a certain dose of the drug with anticancer activity, the growth of the tumor can be inhibited. Assess the anticancer activity of this drug with inhibition rate of tumor weight.

Materials

Animal required: 20 mice, 18 – 20g, inoculate S_{180} neoplasia source and breed 10 – 12 days.

Apparatus required: tissue homogenizer, dissecting scissors, ophthalmic operating curved pincers, Petri dish, injection syringe, beaker, cotton ball (above – mentioned must be steri-lized).

Reagent required: 25% 5 – Fu solutions, sterile saline, tincture of iodine, 70% alcohol.

Methods

1. Preparation of the tumor cells suspension for inoculation   Put the S_{180} neoplasia source mice to death which have been inoculated and breed for 10 – 12 days by cervical dislocation. Fix mice on the wax plate with abdomen upward. Sterilize the sites of tumor and the surrounding skin with tinc-ture of iodine and alcohol in order. Cut it open and take out tumor by aseptic manipulation in sterile chamber. The normal tumor tissue is pink, with a little elasticity and many vessels. In the center of the tumor, usually, necrosis can be seen in pale. Cut down the pink tumor tissue with sterile surgi-cal scissors, clean it with Salin, and weigh it in a petri dish. Then shear to chipping, add sterile Sa-line to tumor tissues (3ml/g), grind carefully in the tissue homogenizer to prepare the uniform cell suspension and preserve it in refrigerator with cover for use. The suspension is better to be ivory with a little pink color. If the red is too deep, the suspension contains too much blood, whose quality is not good.

2. Inoculate mice   Grasp the mice head with left hand while inoculating it, sterilize the skin

under the right forelimb armpit with tincture of iodine and alcohol, hold syringe containing tumor cells suspension with right hand, and stick into subcutaneous tissue of armpit (move needle gently to verify whether the needle stick into subcutaneous tissue), then inject suspension 0.2ml.

3. Grouping and administration　Mark the mice inoculated for 24h and divide them into treatment group and control group at random, 10 mice each group. Inject the mice of treatment group with 0.25% 5 – Fu (0.25mg/10g) by ip., one time every day for 10 – 14 days; inject the control group with Saline 0.1ml/10g by ip. The decrease of animal's body weight should not be more than 15%, when the course is over.

4. Result observation　On the next day after the course of treatment, weigh each mouse and kill them by cervical dislocation. Cut open the mice and take out tumor, weigh the tumor, and check whether they have necrosis or infection.

Results

Record the result in Table 7 – 3, count out the average tumor weight of treatment group and control group, and count out the inhibition rate according to this formula.

$$\text{Inhibition rate} = \frac{\text{ATV of control group} - \text{ATV of treatment group}}{\text{ATV (average tumor weight) of control group}} \times 100\%$$

Deal the result with statistics analysis.

Table 7 – 3　the experimental treatment result of 5 – Fu to mice sarcoma S_{180}

Group	Date of inoculation	Dose and course	Number of animal beginning end	Average weight beginning end	Average tumor weight	Inhibition rate	Significance of difference in average tumor weight
Treatment group							
Control group							

Notes

1. Pay attention to proper sterilization and aseptic manipulation in the process of inoculating tumor, in order to prevent from growing of tumor because of infection.

2. Remove the surrounding normal tissue while striping the tumor.

3. The average tumor weight of the control group should be more than 1g, the lightest tumor must be more than 0.4g, discard it if not so.

4. Repeat this experiment three times to verify its reliability. If the inhibitory rate is above 30%, we can consider expanding tumor spectrum or proceed other pharmacological experiment.

5. Operate rapidly when inoculating and the whole operation should be finished within 30 minutes.

Evaluation

The success rate of tumor graft method is high, and it is more feasible than induced or spontaneous animal tumor method, the rate of false – positive and false – negative erro is lower. This method screen anticancer new drugs from whole body level, and it can be used to observe the anticancer efficiency of drug and colligation reaction of animal to the drug, at the same time. This method is more reliable than *in vitro* methods.

Question

1. How to distinguish the normal tumor tissue and the necrotic tissue when dissecting the load tumor animal? What kind of tissue should be Chosen for inoculation? Why?

2. What problems shall we notice during the course of administration?

3. Why need exactly sterilize when inoculate tumor to mice?

Experiment 7. 5   Human cancer's grafting under kidney capsule of mice (nude mouse)

Objective

Comprehend the method of grafting human cancer into the body of animals (under the capsule of kidney of mice), and screening effective compounds by utilizing it.

Principle

Graft the human cancer cells (as antigen) into the body of nude mouse, observe the growth regulation of tumor in a short period. It is not influenced by different immune activity of the host, and it dose not cause humoral immunity and cellular immunity, so it can be successfully inoculated. There is plenty of nutrition under the membrane of kidney capsule, and it is suitable for the growth of cancer cells. The membrane of kidney capsule is clear, so it is easy to measure the size of tumor by microscope. So the human cancer cells can be grafted under the membrane of kidney capsule.

Materials

Animal required: 12 nude mice or BDF_1, CDF_1 mice, weight 18 – 22g, female and male are all used, fresh tumor tissue of human (such as cancer of lung, mammary cancer, etc) .

Apparatus required: stereomicroscope, operating scalpe, dissecting scissors, ophthalmic operating pincers, $12^{\#}$ or $18^{\#}$ sternal puncture needle, suture needle and nesis, beaker.

Reagent required: 0. 2% cyclophosphamide, diethyl ether, tincture of iodine, alcohol.

Methods

1. Take fresh tumor tissue of human under the condition of sterilization. Shear out envelope and necrotic part which is bleeding, and cut it into 1mm little pieces.

2. Choose healthy nude mouse or BDF_1, CDF_1 mouse, anesthetize them with diethyl ether. Sterilize the operative site on dorsolateral part of the mouse with tincture of iodine and 70% alcohol, then cut open the abdominal cavity and expose the left kidney.

3. Clamp out a little piece of tumor tissue with eye pincers and put it into the needle point of $12^{\#}$ or $18^{\#}$ sternal puncture needle, then inset the sternal puncture needle under the membrane of kidney capsule, and embed the tumor block. Observe the long diameter and short diameter of the tumor block with stereomicroscope, which is assembled by stereomicroscope staff 100 shelf ($0\mu m$, $100\mu m = 1mm$), and sew up the incision after measurement.

4. On the next day after inoculation, divide the mice into two groups in random, six in the treatment group and six in the control group. To the treatment group, inject 0. 2% cyclophospha-

mide 0. 2ml/mouse ip. , once a day, for 5 days. Kill the mice on the sixth day, cut out the kidney with tumor, and measure the diameter of tumor with stereomicroscope (to the nude mouse, administer for 10 days and put them to death at the 11th day).

Results

the volume of tumor $=$ $\dfrac{\text{long diameter} \times \text{short diameter}^2 \ (\text{mm})}{2}$

Measure the volume (mm^3) and weight (g) of tumor in each group, count out average tumor volume $\pm$ standard deviation, and count out inhibition rate with this formula:

Tumor inhibition rate $= \dfrac{\text{ATV of control group} - \text{ATV of treatment group}}{\text{ATV (average tumor volume) of control group}} \times 100\%$

Count out the inhibition rate with tumor weight:

Inhibition rate $= \dfrac{\text{average tumor weight of treatment group (T)}}{\text{average tumor weight of control group (C)}} \times 100\%$

Notes

1. The domestic standard of the evaluation of the effect is $T/C\% \leqslant 60\% - 70\%$, and the result which has significant difference with control group by t test is the positive result. Repeat it three times, only when getting all positive result, can we confirm the effect.

2. The manipulation must be properly sterilized. Deal the tumor source with bacterium cultivation, and cut – out the experiment, if it show contamination.

3. The human tumor tissue, removed in operation, must be inoculated within 4h.

4. The long and short diameter of embedded tumor block should be between 9 and 120μm.

5. Puncture the capsule of kidney gently, to avoid stabbing wound kidney and causing death because of bleeding.

Evaluation

The grafting under kidney capsule of mice method is objective, sensitive, reliable, and has high repetition in the evaluation of effect. The tumor block comes from human body, so it can reflect the character of human tumor much better than other tumor such as S_{180} , and the new anticancer drugs screened with this method have more direct aim. The disadvantage of this method is that the animals such as nude mouse are very expensive, and the method cannot be used in long – term administration to screen chronic anticancer drugs.

Question

1. Why can't the grafting under kidney capsule of mice method be used in long – term administration to screen chronic anticancer drugs?

2. Why to choose the capsule of kidney as tumor grafting site?

Chapter 8　Experiments of contraceptives

Birth control is a national policy of our country. In the early 1960's, steroid contraceptives were invented and then applied widely. Long – term clinical practice shows that it has certain contraceptive effect and high safety, which is superior to other birth control methods. We call the birth of steroid contraceptive drugs as a great revolution of science, medical science and sociology. But the increasing population has not yet been controlled effectively. Hence, the search for safe, effective and convenient contraceptive is still an important aim of pharmacological researchers.

The most fundamental screening method of female contraceptive is anti – procreation experiment, which is to administer female animal in the duration of breeding in the same cage with male animal, and observe the effect on birth. In addition, we can use anti – imbed, anti – early – pregnant, or anti – ovulation experiment, to check the drug affecting on certain stage of the procreation process of female animals.

I. Anti – procreation experiment

1. Short – acting drugs　Take female mice or rats, 10 in a group of common. Give drugs to the treating group for 3 days (chemical drug) or 5 days (preparation of plant drug), then breed with male in the same cage, each two female mate one male, continue to administer in this duration. Take out male animals after 12 – 14 days, and open the abdominal part of female animals to check the conceived percentage of each group, record the embryo number of each pregnant female animals, and notice whether they have dead fetus. Treat the control group with water or solvent, and other treatments are similar to the treatment group. Analyze the result by statistical method (Fig. 8 – 1).

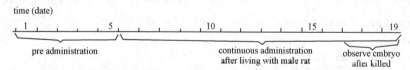

Fig. 8 – 1　Abridged general view of experiment of short – acting female contraceptive drug

2. Long – acting drugs　Administer the experimental animals once beforehand, make them breed with male animals in the same cage three days later, until the female reproduct. Check and record the number of procreative female and the young animal begin from the 19th day after breeding with the male, count out the day number from breeding with female to procreation. The difference of the day number between treat group and control group is contraception time. Dispose the result by statistical analysis. In anti – procreation experiments, if fertility rate of the control group is less than 70%, the result unreliable.

In anti – procreation experiment, we must notice the loss of the weight. Regard the loss of the weight as toxic effect of drug. If initial screening is effective, decrease the dose and test a-gain. Check vulva cork (seed coagulated to white embolism in vagina after copulation) every day. If there has vulva cork, it shows that it has mated. You can also wipe vagina with cotton bud soaked by Saline, smear and look up seed with microscope, while checking whether the rats have mated. In this way, observe the influence of drug to sexual behavior.

Ⅱ. Anti – imbed experiment

Check female animals to see whether there has vulva cork every morning after breeding the fe-male mouse or rats with males in the same cage. Take out the females, which have vulva cork, con-tinue doing it for 5 – 7 days. Divide the females which have vulva corkfemales into 2 groups, 10 in one group in common. Administer once a day from the 1st two 5th day after vulva cork ap-peared. Open the abdominal part of the animals at the 12th day of vulva cork appeared, record the number of embryo in two sides of uterine and conceived percentage. Analyze the result by statistical method (Fig. 8 – 2).

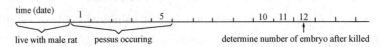

Fig. 8 – 2   Abridged general view of anti – imbed experiment

In this experiment, the date of appearance of vulva cork is different, so in each group, even in the same group, the date of administration and disposal is different, we can only dispose them in batch on time.

Ⅲ. Anti – early – pregnant experiment

The method is similar to anti – imbed experiment. Generally, administer on the 6th – 9th day, after vulva cork appears, constantly for 4 days, put the animals to death on the 12th day, and check the number of embryo and the situation of fetal death. If it present positive result by repeated experiment, you can decrease the day number of administration and repeat again. If the test drug is a long – acting drug, administer once on the 6th day (Fig. 8 – 3).

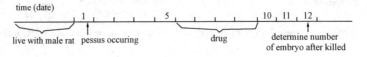

Fig. 8 – 3   Abridged general view of anti – early – pregnant experiment

Note: The commonly used animals in anti – procreation, anti – imbed, and ant – early – pregnant experiment are mice of prime life with body weight of 28 – 35g or rats of prime life 200 – 250g.

Experiment 8. 1   Anti – ovulation effect of norethisterone
(copulation method)

Objective

Observe the inhibitory effect of Norethisterone on ovulation of female rabbits.

Principle

Ovulation of rabbit can be induced the copulation, injecting copper sulfate, copper acetate, or copper gluconic acid, can reduce ovulation. Regard the average ovulated point as index of effect, which present functional relationship with the dose of drug. Regard the ovulation point of control group as 100%, Calculate the inhibition rate of ovulation of the treat group. Calculate the dose, in which the inhibition rate is 50%, and compare inhibitory potency of drugs.

Materials

Animal required: rabbits, 2 – 3kg, 2 females and 2 males.

Apparatus required: gastro – irrigating apparatus of rabbit, forceps, syringe, little beaker, scissor.

Reagent required: benovocylin parenteral solution (1mg/ml), norethisterone suspension (25μg/ml), normal saline.

Methods

Take 2 healthy female rabbits with body weight of 2.0 – 3.0kg, which have been raised separately for three weeks beforehand (confirmed in estrus by vaginal smear, that is most keratino-cyte. sc. Benovocylin 100ug, 36h before copulation, can increase copulation rate). Treat rabbit A with norethisterone suspension (norethisterone 0.25mg/kg) ig., treat rabbit B with saline by the same method. Mate the two female rabbits with two males respectively 12h after administration. 24 h after copulation, kill the female rabbits, cut open and check whether there have ovulation points on the two sides of the ovaries (rabbit ovaries will leave little processus on the follicle after ovulation, on the top of the processus has a bright red point that is ovulation point. Neither dark red apophysis nor apophysis without red points is ovulation point. The normal rabbit ovulates 1 – 10 once). Record the result.

Results

Overview the results of all lab, compare the difference of ovulation between the treatment group and the control one.

Ovulation inhibition rate = (1 – average ovulation point of treat group / average ovulation point of control group) × 100%

Attention

1. The heat period of rabbits changes with season. The copulation rate is over 75% in spring. Transfering the female into the male's cage is easier to cause copulation than the opposite way.

2. Without pure Norethisterone, oral contraceptive tablet NO. 1 can be used. This preparation contains Norethisterone 625μg, Ethinylestradiol 35μg / tablet. Convert the dose according to the Norethisterone in it.

3. While administring by i. p, do not insert catheter into trachea. Before administration, put one tip of catheter into water, pour drug when it has no bubble.

Evaluation

In this method we observe the ovulation effect of Norethisterone by copulation method. The method is convenient, the result is reliable, and the data has high repetition. The method can also be used in the research of contraceptive.

Question

1. Besides inhibition of ovulation, what other procedure can oral contraceptives influence?

2. Try to describe the mechanism of oral contraceptives.

Chapter 9　Experiments of anti-aging drugs

Aging is the degenerative alteration of each organ and tissue in living creature and results from the comprehensive roles played by many pathological and physiological processes. Anti – aging reagents are such kind of drugs that can delay and relieve all sorts of degenerative changes, enhance the vigor of the organism, and increase the life span at the level of tissues, organs, cells and even molecules which are based on the substance and energy metabolism of organisms. Up to now, there have been at least ten sorts of aging theories. it also express various experimental methods about how to research anti – aging drugs and many animal models whose symptoms are the same as that of clinical aging patients. According to some main aging theories, some experimental methods in the research of commonly – used anti – aging drugs will be introduced from the aspects of substance metabolisms in this chapter, immune system and central nervous system and so forth. It is certain that these methods simply reflect one process or one sign. If a drug is effective on some aging model or index, we should not regard the drug as an anti – aging drug directly without comprehensive evaluation through various models and indices.

I . Free radical theory

The free radical theory of aging is the most important theory in biochemical research of aging. The free radicals, formed in oxidation – reduction reaction of metabolic process, can react with nucleic acid, protein and lipid to produce oxide and peroxide. When the lipid of biomembrane is oxidized to peroxide, the penetrability of the membrane is changed and the membrane is damaged, which causes alteration of cell metabolism, function and configuration, resulting in a series of aging processes. Lipid peroxides can be further decomposed by oxidase to malondialdegyde (MDA) which associates with the proteins. Finally, lipofuscin deposits in brain, heart and other important organs, affects the normal growth of cells and accelerate the aging process. The extent of free radical damage can be reflected either by directly determining the amount of free radicals through chemiluminescence method and ESR or by indirectly measuring the amount of oxidation or per – oxidation product such as MDA, LPO. In addition, superoxide dismutase (SOD) is one of the most important enzymes in organism which can catalyze dismutation of free radicals. So activity of SOD in red cells and tissues can be measured and used to evaluate the therapeutic effect of drugs indirectly.

Experiment 9. 1　The determination of lipid peroxide

Objective

Study the method to measure the lipid peroxide and observe the antioxidant effect of drugs.

Principle

Malondialdehyde (MDA), the second derivative of lipid peroxidation, can react with thiobar-

317

bituric acid to produce red product with maximum absorption at 532nm wave – length and can be measured by chromatometry. Tetraethoxypropane can be used as standard material for it can react with lipid peroxide to produce the same product of MDA under the same condition.

Materials

Animal required: a male rat, 250 – 300g.

Apparatus required: centrifuger, tissue homogenate machine, multiuse oscillator, homoiothermy oscillator, 721 spectrophotometer, thermostat.

Reagent required: trichloroacetic acid, thiobarbituric acid (TBA), tetraethoxypropane, normal saline, butanol, 0.1mol/L HCL.

Methods

1. Execute the rat to death after weighing, take the liver out, absorb the remaining blood on it with filter paper, then cut it into very small pieces and weigh them, add Saline to prepare 1% homogenate using tissue homogenate machine.

2. Add 20% trichloroacetic acid 0.3ml to 0.6ml liver homogenerate to precipitate proteins, mix proportionately and keep them still for 20min, add 2ml 0.1mol/L HCl together with 1.0ml 1% TBA and mix together. After boiling the mixture for 15min in 100℃ water, cool it and add 4.0ml butanol to extract, oscillate to mix it together, centrifuge at 3000rpm/min for 15min.

3. Take 4ml upper limpid liquid to determine the absorbance with colorimetric assay at 532nm.

4. Determine the amount of protein in liver homogenerate by Lowry method, use the tetroxide propane as the standard to calculate the lipid peroxide per gram protein.

Results

Calculate by the formula and list the results in Table 9 – 1.

$$C = A / \text{ extinction coefficient } = A/1.56 \times 10^{5} \text{mol/L}$$

C——the concentration of MDA

A——absorbency

L——diameter of light (1cm)

Extinction coefficient——$1.5 \times 10^{-5} \text{m}^{-1} \text{cm}^{-1}$.

Table 9 – 1   Effects of drug on the lipid per – oxidation in live homogenate

Group	Dosage (mg/kg)	Number of test (n)	MDA (nmol/kg) ($\bar{x} \pm SD$)
Control			
drug			

If the content of the test substance is known, thus

$$C = \frac{A}{0.156 \times \text{amount of protein}}$$

Notes

1. The liver must be sheared into small pieces as possible as we can before the preparation of the homogenate. The time and frequency must be kept in consistence when the homogenate is prepared.

2. Each time when homogenate is taken, shake the beaker to make the compound mixed together.

Evaluation

This method is easy to manipulate and the reagent can be easily obtained. Many drugs which are used in clinic are screened by this method. The content of MDA can objectively reflect the degree of aging and it is a definite indicator.

Experiment 9. 2　The assay to determine superoxide dismutase (SOD)

Objective

1. Study the method to determine SOD and understand the relationship between the activity of super – oxidant and the concentration of free radicals.

2. Observe the effect of drugs on the improvement of the activity of enzyme and the clearance free radical.

Principle

Superoxide dismutase (SOD) is an important free radical scavenger in the organism, its function is to catalyse the following reaction:

SOD is decreased during the aging process, so its activity can be used as the quantitative indicator of aging.

The NBT is reduced to formazan by the O^{2-}, which has the maximum absorption at wave – length of 560 nm. The SOD clears the O^{2-} and inhibits the formation of formazan, so we can calculate the concentration SOD of samples by measuring the decrease of the formazan.

Materials

Apparatus required: 721 spectrophotometer, whirling – oscillator, homogenizer.

Solvent required: xathine, nitrobenzene thiocyanate (NBT), xathine oxidase. xathine oxidase: 0. 4U/ml, preserve under the condition of $-20℃$, and dilute with potassium phosphate buffer of pH 7. 8 (50mmol/L) to make the concentration 0. 04u/ml. SOD standard liquid: use 20% alcohol to fill the prescription of 1mg/kg then dilute it to 10μg/ml (58. 52h/ml). Mixed substrate buffer: liquid A is the 0. 2mol/L potassium phosphate buffer (pH 7. 8); liquid B is 0. 4mol/L EDTA – NaOH buffer; liquid C is 10mmol/L xathine that was dissolved in 0. 1mol/L NaOH; liquid D is 7. 5mmol/L NBT dissolved in the 20% alcohol. Take liquid A 135ml, liquid B 0. 188ml, liquid C 4. 5ml and liquid D 3. 75ml, then add water to 240ml to form the mixed substrate buffer.

Methods

1. Extract SOD from red cells　Take 2ml anticoagulant blood with heparin, remove the blood plasma and the leucocytes, use 2 – 3 times the volume of Saline to wash it twice, dilute the erythrocyte with equal volume of cold and warm distilled water to cause haemolysis sufficiently, then rectify the concentration of the hemolytic hemoglobin to 100g/L.

2. Draw 0. 5ml this blood liquid, add 3. 5ml distilled water, 1ml cold alcohol and 0. 6ml chloroform in turn, and mix them together, vibrate for 1min, centrifugate it for 5min with 3000rpm/min to precipitate hemoglobin. Upper limpid liquid contains SOD.

Take three small test tubes with 2. 4ml mixed substrate buffer in each of them, respectively add 0.15ml the extract sample of the erythrocyte in the first tube, 0.15ml SOD standard liquid in the second one, 0.5ml water without ion in the third one. Add water in the first and second tubes to 0.5ml. Place all tubes in 30℃ water for 5 – 15min, during which add xathine 0.3ml every 30seconds (0.04u/ml) one by one. 12min after reaction, calculate the inhibiting percentage of samples with the spectrophotometer and compare them with that of the SOD standard solution, then calculate the concentration of SOD in red cells.

Results

Calculate by following formula and convert the result to the content of SOD (μg) in 1gHb e-rythrocyte.

$$SOD/gHb = \frac{A_3 - A_1}{A_3 - A_2} \times 1 \times \frac{5}{0.15} \times \frac{1}{0.05} = \frac{A_3 - A_1}{A_3 - A_2} \times 666.6$$

A_3——the absorbance with no inhibition by SOD;

A_1——the absorbance of test sample;

A_2——the absorbance of standard SOD;

5——the volume of 5 ml erythrocyte;

0.05——the content of Hb in 100 g/L hemoglobin suspension of 0.5ml blood;

0.15 ml——the volume of SOD extracting liquid.

Notes

1. SOD in blood cell and tissues must be extracted in ice – water bath.

2. Because the color formed in this method is unstable, the assay must be finished in 20min.

Evaluation

1. The reagent is inexpensive, and it can be easily obtained; at one time you can manipulate many tubes, but the sensitivity and precision of this method are not as good as that of o – benzol – tri – phenol.

2. The color is unstable and coefficient of variation is relatively high.

Question

Try to state the relationship between the superoxide dismutase and the free radicals.

II. Effects of drugs on immunological function

In recent years experimental data has indicated that aging is closely related to the state of the immunological function of the organism. As people become senile, the decrease of the secretion of thymic hormone and immunological function lead to the decrease of the resistance to pathogen and the increased incidence of infection and tumor. Some Chinese herbs with effects of complete treatment can regulate the immunological function, improve or regulate the pathologic status resulting from the damage of immunological function to cure the patients. So the effect of drugs on immunological function is a common aspect to observe in the research of the anti – aging drugs.

Experiment 9.3   The assay to weigh the immune organs

Objective

Master the assay to weigh immune organs and observe the effect of drug on the weight of immune organs.

Principle

The weight of immune organs (thymus, spleen) can be increased by immunopotentiators, while immuno – suppressive drugs act in the opposite way. By this method we can observe the antagonistic effect of drugs on the immune organs' weight which are decreased by immuno – suppressive drugs.

Materials

Animal required: 20 mice, 16 – 18g, male or/and female.

Apparatus required: balance

Reagent required: Cyclophosphamide, normal saline, test drug.

Methods

Divide 20 mice into four groups at random: control group (only normal saline is administered), the test group, the cyclophosphamide group, the cyclophosphamide plus the test group. Give the drug once a day for six days. On the forth day after administration, administer 75mg/kg cyclophosphamide intraperitoneally. The next day of the last time for administration, pick out the eyeballs to collect blood and excavate the spleen and thymus for weighing.

Results

Weigh the organs with torsion balance and express the weight in terms of mg/10g body weight, then do the statistical calculation by inter – group t – test and compare the difference of the within groups to see if they have the statistical significance.

Notes

Young mice must be used.

Thymus and spleen must be parted clearly.

Evaluation

1. This method can be easily manipulated, and it can be used to initially screen the traditional Chinese herbs. Many known beneficial herbs have weight – increasing effect on immunological organs.

2. If the results are parallel with other indicators, they must be reliable.

Question

Why do we observe the effect of the test drug after immunological function is inhibited by cyclophosphamide?

Experiment 9. 4　The assay to determine function of the mononuclear phagocytes

Objective

Understand the effect of drug on immunological function of mononuclear phagocyte in mice and further study drug's regulation of immunological function.

Principle

Phagocyte has various functions such as swallowing foreign materials and handling antigen. When some particles of foreign materials enter into blood circulation, they are rapidly removed by mononuclear phagocyte, among which are chiefly the macrophages in the liver and spleen. If the amount of the foreign materials is constant, their clearance rate from blood can reflect the phagocytic capacity of mononuclear phagocyte. The granular foreign material which is frequently used is colloid carbon. In a certain range, the clearance of carbon particles is dose – dependent. That is to say, the rate of phagocytosis is in direct ratio to the concentration of carbon in blood, and it is in inverse ratio to the amount of swallowed carbon particles. Some drugs increasing nonspecific immunological function often improve the phagocytic capacity of mononuclear phagocyte.

Materials

Animal required: 15 mice, 18 – 22g, male or female.

Apparatus required: India ink, stop watch, 721 spectrophotometer, small sippers.

Reagent required: Heparin, 0.1% Na_2CO_3, normal saline.

Methods

1. Divide healthy mice into drug group, negative control group and positive group at random. The ways and routes of administration are varied with different test substances.

2. Prepare colloid carbon suspension of 64mg/ml, melt in boiling water, oscillate and dilute it to 16mg/ml before use.

3. Inject the India ink 30min after the last administration through caudal vein and collect 20μl blood from orbital vein at different time (1, 5 or 2, 10min) after the injection. Dissolve the blood into 0.1% Na_2CO_3 2ml, shake it and determine its absorbance at 600 – 680nm.

4. Execture the mice and weigh the liver and spleen.

Results

1. Draw a diagram by using the logarithm of the absorbance as ordinate and the corresponding time as abscissa, and a line can be got. The slope of the line (K) is used to indicate phago – rate (or clear – up index).

$$K = \frac{\lg A_1 - \lg A_2}{t_2 - t_1}$$

A_1, A_2——the absorbance at different times.

$t_2 - t_1$——time interval between two adjacent samples.

2. Calculate and adjust the clear – up index according to the following formula for the K can be influenced by the weight of liver and spleen.

$$\alpha = \sqrt[3]{K} \text{body weight} / (\text{spleen weight} + \text{liver weight})$$

Notes

1. India ink must be diluted ten times by the Saline, otherwise it will cause the mice dead after injection.

2. The time of collecting blood must be as accurate as possible.

3. If the variance between the weight of liver and spleen of mice is small, we can only calculate K value.

Evaluation

Use the immunosuppressive reagents (such as cyclophosphamide) to cause the inhibition of the

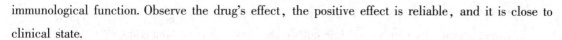
immunological function. Observe the drug's effect, the positive effect is reliable, and it is close to clinical state.

Questions

1. What is the specific immunity and nonspecific immunity?

2. Which kind of the above mentioned immunological function does the experiment belong to?

III. Drug's effect on stress

So – called anti – stress ability reflects the organism's adaptability to adverse environment. Anti – aging drugs, as a kind of drugs used to improve vitality, can normally increase the nonspecific resistant ability of organism to various harmful stimuli, and revert disorder function to normal, which is called adaptor – like action in the traditional Chinese herbs. Mouse is often used in anti – aging experiments to observe the effect of various stimuli on the survival time of mice.

Experiment 9.5   Hypoxia tolerance test of mice

Objective

Master the method to do hypoxia tolerance test of mice and observe the effect of drug on hypoxia tolerance of mice.

Principle

Hypoxia, a kind of tension stimulus, can cause various kinds of irritability actions. Hypoxia of brain and heart is the main cause of death. Many anti – aging drugs can lengthen the survival time of mice in anoxic condition by improving myocardial energy metabolism and increasing blood supply in the heart or reducing oxygen consumption.

Materials

Animals required : 30 mice, 18 – 20g, male or female.

Apparatus required: 150ml wide – mouthed glass bottle, stopwatch, balance, Reagent required: vaseline, sodium lime.

Reagent required: propranolol.

Methods

Divide the mice into three groups with 10 mice in each, put them respectively into tightly sealed wide mouthed bottle of the same volume (150ml) with equal sodium lime (25g) in it to absorb water and carbon dioxide. The lid of the bottle is smeared with vaseline. After putting the mice in, close tightly the lid and calculate the time of respiratory arrest by using stopwatch. Set controls of negative group and positive group (propranolol 20mg/kg, ip) for each experiment.

Results

Calculate the average dead time of each group ($\bar{x} \pm S$), do statistical t – student test to see significance between groups.

Notes

1. The containers must be sealed tightly without air leak, and they must have equal volume.

2. In order to prevent the sodium lime from being affected with damp, the container must be

sealed in each experiment.

3. Experimental data varies with different weight, sex and room temperature.

Evaluation

1. This method is easily manipulated, and it can be used for initial screening as basic approach.

2. Without high specificity, it turn out positive findings for some sedative and hypnotic, vasodilated drugs, drugs which have complete effect and the activate – blood and clear – clot drugs.

Questions

1. What is the function of sodium lime in the experiment?

2. Why does the experiment have poor specificity?

Experiment 9.6 The cold – resistant test of mice

Objective

Study the cold stimulation method, observe the effect of drugs on strengthening the cold hardiness.

Principle

The cold stimulation is a type of physical stimulation, when the body is stimulated by it, a series of protective action, such as vasoconstriction of the skin, reflex tremor and hypermetabolism, may take place. Then the adrenal cortical hormone is secreted profusely, which is good to anti – stress. When the adrenal cortical hormone is used up, it may be recovered with the help of the anti – aging drugs, so the drugs can enhance the ability of anti – stress.

Materials

Animals required : 30 mice with the same sex, 18 – 20g.

Equipments required: The refrigerator, the balance, and the hydroscope.

Methods

Adjust the refrigerator or the cryogenic refrigerator to make its temperature at −5℃ ±1℃. Divide the mice into groups, 1hour after administration, put the cage in the refrigerator, and observe the death rate for 50 minutes or 60 minutes, or observe the living time of each mouse until they are all dead.

Results

Calculate the average death rate in 50 minutes or 60 minutes or the average living time, and make a comparison between the groups.

Notes

The mouse should have the same sex, and their weight should be similar in order to avoid too much variance of the result.

Evaluation

1. It is easy to manipulate, but it is lack of the specificity.

2. Anti – hyperthermia test can be done while performing this test (temperature at 45℃ ±1℃, the other conditions are the sane with the cold – resistant test).

Questions

What is the adjustment of the drugs?

Experiment 9.7　The swimming test of mice

Objective

To know the method of the swimming test of mice, and observe the anti – tiredness effects of drugs.

Principle

Take the swimming time as the index of the tiredness of the mice, the drugs that have the anti – tired effect can prolong the swimming time.

Materials

Animals required: 30 mice, 18 – 22g, male.

Equipments required: The glass jar, the calorstat, the hydroscope, the mud (or the aluminium blade), and some rope.

Reagent required: normal saline, test drug.

Methods

Divide 30 mice into 3 groups randomly, give the test drugs to the first group, give the drugs which are used as the positive control to the second group, and give the normal saline which is used as the negative control to the third group. At a certain time after administration, put the mice in the glass jar to start the swimming test, adjust the temperature to $30\ ℃ \pm 1\ ℃$ and the depth of the water to 25cm. To shorten the observation time, the tails of the mice can be loaded with some thing whose weight is 5% of the mouse's weight, calculate the time when the nose sinks with the stopwatch.

Results

Record the swim duration of each mouse, calculate the mean of the durations, and make the significance test between the groups. Observe if the drugs have some anti – tiredness effects.

Notes

1. Control the water temperature strictly.

2. Only one mouse can be used to swim in one glass jar. Too many mice in one jar may lead to mutual movements including climbing and pushing, which will affect the results.

Evaluation

1. The method is easy, but the variance of the results is big.

2. The big difference of the weight may affect the results.

3. Cold water can be used in this test (it is called cold – water swimming test). The result obtained is the integrated index of the physical strength and the stress reaction.

Questions

What is the possible mechanism of the anti – tiredness drugs?

IV. The effects on the central nervous system

Biological researchers pay more and more attention to the relationship between the central nervous system and the senium of the body. The senium can cause the central catecholamine decrease, which lead to the biochemical damage of the brain, including the degeneration of the nervous system, and the change of the independent behaviour and act. In 1980, Fowler found that the activity of the monoamine oxidase – B (MAO – B) is increased with the age, it had a close relationship with the senium, many anti – aging drugs show effect by decreasing the activity of the MAO – B and the biochemical damage caused by the central catecholamine.

Experiment 9. 8   The test of the activity of the monoamine oxidase – B

Objective

Study the method to test the activity of MAO – B and observe the inhibition of MAO – B by the drug.

Principle

Make the bridal to be the substrate, its made from the benzaldehyde with the help of MOA – B, extract the product by cyclohexane, and detect the A at 242nm.

$$RCH_2 - NH_2 + O_2 + H_2O \rightarrow RC$$

Materials

Animal required: mice.

Reagent required: 0. 2mol/L phosphoric acid buffer, 8mmol/L bridal, 60% perchloric, cyclohexane.

Methods

1. Take out the whole brain of the mice, put it in to a container, add the cool phosphoric acid buffer (0. 2mol/ml) 10 times of the volume to prepare the homogenate by sonication, and centrifuge it (5000r/min), abandon the deposit.

2. Centrifuge the supernatant (17000r/min) for 30 minutes, take out the deposit, suspend it with the phosphoric acid buffer, that is the coarse enzyme.

3. Add 0. 3ml bridal (8mmol/L) into the suspension (0. 5ml), add 0. 2mol/L phosphoric acid buffer (pH 7. 4) to 3ml, warm the reactive system at 37℃ for 3 hours, shake it every 15 minutes, then add 60% perchloric 0. 3ml to stop the reaction.

4. Extract it by 3ml cyclohexane, centrifugate it at 3000r/min for 10 minutes, take out the suspension to detect the A at 242nm.

The operations of 3, 4 are as followers:

	The blank tube	The test tube
Enzyme	—	0. 5ml
8mmol/L bridal	—	0. 3ml
0. 2mol/L phosphoric acid buffer	3. 0ml	Add to 0. 3ml
3 hours at 37℃		
8mmol/L bridal	0. 3ml	—
60% perchloric	0. 3ml	0. 3ml
Cyclohexane	3ml	3ml

Results

Observe the activity of the enzyme with the productive benzaldehyde in 3 hours, or consider

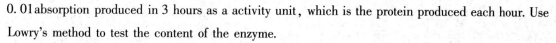
0. 01absorption produced in 3 hours as a activity unit, which is the protein produced each hour. Use Lowry's method to test the content of the enzyme.

Notes

Don't add the bridal in the blank sample before warming in order to avoid the interferences of the monoamine in the enzyme solution.

Evaluation

It is complicated to process the samples and its sensitivity and accuracy are less than the isotope test.

Questions

Describe the relationship between the activity of MOA – B and aging.

Chapter 10　Evaluation of drug safety

Ⅰ. Drug toxicity test

The toxicity research should be carried out carefully and seriously before the new drug is recommended to clinical trial in order to evaluate its safety completely. Its purposes are: ① Rejectthe drug with unacceptable toxicity and locate the target organs and tissues related to side effects. ② Define the relationship between the side effects and the dose and therapeutic course. ③ Determine whether the toxic effect is reversible and how to prevent. According to related regulations of State Drug Administration, the evaluation of drug safety involves the acute toxicity, the chronic toxicity and the special toxicity which include the mutagenesis test, the reproduction toxicity and the carcinogenesis toxicity. In addition, dependence test should be done if the drug affect the central nervous system. Skin irritation and hypersensitivity tests need to be done if the drug is administered through skin.

Acute toxicity test

Acute toxicity test it defined as the rapid and severe toxic reactions after the animal is administrated with large dose of a certain drug once or several times in a short time (24h). The reactions include death, which is the first gate for assessing the safety of a drug. Its purposes are: ① Determine the 50% lethal dose (LD_{50}) and related parameters of a drug. ② Reveal the target organs and its specific action mechanism of the drug toxicity by the toxicity symptoms. ③ Provide the evidence for determining the dose in the long term toxicity test. Mice or rats sometimes are used in the experiment. It always takes $1-2$ weeks according to the time when the toxicity occurs. For the drug to be used clinically, two routes of administration should be adopted and at least one route should be consistent with the clinical use and the observing time is 14 days.

Experiment 10.1　Acute toxicity test of procaine

Objective

Study the method, procedure and calculation of LD_{50} determination.

Principle

The lethal dose is usually used to evaluate the degree of acute toxicity of the drug. Half lethal dose is one of the indicators because it is the highest sensitivity point on the dose – reaction curve. Long tail "S" like curve (Fig. 10 – 1) is drawn by using death rate as the ordinate and the dose as the abscissa for certain relation between dose and biological reaction. There are a maximum slope in 50% death rate and two mind ends which the right is longer than the left on the curve, and it is because the number of the animals selected randomly which have high sensitivity or have no sensitivity is completely small, while the sensitivities of majority of animals are close to each other while.

The curve Fig. 10 – 1 is transformed to the following curve (Fig. 10 – 2) with features of the symmetry of the left and right and the point of symmetry in 50% death rate by using logarithm trans-

扫码 "学一学"

formed dose as abscissa. At the point, the slope is maximum and the change is obvious. That is to say that the reaction of the animal to the drug dose is most sensitive, and dose is the most accurate and error is mininum.

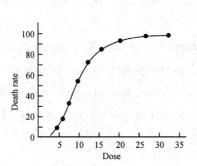

Fig. 10 – 1   The relationship
between death rate and dose

Fig. 10 – 2   The relationship between
death rate and logarithm dose

Probit, a kind of function in mathematics, is the transform of the death rate, and it has a line relation with the logarithm dose (Fig. 10 – 3).

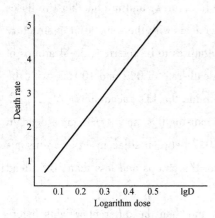

The transformation is called probit method and LD_{50} can be calculated by diagram or formula.

Materials

Animal required: 50 mice, 18 – 22g, half male and half female.

Equipment required: mouse cage, balance, and syringe

Solution required: 1% procaine, carbazotic acid for marking the mouse.

Fig. 10 – 3   The relation between
probit and logarithm dose

Methods

1. Separate the male from the female, and weigh them respectively. Put the mice of the same weight class (eg, 18. 0 – 18. 9g) into the same mouse cage.

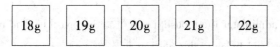

2. Female and male mice are divided into 5 groups (10 mice in each group), according to weight (from high to low or the other way around) and subsequent stratified – randomization method. The aim is to make different sexes and weights distributed to each group evenly.

Number of group	1#	2#	3#	4#	5#
Number of mice	①	2	3	4	5
	5	①	2	3	4
	4	5	①	2	3
	3	4	5	①	2
	2	3	4	5	①

3. Inject intraperitoneally 1% procaine to the mice in each group with the dose of 130mg/kg, 153mg/kg, 180mg/kg, 212mg/kg and 249mg/kg respectively using 1 : 0.85 as the ratio between adjacent groups. Observe the response and record the number of dead mice within 30min.

4. Calculate LD_{50} and 95% confidence interval by improved Kou' method and Bliss method.

Results

Experiment report should cover: ① the batch number, specification, manufacturer, physical and chemical properties, concentration of the drug and the temperature in the laboratory. ② the species, sex, weight range, groups, route of administration, dose, time of administration, toxic symptom, death time and death rate of the animal. ③ the calculating process and result of LD_{50} (including 95% confidence interval of LD_{50}).

Notes

1. The mice selected should be healthy, in the similar weight (18 – 22g), no pregnancy, and the sex should be half male and half female or of the same sex.

2. The proper dose range of the certain drug should be tested before determining its LD_{50} accurately, which means the doses that can cause the death rate of near 0% and 100% can be obtained. If the drug to verify is known, find out the LD_{50} in the literatures, and use another two doses bigger or smaller than LD_{50}. If the drug is new, LD_{50} of the chemicals with the same kind of structure can be referred. If it is a unknown drug or the drug without literatures to be referred, 3 – 4 groups of 2 – 3 mice each should be used to test the dose causing the death rate of 0% and 100%, with the dose of 2 : 1 between adjacent groups. This is the clue to determine the LD_{50} accurately.

3. Several proper doses are chosen in the range of doses causing 0% and 100% mice dead in the pre – testing. Four to five doses with ratio of 1 : 0.8 – 1 : 0.7 between adjacent doses are usually used for mice. It is better to make over 50% dead in half of the groups and less than 50% dead in another half of groups.

4. When dividing the mice, set apart the different sexes and then the different weights before dividing the mice at random. This is called random division class by class.

5. Better to give the drug to the mice from the middle dose firstly in order to judge whether the maximum and minimum dose are proper or not by observing the reaction. If not, they can be adjusted at any moment.

6. Try to weigh and administer the mouse as accurate as possible. The pH and osmotic pressure of the drug should be involved in physiological range.

7. Try to maintain the hungry state of the animals, temperature in the lab, experimental time as constant as possible, for they can influence the results of the experiment.

Appended: Calculating method

1. Improved Kurber method by Sun   In 1931, original Kurber method raised by Kurber was ignored because of the error in it, and it was improved by Finney in 1952. In 1963, Improved Kurber method, a simple and relatively accurate one, came by combing the advantages of both Kurber method and probability unit according to linear equation related point and slope by Sun Ruiyuan.

(1) Basic requirements

1) Data should be consistent with or near logarithm normal distribution.

2）The ratio of the nearing doses should be equal.

3）The number of animals in each group should be same or similar. 10 animals are often used.

4）Death rate of 0% and 100% are not necessary but the sum of deeth rates of the minmum and maximum doses should be better in the range of 80% – 120%.

（2）Calculating formula

1）The following formula can be used to calculate LD_{50} when death rates in the group with the minimum dose is 0% and that with the maximum dose is 100%.

$$LD_{50} = lg^{-1} [X_m - i (\Sigma p - 0.5)] \tag{10-1}$$

X_m——the logarithm of maximum dose;

p——death rate in each group (expressed with decimal);

Σp——the total addition of death rate in every group $(p_1 + p_2 + p_3 \cdots \cdots)$;

i——the minus of logarithm doses between the nearing groups.

2）The following correcting formula can be used to calculate LD_{50} when death rates in the group with minimum dose is over 0% and below 30%, or when death rates in the group with maximum dose is below 100% and over 70%.

$$LD_{50} = lg^{-1} \left[X_m - i \left(\Sigma p - \frac{3 - P_m - P_n}{4} \right) \right] \tag{10-2}$$

P_m——the death rate in group with maximum dose;

P_n——the death rate in group with minimum dose.

3）The standard error of LD_{50} can be calculated by following formula.

$$S_{lgLD_{50}} = i \cdot \sqrt{\frac{\Sigma p - \Sigma p^2}{n-1}} \tag{10-3}$$

n——number in each group.

4）95% confidence interval of LD_{50} can be calculated by the following formula.

$$lg^{-1} (lgLD_{50} \pm 1.96S_{lgLD_{50}}) \tag{10-4}$$

（3）Example   Divide 50 mice (18 – 22g, half male half female) into 5 groups with 10 mice each randomly. Administer intraperitoneally PAM with the dose in the table. The ratio of dose in adjacent groups is 1 : 0.8. The number of the death in 3 days is listed in the Table 10 – 1. Calculate the LD_{50}, the standard error and 95% confidence interval by using improved Kurber method.

Table 10 – 1   Effect of PAM abdominally administrated on mice

Group	Number	Dose (mg/kg)	Logarithm dose	Number of the dead	Death rate (p)	p^2
1	10	300	2.48	10	1	1
2	10	240	2.38	8	0.8	0.64
3	10	192	2.28	5	0.5	0.25
4	10	154	2.18	3	0.3	0.09
5	10	123	2.08	0	0	0
					Σp 2.6	Σp^2 1.98

Calculate LD_{50} by formula （10 – 1），

$X_m = 2.48$, $i = 0.10$, $\Sigma p = 2.6$

$$LD_{50} = \lg^{-1} [2.48 - 0.10 (2.6 - 0.5)]$$
$$= \lg^{-1} 2.27 = 186 \text{mg/kg}$$

Calculate standard error of LD_{50} by formula (10 – 3),

$$n = 10, \quad \sum p^2 = 1.98$$

$$S_{\lg LD_{50}} = 0.10 \sqrt{\frac{2.6 - 1.98}{10 - 1}} = 0.026$$

Calculate 95% confidence interval of LD_{50} by formula (10 – 4),

$$\lg^{-1} (\lg 186 \pm 1.96 \times 0.026) = \lg^{-1} (2.22 - 2.32)$$
$$= 166 - 209 \text{mg/kg}$$

LD_{50} of the drug PAM administrated intraperitoneally is 186mg/kg, and 95% confidence interval of LD_{50} is 166 – 209mg/kg.

2. Bliss method

(1) Bliss method, which is also called probit method, was designed by Bliss by using the linear relation between logarithm dose and change – over number (probit). It is the most rigorous method mathematically among many calculation methods of LD_{50} and is recommended in the method of examination and approval of new drugs. Its advantages are: ① $LD_5 - LD_{95}$ can be calculated. ② Dose is flexible and only death rate both above 50% and below 50% is needed. ③ Accurate results. However, its disadvantages are: ① Complex calculation. ② The table of weight is acquired. Because of the wide use of the computers, with the development of many softwares, Bliss method is used in great convenience and overcome completely the shortcoming of the complex calculation. Now take a look at the example below.

(2) Example   Divide 50 mice (18 – 22g, half male and half female) into 5 groups with 10 mice each at random. Administer intravenously total saponin of Sanchi with the dose in the table. The ratio of dose in nearing group is 1 : 0.85. The number of the dead in 7 days is listed in the Table 10 – 2. Calculate the LD_{50}, LD_5, LD_{95} and 95% confidence interval through Bliss method using softwaves.

Predicted probit unit (Y) can be read out from the provisional line in Fig. 10 – 3 (the provisional line comes by drawing a diagram using logarithm dose as abscissa and ye as ordinate).

Weight coefficient (w) can be got in Table 10 – 4.

Table 10 – 2   Effect of intravenously Administrated total saponin of Sanchi on mice

Dose (mg/10g)	Logarithm dose	Number of the dead/number in total	Death rate %	Experimental probit unit	Predicted probit unit	Corrected probit unit	weight coefficient	weight				
D	X	r/n	p	ye	Y	y	w	Nw	nwx	nwx²	nwy	nwxy
9.0	0.9542	10/10	100		6.5	7.02	0.269	2.69	2.5669	2.4495	18.8838	18.0197
7.6	0.8208	8/10	80	5.84	5.8	5.84	0.503	5.03	4.4305	3.9024	29.3752	25.9741

continue

Dose (mg/10g)	Logarithm dose	Number of the dead/numberin total	Death rate %	Experimental probit unit	Predic-ted probit unit	Correc-ted probit unit	weight coeff-icient	weight				
6.5	0.8129	5/10	50	5.00	5.1	5.00	0.634	6.34	5.1539	4.1897	31.7000	25.7694
5.5	0.7403	3/10	30	4.48	4.4	4.48	0.558	5.58	4.1312	3.0586	24.9984	18.5879
4.7	0.6721	1/10	10	3.72	3.8	3.72	0.370	3.70	2.4868	1.6713	13.7640	9.2508
				Table 10 – 3	(comes from the Provisio nalline)	Table 10 – 4	Table 10 – 4	23.34	18.7693	15.2715	118.7214	97.4218

Note: Experimental probit unit (ye) can be looked up in Table 10 – 3.

The standard error of LD_{50} can be calculated by following formula:

$LD_{50} = \lg^{-1} 0.7963 = 6.26 \text{mg/10g}$ (confidence limit is 5.74 – 6.81 mg/10g)

$LD_5 = \lg^{-1} 0.6467 = 4.43 \text{mg/10g}$ $LD_{95} = \lg^{-1} 0.9459 = 8.83 \text{mg/10g}$

Table 10 – 3   Probit table

Reaction rate	0	1	2	3	4	5	6	7	8	9
0	—	2.674	2.949	3.119	3.249	3.355	3.445	3.524	3.595	3.659
10	3.718	3.773	3.325	3.874	3.920	3.964	4.006	4.046	4.085	4.122
20	4.158	4.194	4.228	4.261	4.294	4.326	4.375	4.387	4.417	4.447
30	4.476	4.504	4.532	4.560	4.587	4.615	4.642	4.668	4.695	4.721
40	4.747	4.773	4.798	4.824	4.849	4.874	4.900	4.925	4.950	4.975
50	5.000	5.025	5.050	5.075	5.100	5.126	5.151	5.176	5.202	5.227
60	5.253	5.279	5.305	5.332	5.358	5.385	5.413	5.440	5.468	5.496
70	5.524	5.553	5.583	5.613	5.643	5.674	5.706	5.739	5.772	5.806
80	5.842	5.878	5.915	5.954	5.995	6.036	6.080	6.126	6.175	6.227
90	6.282	6.341	6.405	6.476	6.555	6.645	6.751	6.881	7.054	7.326

Table 10 – 4   Table of weight coefficient and corrected probit

Xx – pectcd problt Y	Maxlmum Conectcd Problt Y + Q/Z	Ranac 1/Z	Mlnlmum Cenccted Cncccted Problt Y – P/Z	Wolght – lng coemdent Z/pq	Maxtmurn conected Problt Y + Q/Z	Range 1/Z	Mlnlmum Cotrcctod Problt Y – P/Z	Xx – problt Pectod Y
5.0	6.253	2.507	3.747	0.6366	6.253	2.507	3.747	5.0
5.1	6.259	2.519	3.740	0.6343	6.260	2.519	3.741	4.9
5.2	6.276	2.557	3.719	0.6274	6.281	2.557	3.724	4.8
5.3	6.302	2.622	3.680	0.6161	6.320	2.622	3.698	4.7
5.4	6.336	2.715	3.620	0.6005	6.360	2.715	3.664	4.6
5.5	6.376	2.840	3.536	0.5810	6.464	2.840	3.624	4.5
5.6	6.423	3.001	3.422	0.5579	6.578	3.001	3.577	4.4
5.7	6.475	3.203	3.272	0.5316	6.728	3.203	3.525	4.3
5.8	6.531	3.452	3.079	0.5026	6.921	3.452	3.469	4.2
5.9	6.592	3.758	2.834	0.4714	7.166	3.758	3.408	4.1
6.0	6.656	4.133	2.523	0.4386	7.477	4.133	3.344	4.0

continue

Xx – pectcd problt Y	Maxlmum Conectcd Problt Y + Q/Z	Ranac 1/Z	Mlnlmum Cenccted Problt Y – P/Z	Wolght – lng coemdent Z/pq	Maxtmurn conected Problt Y + Q/Z	Range 1/Z	Mlnlmum Cotrcctod Problt Y – P/Z	Xx – problt Pectod Y
6.1	6.723	4.590	2.132	0.4047	7.867	4.590	3.277	3.9
6.2	6.793	5.150	1.643	0.3703	8.357	5.150	3.207	3.8
6.3	6.865	5.835	1.030	0.3350	8.970	5.835	3.135	3.7
6.4	6.939	6.679	1.621	0.3020	9.739	6.679	3.061	3.6
6.5	7.016	7.721	—	0.2691	—	7.721	2.934	3.5
6.6	7.094	9.015	—	0.2375	—	9.015	2.906	3.4
6.7	7.174	10.633	—	0.2077	—	10.633	2.826	3.3
6.8	7.255	12.666	—	0.1799	—	12.666	2.745	3.2
6.9	7.338	15.340	—	0.1544	—	15.340	2.662	3.1
7.0	7.421	18.522	—	0.1311	—	18.522	2.579	3.0
7.1	7.506	22.736	—	0.1103	—	22.736	2.494	2.9
7.2	7.592	28.189	—	0.0918	—	28.189	2.408	2.8
7.3	7.679	35.302	—	0.0756	—	35.302	2.321	2.7
7.4	7.766	44.654	—	0.0617	—	44.654	2.234	2.6
7.5	7.854	57.05	—	0.0498	—	57.05	2.146	2.5
7.6	7.943	73.62	—	0.0398	—	73.62	2.057	2.4
7.7	8.033	95.96	—	0.0314	—	95.96	1.967	2.3
7.8	8.123	126.34	—	0.0246	—	126.34	1.877	2.2
7.9	8.213	168.00	—	0.0190	—	168.00	1.787	2.1
8.0	8.305	225.6	—	0.0146	—	225.6	1.695	2.0
8.1	8.396	306.1	—	0.0110	—	306.1	1.604	1.9
8.2	8.488	419.4	—	0.0083	—	419.4	1.512	1.8
8.3	8.581	580.5	—	0.0061	—	580.5	1.419	1.7
8.4	8.673	811.5	—	0.0045		811.5	1.327	1.6

Evaluation

The way is simple and LD_{50} is one of the important signified parameters. Therapeutic Index (TI), an indicator of drug safety, can be calculated by the following formula with the data coming from the same species of animals and same route of administration.

$$TI = LD_{50}/ED_{50}$$

ED_{50}, half effective dose, refers to the dose that cause effects on half of animals.

The bigger the TI is, the safer the drug is. It can be potentially used only when the TI is bigger than 3 and TI of the drugs used clinically is over 10.

Neither LD_{50} nor TI can reflect the mechanism of special toxicities absolutely and completely. Because causing death is a process of quality response, bi – curve function in mathematics (S – like curve) between probability of accumulating reaction and dose exists and linear relation exists between probability of accumulating reaction and logarithm dose. The slope in the latter curve reflects the relation between death and dose and sometimes is more important than LD_{50}, especially in comparing the safety of same series of compounds. Different toxic symptoms of two drugs with the same or similar LD_{50} but different slopes of the curve occur in the same range of doses (Fig. 10 – 4 drug A and B). However, two drugs with different LD_{50} but the parallel dose – effect curve have the similar toxicity mechanism Fig. 10 – 4 (drug A and C). The smaller the slope is, the safer the drug is. LD_1, LD_{10} and ect can be calculated by dealing the curve to low dose side.

TI is only used to compare two drugs which the dose – effect curves of therapeutic effects and death effects are parallel. And other parameters like Safety Index (SI), Certain Safety Factor (CSF) should be referenced if the slopes of two drugs are different.

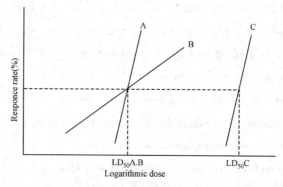

Fig. 10 – 4   The relations between toxicity and dose in different drugs

$$SI = LD_5/ED_{95}$$

SI, although less used than TI, is paid much attention to recently, because it indicates the safety clinically.

$$CSF = LD_1/ED_{99}$$

CSF and TI are not always parallel. As the Fig. 10 – 5 indicates that drug A prefers to drug B in term of TI, but the former already has toxicity in the dose of 99% effect for the CSF is below 1, however, the latter is in converse for its CSF is over 1.

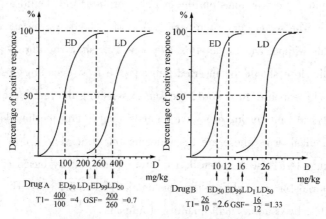

Fig. 10 – 5   The relation between evaluation of

safety and causing death dose and effective dose

Questions

1. What is LD_{50}? What is the meaning and basis to determine LD_{50}?

2. Discuss the basics and advantages of Bliss method and improved Kou' method, both of which are used to calculate LD_{50}?

Long – term toxicity test

The aim of long – term toxicity test is to observe the toxic response caused by continuous administration, to judge whether or not a new drug is worth researching and developing further by toxicity data of animals, and to provide reference for the selection of clinical original dosage.

The objective and significance of long – term toxicity test determine that the basic Principle of the test design should be comprehensive, precise and reasonable. During the course of the whole test, the conditions must be strictly controlled, and other effects beside the test drug should be eliminated to the least; the observational indices should specifically reflect the toxicity of test drug, and the results can be used to explain the possible toxic response, action characteristics and safe range of test drug when it is applied to long – term utilization.

In general, long – term toxicity test should be conducted on at least two species of animals of both sexes. Three dose groups – high, middle and low – should be established besides the blank control group. Solvent reference is established when necessary. Some important aspects of long – term toxicity test design are discussed particularly as follows:

(1) Animals   The test requires at least two species of animals including rodent and non – rodent. The first choice of the rodent is rat, at least six weeks old. The test usually begins after the animals are raised and observed for one week. The number of animals is not less than 15 each sex. The first choice of the non – rodent is dog, at least 6 – 12 months old. Every dose group requires more than 5 male and female respectively.

All kinds of test animals should be marked with source and strain. Raising condition must be strictly controlled and be constant, such as room temperature, moisture, illumination, ventilation, drinking quality and nutrition – balanced diet.

(2) Dose   The most difficult task in long – term toxicity test is to select the dose level without the obvious toxic response. Generally, three different doses are needed. The first dose should be high enough to cause definite toxic symptoms but the mortality of the group should not exceed 10% at the end of the experiment. The second one, the basic safe dose, should be higher than the optimal effective dose of animals without causing any toxic response. To show the dose – effect relationship of toxic action, a middle dose should be inserted between the two preceding doses which can cause slight or moderate toxic response. In a word, the aim of selecting the high dose is to obtain explicit information of toxicity without causing excessive animals' death, and the low dose should be higher than the expectant clinical dose. These are the fundamental Principles of dose design. In practice, the parameters of long – term test are often derived from acute toxicity based on acute toxicity test, pharmacokinetic materials or some short – term accumulative toxicity tests. The best way is to conduct dose – groping test by using a small quantity of animals.

(3) Route of administration   The route of administration in long – term toxicity test should be consistent with that of expectant clinical application in every possible way. Intravenous or intramuscular injection in clinical usage can be replaced by intraperitoneal or subcutaneous injection, and oral administration can be superseded by oral injection or feeding mixed with the drug.

(4) Test period   The period of long – term toxicity test of new drugs is regulated differently in various countries. In China, Method of Examination and Approval of New Drug points out that

continuous administration period of animal test must be three – four times that of clinical test, as is listed below.

	Clinical test	Long – term toxicity test
	1 – 3 days	2 weeks
Administration	7 days	4 weeks
Period	20 days	12 weeks
	> 30 days	half a year

(5) Observational indexes　During the whole test, a detailed observational record should be made every day or every two days. The main content of general daily observation contains the behaviors, activity appearance and feces of animals. Everyday food consumption should be recorded, and the weight should be recorded every one or two weeks. 24 hours after the last administration, 2/3 – 1/2 animals are killed to carry out hematological (erythrocyte or reticulated corpuscles counting, hemoglobin, total leucocytes counting and classification, blood platelets, coagulation time) and blood biochemical (aspartate aminotransferase, alanine aminotransferase, alkaline phosphatase, urea nitrogen, total proteins, albumin, blood glucose, total bilirubin, inosine, total cholesterol) examination and systemic necropsy. Then major organs should be removed at systemic necropsy to undertake visceral coefficient determination and histopathologic examination. The rest of the animals should be observed for another 2 – 4 weeks, killed for examination in order to learn the reversible degree of toxic response and other possible delayed toxic response. If the test period is more than three months, a small quantity of animals (in high – dose group and control group) can be killed to examine each index in the middle of the test.

Specific toxicity test

Specific toxicity test includes genetic toxicity test, reproductive toxicity test and carcinogenesis test. These toxic responses usually appear through relatively long incubation or in some special cases. In spite of the low incidence rate, the outcomes they cause are serious and hard to reverse. Therefore, specific toxicity test is attached more and more importance.

(1) Genetic toxicity test　The aim of genetic toxicity test, aslo named mutagenesis test is to verify whether the drug has the potential to damage the genetic mechanism of human or mammals and cause mutation. Because mutagenesis tests are various, convenient, fast, economical and the results have certain relations with carcinogenesis test; it becomes the short – term screening method of the carcinogenesis test. Based on the distinction of chemical structures, physical and chemical properties and effect terminals on genetic substances (gene mutation and DNA damage) of the test drug, microbial reverse mutation assay, chromosome aberration test of cultured mammalian cell and micronucleus assay of animal are required for new drugs. The former two are in vitro tests and the latter one in an in vivo test. Because of their own advantages and disadvantages respectively, they can reinforce and cite each other. If the results of the preceding tests are positive or suspected positive, other tests can be selected to research and analyze further, such as gene mutation assay of cultured mammalian cell or sex – linked recessive lethal assay of drosophila, dominant lethal assay of rodent or chromosome aberration test of spermatogenous cell, unscheduled DNA synthesis test or

SOS color – displaying test.

（2）Reproductive toxicity test　Reproductive toxicity test is divided into Ⅰ stage reproductive test, Ⅱ staye teratogenesis test and Ⅲ stage perinatal toxicity test.

In Ⅰ stage reproductive test, animals are administrated before mating to evaluate the effects on embryo, foetus, perinatal stage and ablactation stage after reproductive cells contact the drug. Mouse and rat are usually selected as experimental animals. Male should be administrated continuously for 60 – 80 days before mating, and female from 14 days before mating to organogenesis period after gestation. General condition, weight alteration, pregnancy rate, quantity of dead and living foetus, weight of living foetus, appearance and alteration of viscera and bones should be observed. Histological examination is conducted when necessary.

In Ⅱ staye teratogenesis test, animals are administrated during organogenesis period to observe whether or not the test drug has embryotoxicity and teratogenesis after the maternal receiving the drug. The first choice of experimental animal is Wistar or SD rat. Mouse or rabbit can also be used. 2 – 3 doses should be chosen. The high dose should be able to cause maternal toxic response or be maximum administration dose. The low dose should cause no toxic response of maternal and embryo. Besides, solvent reference should be established and positive control when necessary. The animals should be administrated continuously during organogenesis period of embryo. The time of rat is 6 – 15 days, mouse 6 – 15 days and rabbit 6 – 18 days. All the animals are dissected and examined in the late trimester of pregnancy to observe the establishment of pregnancy and the situations of fetal death, absorbing foetus and development of living foetus in uterus. Then 1/2 foetus should be fixed in Bouin's solution to examine viscera and another 1/2 in alcohol to check deformity of bones. All the data should be collected in a list. The embryotoxicity and teratogenesis potential of the drug are judged after the data are statistically disposed.

In Ⅲ staye perinatal toxicity peripostanal test, animals are administrated during and after postnatal period to examine the drug actions on late period of embryo growth, birth process, delivery, lactation, neonate survival and growth development. Rat and rabbit are generally used. Rat should be administrated from 15 days after pregnancy to 28 days after delivery, and rabbit from 22 days after pregnancy to 31 days after delivery. Then general condition, quantity of foetus, developmental status and appearance of animals should be observed and recorded. A certain number of foetuses should be taken to coupled breeding to observe their survival, growth and development including the behavior, reproductive function and other abnormal symptoms. Motor and learning ability should be studied on F1 animals when necessary. According to the results plus histopathologic examination, toxic actions and degree in peripostnatal period can be judged and evaluated comprehensively.

（3）Carcinogenesis test　Carcinogenesis test is the most expensive and time – consuming animal test in specific toxicity test, so it is only required when the result of mutagenesis test shows positive, or when cytotoxicity and abnormal activation of tissues are detected in long – term toxicity test, or when the chemical structure of the test drug is related or similar to some known carcinogens. Carcinogenesis test is divided into short – term and long – term carcinogenesis test.

Short – term test includes cultured mammalian cell mal – transformation test and animal short – term carcinogenesis test. The former is an in vitro test. The cultured cells are activated through metabolism and the result is judged from mal – transformation rate of cells. The latter is an in vivo test. Short – term lung tumor induced test of mouse is usually adopted. A series mouse is recommended as experimental animal. High, middle and low doses should be established. The animals of the high dose group should be administrated three times a week with maximum tolerant dose for eight weeks continuously. Negative reference group is also needed and the time for observation is 30 – 35weeks or less. Positive conclusion can be drawn if the results conform to the conditions as follows: ①The average amount of lung tumor in test group is remarkably more than control group. ②Dose – effect relationship exists. ③The average amount of lung tumor in negative control group corresponds to the incidence rate of lung tumor in same – aged normal mice reported in literature.

Long – term carcinogenesis test is a rather lasting animal test, so the test design should be detailed and well considered before the test. The problems including animal requirement, dose design and grouping, route of administration, observational period and indices are discussed below.

1) Animal: Requirements of animals are as the following: high sensitivity; moderate longevity; able to complete whole – life test within a relatively short time; strong disease – resistance; low incidence rate of spontaneous tumor; small habitus; easy to meet the required quantity of test. The first choice is the rodent such as mouse, rat and hamster. With regard to the age, it is generally believed that the weanlings or saplings are preferred because they are more sensitive to some carcinogens.

2) Dose design and grouping: Dose design is the key step of the whole test. Too low dose may lead to false – negative result, which makes conclusion hard to be drawn. Too high dose may result in death of animals, which hinders the test process or makes it impossible to use the data of the high dose group.

Although more dose groups are fine, more manpower and financial resources are required meanwhile. In general, the high dose can be determined by pre testing of LD_{10} for 3 – 8 weeks with the requirement that 10% – 20% of the animals appear mild chronic intoxication (no animals is dead) which often shows mild inhibition of weight increase or alteration of serum enzyme (the conditions indicate that the dose is suitable). The low dose can be converted in accordance with clinical proposed dose. It should not be lower than 10% of the highest dose and not influence normal growth, development and longevity of animals. A reasonable middle dose can be inserted between the high and low dose. In addition, positive, solvent and blank control groups are also needed. In every group, the number of male and female animals should be at least 50 respectively in respect that the quantity is enough to undertake biometrical disposition ultimately.

3) Route of administration: The Principle is the same as that of long – term toxicity test. That is, to select the route consistent with that of clinical application. The routes include feeding, oral injection, daubing on the skin and subcutaneous or intramuscular injection.

4) Observational period: It is generally required that administration period should occupy the longevity of the animals in a great measure so that the carcinogens with relatively weak carcinogenic action and long incubation are offered opportunities to display their carcinogenic activity. On balance, carcinogenesis test can be ended when there is obvious distinction between tumor incidence rate of administration group and that of negative control group.

5) Observational indices and pathological examination: The behavior, activity and ingestion volume of animals should be observed at least once a day. The animals should be weighed one time every week at the beginning and one time four weeks at least 13 weeks later. All the animals should be dissected and blood routine examination is required. If tumoral or suspected lesion is observed by naked eye, the organs requiring pathological examination are as follows: skin, mammary gland, lymph node, salivary gland, breast bone, vertebra, thigh bone, thymus gland, trachea, lung, bronchus, heart, thyroid gland, lingua, esophagus, stomach, duodenum, large intestine, liver, pancreas, kidney, adrenal gland, testicles, ovaries, gonad, eyeball, pituitary body, spinal cord and so on.

6) Result evaluation: The result is judged to be positive if it confirms to one of the conditions below: ① positive in test group and negative in control group. ② in spite of occurrence of tumor in both test and control groups, the tumor incidence rate in test groups is higher than control group. ③ in spite of no obvious distinction between test and control group, the incidence time of tumor in test group is earlier (incubation is shorter).

II. Safety limit of preparation experiment

In order to control the quality of preparation to ensure the safe drug – using, quality examination from the view of pharmacology should be done on the drug beside the necessary physicochemical examination, and these examinations are called safety limit experiment. Limit experiment is mainly used to examine injections, which usually involves the following: pyrogen test, irritation test, anaphylaxis test, hypotense material test and hemolysis test, etc. In practice, items of examination are usually determined complying to pharmacopeia or the demand of production standard for routine preparations and to the property of drug and production specification of preparation for new preparations and Chinese herbal medicine preparations. The experimental methods described below are for references only. To declare for new drugs, please refer to relevant regulations and policies issued by national drug administration department.

Experiment 10.2   Pyrogen experiment

Objective

Study the method and judge standard of examining pyrogen in injections with rabbits.

Principle

After the remains or metabolites of some microbes (especially gram – negative bacilli) into the body (especially through intravenous injection), fever – like reactions will appear. The substances that can cause the reaction are called pyrogens whose chief chemical components are proteins, lipopolsaccharides (LPS), nucleoproteins and their hydrolysates.

Materials

Animal required: 3 rabbits, weigh 1.7 – 3.0kg.

Equipments required: Rabbit – fixed box, platform balance, rectal thermometer, small aluminium case, syringe, syringe needle, forceps, alcohol – cotton , dry cotton ball.

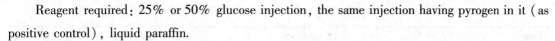
Reagent required: 25% or 50% glucose injection, the same injection having pyrogen in it (as positive control), liquid paraffin.

Methods

(1) Preparation of appliance   syringe and all the other apparatus that have direct contact with test materials used in the experiment should be given depyrogen treatment beforehand. The method is : syringe, needle and forceps alike can be put into aluminum case and be heated for 30minutes at 250℃ in an oven or 2 hours at 180℃, wait – to – be used after cooling.

(2) Selection of rabbits   Body temperature measurement should be done on those rabbits which have not been used in the pyrogen examination, within 7 days before experiment for selection. Measure the temperature 4 times with thermometer every other half an hour in 2 – 3 hours after fasting. If the 4 times' temperatures are all between 38. 3 – 39. 6℃ and the difference between maximum and minimum is within 0. 4℃, then the rabbit is thought to be fit for the pyrogen examination. For those rabbits that have been used in the pyrogen examination, can be used again after more than 2 days if the tested drug used last time is decided to be up to standard but they can't be used again until at least 2 weeks later if the tested drug used last time is decided not to be up to standard.

(3) Preparation before experiment   The rabbits that enter the experiment should be in a condition of the same temperature, deprive them of food 2 – 3 hours before experiment. Measure their temperature 2 – 3 times with rectal thermometer every 30 minutes, and the difference of last 2 times should be within 0. 20℃, take the mean temperature of the last 2 times as normothermia of the rabbit . The normothermias of all the rabbits that enter the experiment should be limited in 38. 3 – 39. 6℃ and the differences of them should be less than 1℃.

(4) Method of detection   Take 3 rabbits fit for using, inject tested solution that has been heated to 37℃ in them slowly through side – auricular vein within 15 minutes after measuring their normothermias. Then measure their temperatures 3 times in the same way as before every 1 hour. Minus the normothermia form the maximum of the 3 times temperatures; the result is temperature elevation degree of the rabbit.

Results

1. If the increased temperature of all the 3 rabbits are less than 0. 6℃ and the sum of them is less than 1. 4℃, the tested drug fits the standard.

2. If only one of the three rabbits' temperature elevation degree is 0. 6℃ or more than it or all the three are less than 0. 6℃ but the sum is 1. 4℃ or more, take another 5 rabbits to retest. If no more than 1 rabbit's temperature elevation degree is 0. 6℃ on more, and the sum of temperature elevation degree of the 8 rabbits entered the two tests is less than 3. 5℃, the tested drug also should be taken as up to standard.

3. If among the 3 rabbits in the preliminary examination, there are over 1 rabbit whose temperature elevation degree is 0. 6℃ or more; or among the 5 ones in the retrial examination, there are over 1 rabbit whose temperature elevation degree is 0. 6℃ or more; or among the total of 8 ones in the two tests, the total of the temperature elevation degree exeed 3. 5℃, the subject is considered unacceptable.

4. Take report according to Table 10 – 5.

Table 10 − 5 experiment result of pyrogen examination in injection

Date		temperature		examiner	
Drug name		description and content		batch number	
Number	1	2	3	4	5
Weight					
First measurement					
Second measurement					
Mean temperature					
Time of injecting					
First measure					
Second measure					
Third measure					
Difference between before					
And after injecting					
Result					

Notes

1. The rabbits that enter the experiment should be healthy without any injury, weigh 1. 7 − 3. 0kg . no pregnancy if female, feed them with same forage from 7 days before experiment. In this period, weights of them shouldn't lessen, and there should be no unusual state of mind, appetite and excretion.

2. Measure temperature gently to avoid stimulating rabbits, and smear liquid paraffin on the mercury ball of thermometer before inserting it into anus of the rabbit. The depth of insertion in every rabbit should be the same, usually about 5 cm, wait for 1. 5 minutes.

3. Use one rectal thermometer on one rabbit to reduce error in measurement.

4. Inject tested drug in rabbits quickly to avoid their struggling which can cause temperature change. Inject it at a low speed, 5 − 10 minutes for the large dosage. The injection dose: Isotonic large scale transfuse 10ml/kg; Chinese medicinal herb parenteral solution 1 − 2ml/kg.

5. There are many factors that can affect pyrogen examination, so the experiment should be carefully done. Do it at best in the condition of 15 − 25℃, the range of the room temperature change should be limited in 5℃ throughout the experiment.

6. Drugs that usually need pyrogen examination and their dosages are listed in Table 10 − 6.

Table 10 − 6 Drugs need pyrogen exanimation and their dosages

Drug	Injection dose
Water for injection	Add no − pyrogen sodium chloride to it to make 0. 9% solution, inject 10ml/kg through Intravenous
Sodium chloride or compound injection of sodium chloride	Inject 10ml/dh through intravenous
Glucose sodium chloride injection	Inject 10ml/kg through intravenous
25% or 50% glucose injection	Inject 10ml/kg through intravenous
Sodium citrate injection	Make 0. 5% solution with water for injection, Inject slowly (10ml/kg)
Heparin injection	Make 100U/ml solution with sodium chloride injection, inject 5ml/kg through intravenous
Oxytetracycline hydrochloride for injection	Make 5000U/ml solution with sodium chloride injection, inject 1ml/kg through intravenous

Evaluation

Injections, especially major injections such a glucose injection, normal saline and so on, pyrogen examination has become a routine work in production process. Generally, intravenously injected drugs that are more than 5 – 10ml need to be examined; Chinese herbal medicine injections need a long time to be compounded, so they are more probable to be contaminated and also need to be examined. At present, pyrogen examination, according to pharmacopeia, is to inject a certain dose of the tested drug into the rabbit's body through vein. Observe the rabbit's temperature elevation in a set period to decide if the pyrogen in the tested drug is within the limitation. Another method of pyrogen examination is limulus test, it can be carried on in test tubes with less materials and time and with high sensitivity, so it can be applied when requirements are provided.

Questions

1. What is pyrogen and what is its chemical nature? Which method can you use to get rid of the pyrogens on utensils?

2. What are the requirements of animals while performing pyrogen test in rabbits? Which factors can influence rabbits' temperature? What should be paid attention to in the experiment?

Experiment 10.3　Irritation test

Objective

Comprehend the significance of irritation test, and grasp the experimental method and the criterion of judgment.

Principle

Generally, new productions of hypodermic or intramuscular injection, or preparations of eye drops, nose drops and suppositories, etc need irritation test. The method is to apply drugs on local tissue, observe if it can cause irritation symptom to the tissue such as red swelling of the skin, bleeding, degeneration, necrosis and so on. The result can be used for finding out the toxicity of the drug and as a reference to select the reasonable method of application.

Materials

Animal required: 2 rabbits, 2.0 – 3.0kg, no sex restriction.

Equipments required: Syringes and needles, dropping pipette, scalpel, surgical scissors, rabbit – fixed box, alcohol – cotton.

Reagent required: 1% potassium antimony tartrate injection, sterile normal saline.

Methods

1. Method of Rabbit quadriceps muscle of thigh　This method can be used to examine the irritation of those preparations for intramuscular injection. Quadriceps muscle of thigh is in the front of thigh, in the center of it is musculus rectus femoris, beneath which is musculus vastas intermedius, medial and lateral of which are musculus vastus medialis and musculus vastus lateralis respectively, four muscles are jointly named quadriceps muscle.

In experiment, take 2 healthy rabbits, both of them are injected 1% potassium antimony tartrate injection 1.0 – 2.0ml in quadriceps muscle of thigh of one side and are injected sterile normal saline in the counterpart of the other side to make a control. Kill the rabbits by bloodletting 48 hours later, dissect them and extract their quadriceps muscle of thigh, longitudinally incise it to observe the reaction of muscular tissue in injection site.

The reaction of muscular tissue is generally divided into 6 degrees:

0 Degree (−): There is no distinct difference between muscular tissue that is injected the tested drug and its control part.

Degree 1 (+): There is hyperemia in the muscular tissue being injected the tested drug, and the diameter of it is less than 0.5cm.

Degree 2 (+ +): There is aula – swelling and hyperemia in the muscular tissue being injected the tested drug, and the diameter is about 1cm.

Degree 3 (+ + +): There is aula – swelling, purple and luster – losing, and necrosis plaque can be seen in the muscular tissue.

Degree 4 (+ + + +): There is aula – swelling, purple and luster – losing, and the diameter of necrosis plaque is about 0.5cm.

Degree 5 (+ + + + +): There are more serious reactions and massive necrosis in the muscular tissue.

Drugs whose mean reaction degree of the 2 rabbits is blow degree 2 can be used as intramuscular injection, and those whose mean reaction degree is between 2 and 3 should be retested or be considered with other aspects to decide their clinical application. Those can't reach the set standard of intramuscular injection also can't applied by hypodermic injection or through mucosa and surface of wound.

2. Method of rabbit conjunctiva　This method is mainly used to test the irritation caused by eyedropper and other mucosa – applied drug. In experiment, take 1 healthy rabbit, put it into fixable box, and observe the normal color and lustre and distribution of vessels of its conjunctiva after it calms down. Draw the inferior eyelid into a circle, and also press the nasolacrimal duct with your fingers (to prevent absorption through drug flowing into the nasolacrimal duct). Drop to be tested liquid drug and normal saline 0.1ml (or 2 drops) into the conjunctival sac of left eye and right eye respectively. If the tested drug is an unguentum, crush 0.1g of it into conjunctival sac and crush the same amount of ointment base into the sac of the other side to make a control.

Detect the secretion of tears every 5 minutes within 30 minutes after drug application. Turn open the eyelid slightly to observe the reaction of conjunctiva every 1 hour. Within 3 hours after drug application. The tested drug is up to standard if there is no distinct irratation symptom such as hyperemia, lacrimation, photophobia and hydrops, etc.

3. Method of rabbit auricular concha　The auricular concha of rabbit is comparatively thin, so after injecting drugs into hypodermic of its auricular concha, the irritation reaction can easily be seen by transillumination. This method needn't to kill the animal so it is fit for primary test for irritation of injections.

In experiment, take 1 healthy rabbit, put it into fixable box and detect the normal state of auricular concha by transillumination. Choose the site near basal portion of auricular concha where there is less vessel to inject the tested drug 0.1 − 0.2ml through hypodermic in it. Inject the same amount of sterile normal saline in the according site of the other side to make a control. Observe the ears of rabbit every 10 minutes within 30 minutes to see if aula – swelling appears and its influence extent. Observe it every 1hour after the 30 minutes until 3 hours after drug application. Detect if there is tissue – necrosis phenomenon on the site of drug application after 24 hours. The tested drug is up to standard if there is no distinct irritation reaction.

Results

Make reports according to the follows:

1. Name of the tested drug, content of basic remedy, physicochemical property, product unit and lot number.

2. Sex, weight and body condition of rabbit.

3. Method of experiment, the way of application and dose, time of application, result observation and conclusion of the experiment.

Notes

1. In the method of rabbit quadriceps muscle of thigh, sterilize strictly before injection to prevent infection. For syringes and needles, use high pressure to sterilize them. Sterilize the administration site with iodine tincture and alcohol. Take a small piece of tissue for pathological analysis to detect if there is inflammation phenomenon, if necessary.

2. In the method of rabbit conjunctiva, observation should be kept on until the effect of drug completely vanishes and the conjunctiva has completely recovered for those drugs with irritation.

3. In the method of rabbit auricular concha, keep away from small vessels when injecting. Keep on observing until the effect disappears completely and the injection site recovers completely when there is irritating reactions.

Question

Which kinds of preparations are used in the method of rabbit quadriceps muscle of thigh, conjunctiva and auricular concha fit for respectively in irritation test? What are their method and index of judgement?

Experiment 10. 4   Hypotensive substance test

Objective

Study hypotensive substance test method for injections.

Principle

In some biochemical preparations (such as antibiotics) and animal visceral preparations, there is contamination of histamine, putrescine, cadaverine and other hypotensive substances during process of production. So, these kinds of preparations, especially those for injection, must pass hypotensive substance test.

Materials

Animal required: 1 cat (dog), weight 2 – 3kg (dog about 10kg), female (no pregnant) and male is for use.

Equipment required: Operation table, operating scalpe, surgical scissors, hemostat, tracheal cannula, arterial cannula, venous cannula, artery clamp, pressure transducer, physio – pressure monitor, injection syringe, iron cage, screw clips, double fovea clips, cotton line, carbasus, infant scale, rubber channel.

Reagent required: Histamin (0.5μg/ml), estreptomicina (15k Unit/ml), 3% sodium pentobarbitone solution (for anesthesia).

Methods

1. Operation   Treat the cat by ig. 3% sodium pentobarbitone solution (1mg/kg), then fix it on operation table. Cut open trachea, insert tracheal cannula for artificial respiration when necessary. Separate vein, insert venous cannula and connect with transfuse instrument for infusion. Separate common carotid artery, insert arterial cannula full of anticoagulant and connect with pressure transducer, physio – pressure monitor for tracing blood pressure.

2. Tracing normal blood pressure   Adjust zero to measure normal – pressure, then open artery clamp, tracing a segment of normal blood pressure.

3. Sensibity test   Inject different doses of histamine contrast dilution by weight in several times. 0.05μg/kg, 0.1μg/kg and 0.15μg/kg, each dose is administered three times after the blood pressure is stable. If the dose 0.1μg/kg cause the decrease of BP surpassing 2.7kPa, at the same time, the reactions caused by different doses differ, and the difference is large for the largest difference of reactions caused by each dose, sensibity test is qualified. The test can begin.

4. Administration   The iv. group treated with histamine 0.1μg/kg (dS), according to pharmacopeia, the injection volume of test drug (dT) and control drug is identical. Inject 8 doses according to following sequence: dS_1, dT_1, dT_2, dS_2, dS_3, dT_3, dT_4, dS, there is 5 mins between 2 doses. Compare the reactions caused by dS_1/dT_2, dT_1/dS_2, dS_3/dT_4, dT_3/dS_4.

Results

If the reactions caused by dT are all smaller than that caused by dS, the hypotensive substance limitation of the test drug accords with regulation. If the reactions caused by dT are all larger than that caused by dS, the hypotensive substance limitation of the test drug does not accord with regulation. If the reactions caused by dT are not all smaller than that caused by dS, take other animals to test again. If the result of the 2nd test is still the same, the hypotensive substance limitation of test drug does not accord with regulation.

Record following observations in experimental report:

1. Test drug name, main content of drug, physicochemical properties, origin of product and batch number.

2. Species, sex, weight and health status of experiment animals.

3. Attrnuant degree of histamine control and test solution, BP descent worth caused by injections of histamine control and test solutions. Check conclusion. The results are showed by integra graphs.

Notes

1. Injection speeds should be similar. Inject a certain volume saline after each injection. Interval time of two adjacent doses should be constant, but each injection should be injected after the reaction caused by last injection is recovered.

2. When histamine control and test solutions are dispensed with histamine phosphate, the doses should be calculated according to histamine. Dispense to 1.0 mg/ml solution with water. Divide and store at $4-8℃$, use in 3 months if no deposit appears. Dispense to 0.5mg/ml dilution with saline while using. .

3. The test drug should be dispensed to proper concentration. Its injection volume should be e-qual to the volume of control dilution.

Evaluation

In the test, a certain volume of test drug and histamine control solutions are injected into vein of cat (dog) in turns to compare the degrees of BP decrease. Judge whether the hypotensive sub-stance limitation test of drug accords with regulation. It is a commonly used method at present.

Question

1. Which hypotensive substances may be mixed in the preparation? Which kind of preparation should be regarded to carry out hypotensive substance test?

2. Why four dS and four dT should be injected in turn?

Experiment 10.5　Haemolyticus test

Objective

Study haemolyticus phenomenon from the experiment and grasp basic operation of haemolyticus test.

Principle

Hemolysis is a phenomenon of RBC disruption and lysis. There is presence of saponin in many Chinese medicinal herbs such as tangshen, platylodon root, oleander, siberian milkwort root, san-chi, etc. Saponin, a kind of surfactant, has strong emulsification and haemolytic effects. In addi-tion, the injection of hypotonic solution in high dose or some steroid compound should cause hae-molysis. Whether there is erythrocyte agglutination should be observed in the test.

Materials

Animal required: 1 rabbit, 2.5 – 3kg, female or male (for collecting blood).

Equipments required: Beaker, bamboo pick (for removing Fibrin), test tube, test tube rack, drip tube, straws, centrifugal apparatus, thermostatic bath.

Reagent required: 5% siberian milkwort root decoction or 4% platylodon root sheet decoction, normal saline, distilled water.

Methods

1. Preparation of 2% erythrocyte suspension　Get fresh rabbit blood 10 – 20ml, stir with bamboo pick to get rid of fibrin, then flush it 3 – 5 times with saline. Add saline 5 – 10ml every time, mix thoroughly and centrifuge, abandon supernatant, and add saline to centrifuge again, until supernatant is no red. According to the volume of erythrocytes obtained, dispense to 2% suspension with saline.

2. Get 7 test tubes (15 × 150mm), number them, add various kinds of solutions into tubes in turn according to following Tab. Don't add any test solution into No.6 tube as a control tube. Don't

add any test solution into No. 7 tube and replace saline with distilled water as complete hemolysis control tube. Weave thoroughly, then keep warm at 37℃ thermostatic bath, observe hemolysis in every tube at 0.5, 1, 2, 3 hours.

Test tube	1	2	3	4	5	6	7
Siberian milkwort root solution（ml）	0.1	0.2	0.3	0.4	0.5	—	—
Normal saline（ml）	2.4	2.3	2.2	2.1	2.0	2.5	distilled water 2.5
2% erythrocyte suspension（ml）	2.5	2.5	2.5	2.5	2.5	2.5	2.5

Results

1. Entire hemolysis：solutions are limpid, red, and have no erythrocyte remained in bottom of the tubes.

2. Partial hemolysis：solutions are limpid, red or brown, and have a little erythrocyte remained in bottom of the tubes. RBC are rare or deformed in microscopic examination.

3. No hemolysis：all RBC sink. Supernatant colorless and limpid. RBC not agglutinative in microscopic examination.

4. Agglutination：No hemolysis, but there is erythrocyte agglutination, it can't be divergent by shaking, or it appears as precipitation.

In general, if there is hemolysis, partial hemolysis or agglutination in No. 3 tube or the former ones, the test preparation can't use for vein injection.

Record following content in experiment report：Name, content, physiochemical properties, origin of product and batch number, result of every tube after keeping warm and experiment conclusion.

Notes

1. The animals for collecting blood include rabbit, goat, dog and rat.

2. 2% erythrocyte suspension used in the test can be replaced by 2% blood saline suspension. The two results are similar, but the former is limpid and easy to observe, the latter is operated conveniently.

3. If the solution is limpid, yellow or brown, and there is brown flocculent deposit within 0.5h, the solution should have the factor that can agglutinate blood cell protein. Drop the solution onto the carry sheet glass, observe RBC agglutination in microscope, drop saline at the edge of cover glass, agglutinated RBC which can be broken up is pseudo – agglutination, otherwise, it is real agglutination. The latter can't be used for clinical injection, the former can be considered cautiously to be used according to local stimulation test.

Evaluation

The test is a commonly – used method for evaluating hemolysis and agglutination effects of drugs. To assure safety application of drugs, the injection prepared from Chinese traditional herbal, especially intravenous injection should be considered to test for its haemolyticus.

Questions

1. What is hemolysis? Which factors relate to drugs which can cause hemolysis?

2. How to perform haemolyticus test? How to judge its results?